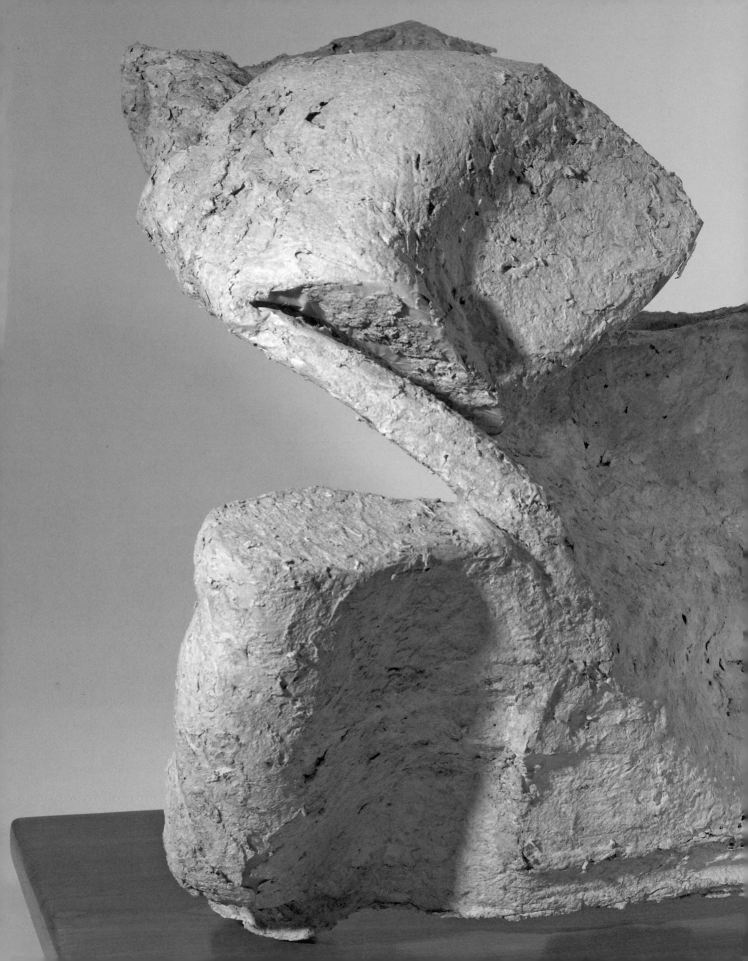

Surviving Cancer: Our Voices & Choices

A Collaboration
Compiled and Illustrated
by Marion Behr

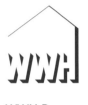

WWH Press

ISBN 13 978-0-61585600-1
Library of Congress Control Number: 2013946669

This book is a compilation made possible by each author's
contribution. The opinions expressed in each article are those
of its author. The publisher does not specifically endorse the
opinions and/or information presented by these authors or
that of the external websites linked herein, or the services,
information, format and content they provide. This book is not
intended as a substitute for the medical advice of physicians.
The reader should regularly consult a physician in matters
relating to his/her health and particularly with respect to any
symptoms that may require diagnosis or medical attention.

All efforts have been made to ensure that web references are
accurate at the time of publication.

To Lancaster Public Library,
Hope our book helps every
reader.
Best wishes always,
Marion

This book is dedicated
to
everyone who has been touched by cancer,
to
my husband, Marc Behr,
who has helped me
endlessly,
to
Carol Howard,
a dear friend,
to
Vasumati B. Solanki,
to
Elias Ventura Cohen
and to
Michael Luft S.
Love to all

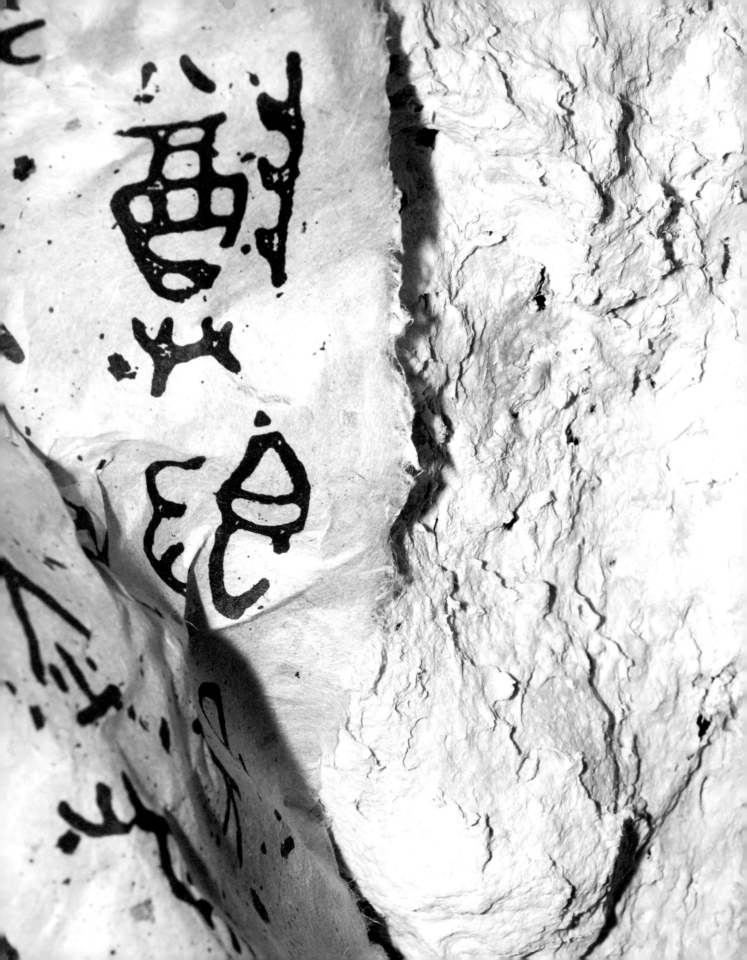

12   LIST OF ILLUSTRATIONS

15   FOREWORD
       Professor Eitan Yefenof, Ph.D.
       Director, Lautenberg Center for Immunology and Cancer Research

16   PREFACE

18   ACKNOWLEDGMENTS

20   A Set of Questions to Help Define What You May Need to Know

I   First Steps—*Facing a diagnosis and assembling your team*

25   How to Find the Medical Team for You
       Kathleen Toomey, M.D.

26   I Was Only Twenty-Seven
       Pamela Adams

27   Focusing Beyond the Cancer
       Marion Behr

30   The Primary Care Doctor on the Cancer Team
       Barrie L. Raik, M.D.

33   Denial
       Joyce Greenberg Lott

37   Concerns of a Family Physician
       Julie Ann Juliano, M.D.

II   Hand in Hand—*Additional partners on the road to wellness*

41   Your Oncology Nurse Practitioner
       Debra A. Walz, R.N., M.S., W.H.N.P.-B.C., A.O.C.N.P., STAR/C

43   My Experience as a Cancer Study Participant
       Sushma Prasada

46   Will I Live?
       Peggy S.

47   The Role of the Gynecologist in Breast Cancer
       Susan N. McCoy, M.D.

51   Experiencing Ovarian Cancer
       Pam Cooper

III   The Diagnostic Process—*Defining the condition*

55   My Daughter Was Only Two and a Half
       Meera Bagle

58   Family History and Genetic Susceptibility
      Ruth Oratz, M.D., F.A.C.P.

61   My Mother Died of Breast Cancer at Forty-Two
      Nora Macdonald

63   Lumps and Bumps in the Male Breast: Men Can Get Breast Cancer Too
      Dawn Behr-Ventura, M.D., M.P.H.

66   Male Breast Cancer Is Real
      Rich Loreti

70   Scars of Life and Love
      Dawn Meade

73   Another Yearly Mammogram
      Sondra Schoenfeld

74   Mammography, Ultrasound and MRI
      Jane Tuvia, M.D.

79   A Radiology Technologist's Advice
      Sandra Scott, R.T.(R.)(M.)

83   The Self-Exam
      Keshia D. Hammond-Merriman

84   Watchful Waiting
      Anne M. Johnston, Ph.D.

89   Of Underlying Concern
      Wilbur Dexter Johnston, Ph.D.

IV   A Different Kind of Challenge—
      Lack of diagnostic support in a developing country

91   A Hard Place in My Breast
      Men Salath

92   What Happened To and In Me?
      Naov Davin

94   Cancer in Cambodia: A Doctor's View
      Sedkai Meta, M.D., *told by Charulata Prasada*

V   Major Treatments—*Explained by specialists and described by survivors*

97   Medical Options
      Richard Margolese, M.D., C.M., F.R.C.S.(C.)

101   Uphill Imperative
      Monica Becker

104   A Breast Surgeon's View
      Christine Rizk, M.D., F.A.C.S.

111   Breast Reconstruction
       William L. Scarlett, D.O., F.A.C.S., F.A.C.O.S., F.A.A.C.S.

114   Breast Cancer and Lymphedema
       Marcy McCaw, B.Sc.P.T., C.L.T.

118   Chemotherapy: What Is It and How Should You Prepare for It?
       Myra F. Barginear, M.D.

121   The Port Is a Great Invention
       Annelise DeCoursin

123   When Pink Was Just a Color
       Paula Flory

126   The Grace of Caregiving
       Tobias D. Robison

129   Radiation Therapy
       Mitchell K. Karten, M.D.

131   Surviving Cancer
       Evie Hammerman, M.S.W.

136   *Heart*
       Michael Carr

137   *The Man in the Vinyl Chair*
       Michael Carr

VI   Further Guidance—*Essential advice for the road to recovery*

139   Oncology Social Workers and How We Help
       Vilmarie Rodriguez, M.S.W., L.C.S.W.

143   The Importance of a Nurse Navigator
       Sherry Melinyshyn, R.N.(EC)., B.N.Sc., C.O.N.(C.), P.H.C.N.P.

145   The Contributions of a Patient Navigator
       Cheryl Kott

146   Look Good—Feel Better
       Michele Capossela

147   Nutrition and Cancer
       Karen Connelly, R.D., C.S.O.

151   Understanding Cancer-Related Fatigue
       Meryl Marger Picard, Ph.D., M.S.W., O.T.R.

VII   The Whole Person—*Addressing the mind, body and spirit*

157   Breast Cancer and Spiritual Care
       Nomi Roth Elbert, M.Ed., Spiritual Care Provider

159   The Role of the Oncology Social Worker
      Elisabeth (Elsje) Reiss, M.S.W., L.C.S.W.

163   Complementary Medicine
      Richard Dickens, M.S., L.C.S.W.-R.

168   Using the Mind–Body Connection to Get Physical and Emotional Relief:
      Jin Shin Jyutsu, Gentle Self-Acupressure
      Kerry Kay

VIII   Financing Your Wellness—*Cancer and money management*

173   Affording Cancer Treatment
      Megan McQuarrie

177   Medical Insurance
      Stuart Van Winkle, C.F.P.®

180   The Road to Financial Wellness
      Richard A. Fontana, C.F.P.®

183   Essential Help from the Women's Health & Counseling Center
      Christine Bonney

186   COBRA: Health Insurance after Job Termination
      Omri Behr, Ph.D., J.D.

188   NBCCEDP: A Path for Patients without Insurance or Funds
      Omri Behr, Ph.D., J.D.

IX   Finding Community and Compassion—
Interactions between cancer support organizations and survivors

191   My Cancer Story
      Mariann Linfante Jacobson

194   Cancer Support Community
      Ellen Levine, M.S.W., A.C.S.W., L.C.S.W., O.S.W.-C.

197   The Most Painful Trial of My Life
      Lucinda (Cindy) Newsome

199   Sisters Network: Founding a Chapter
      Dorothy Reed

200   When Life Pulls Out the Carpet from Beneath Us… Do Flips!
      Pamela Schwartz

203   Seventeen-Year Breast Cancer Survivor
      Kathi Edelson Wolder

207   Formation of a Chapter for the Susan G. Komen® Organization
      Kathi Edelson Wolder

209 Cancer Hope Network Volunteer
    Linda Kendler

210 Cancer Hope Network: All About Hope
    Joe Wojtowicz

212 In The Pink: Early Cancer Detection and Education Program
    Aretha Hill-Forte, M.P.H.

213 Why?
    Jeanette Joyce

215 Breast Cancer Prevention Institute
    Angela Lanfranchi, M.D., F.A.C.S.

x Searching for Answers—
    Two perspectives on research and programs that look to the future

219 Growth Hormone-Releasing Hormone and Its Analogs in Cancer
    Andrew V. Schally, Ph.D., Nobel Prize Laureate

221 Good Treatment and Good Science
    Richard Margolese, M.D., C.M., F.R.C.S.(C.)

xi Summing It All Up—*Inspiration and information*

225 A Relay for Life
    Alicia Rockmore

225 What Kept Me Going
    Lori Cohen

227 Avon Walk
    Tracy Redling

230 Inspiring Hope
    Angela Lanfranchi, M.D., F.A.C.S.

233 Mammogram Math
    Lora Weiselberg, M.D.

235 The Beginning…

236 Information and Resources for Cancer Patients

240 Contributor Biographies

252 Glossary

260 Index

List of Illustrations

These illustrations are of sculptures whose armatures are actual Alpha® radiation cradles, used by radiation patients. The identity of their users is not known. They were donated by St Barnabas Hospital, Livingston, NJ.

1	*KIMONO DANCE* (DETAIL)
2–3	*COURAGE*
6	*KIMONO DANCE* (DETAIL)
14	*NAILED IT* (DETAIL)
28	*NAILED IT*
36	*CONDUCTING*
48	*NESTING*
56	*FRIENDSHIP*
60	*CONDUCTING* (DETAIL)
68	*CONTEMPLATION*
72	*KIMONO DANCE* (DETAIL)
78	*MAMMOGRAM MOMENT*
82	*PULLING ONESELF TOGETHER*
86	*PULLING ONESELF TOGETHER* (DETAIL)
88	*KERNEL OF CONCERN*
98	*MOMENT OF ANXIETY*
102	*TOXIC*
108	*KIMONO DANCE* (DETAIL)
112	*PRERECONSTRUCTION*
122	*EXERCISING*
128	*IMAGE EARLY* SCULPTURE (DETAIL)
134	*CANCER SCARES*
140	*KIMONO DANCE*
148	*OVER THE BARRIER*
154	*REACHING OUT* (DETAIL)
158	*PRAYING*
162	*MUTUAL SUPPORT*

174   *THE PRICE IS HIGH*

182   *LIGHT COMING THROUGH BLUE*

184   *THE PRICE IS HIGH* (DETAIL)

192   *FAMILY MATTERS*

198   *COURAGE*

204   *CANCEL CANCER*

216   *QUITTING TIME*

226   *DETERMINATION*

232   *IMAGE EARLY* MONOPRINT

239   *JUMPING FOR JOY (THE TREATMENT IS OVER!)*

262   *CONDUCTING* (DETAIL)

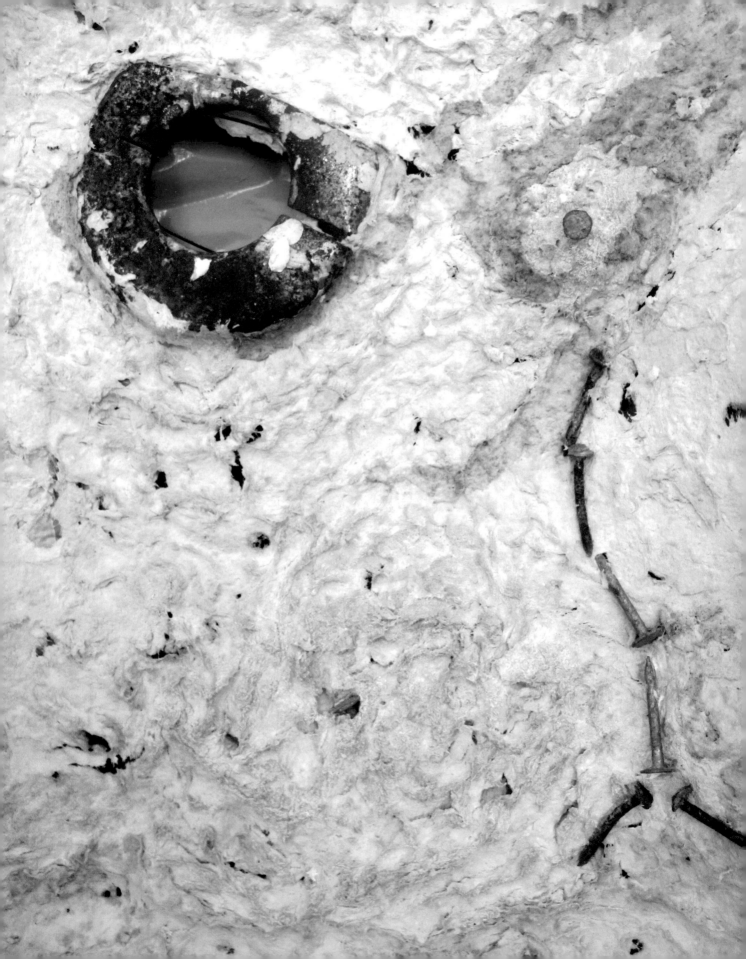

Foreword

My colleagues and I are often hailed by our peers for the great progress we have made in researching the molecular basis of malignant diseases. Such compliments should have left me with a strong feeling of satisfaction, yet when I hear that a family member or friend has contracted cancer, my conscience is filled with a sense of guilt. As a cancer researcher I take the blame upon myself.

This emotional contradiction becomes clear when reading *Surviving Cancer: Our Voices and Choices*. It highlights the various sides of cancer patients in bright and dim colors. Their suffering, hope, frustration, faith, depression and optimism rise up to the surface in loud and clear voices. Their feelings are expressed in sharp contrasts. "Why? Why? Why?" asks Sushma Prasada. "So much love to give, done a lot, so much more to do, so little time left." "Will I Live?" asks Peggy, and no one can give her a definitive answer.

It is a cry from the heart to all professionals who deal with cancer. Decades of investment in basic cancer research did not yield the coveted cure for this dreadful disease. One out of every three individuals will have to face cancer—it is a reality that our society should not tolerate. To my fellows and students I say: "read *Surviving Cancer*. It is a personal account of cancer patients that should motivate you to try harder and research deeper. There are people beyond the laboratory bench who need you and the work that you are doing. They desperately ask for a remedy to a devastating illness. Don't let them down."

The personal stories are ornamented with daring images of unusual sculptures. Radiation cradles belong in hospital wards; patients seek to avoid and forget them. Marion Behr is challenging the reader with restructured and painted cradles that radiate out the message of the book: "Cancel Cancer." One image is worth a thousand words.

Eitan Yefenof, Ph.D.

Professor and Director
Lautenberg Center for Immunology and Cancer Research
Bertha & Max Densen Chair of General and Tumor Immunology
Hebrew University Faculty of Medicine

PREFACE

"You have cancer," I heard the doctor say.

Next I felt a barrage of emotional jolts: fear for the future, dread of a disease I could not comprehend and anger because something was growing inside of me that had no right to be there. Would it destroy me? All these feelings were followed by a very basic animal instinct: I was determined to survive, but how? I didn't know where to begin. What kind of hurry was I in? How much time would it take to find a solution? Where could I find the necessary doctors? The questions seemed endless. The Internet provided many facts, as did other sources, but how could I discover the right path to follow to get well?

Despite the joint efforts of my family, gathering information took time. Some issues remained confusing or unresolved. While speaking with other cancer patients, who all had unique personalities and a vast variety of needs, it became evident that many of us felt overwhelmed.

Surviving Cancer: Our Voices and Choices is a source book, written in part by cancer survivors of different ages who provide insight into personal experiences and choices to ease the way for new cancer patients. Dr. Kathleen Toomey presents the concept of a "cancer team" and other doctors and health care professionals share pertinent information in their areas of expertise. The doctors' articles are arranged to correspond with the usual order of visits experienced by most cancer patients. The medical articles are interspersed with personal narrations by cancer survivors, which often relate to the issues discussed in the doctors' articles.

Cancer organization leaders describe how their groups are beneficial to cancer patients. These articles follow narrations by survivors who were helped by their programs. Different cancer organizations suit different personalities. A Nobel Prize recipient, recognized for his work in cancer research, introduces us to some of his ideas. There are also insights concerning clinical trials, caregiving, financial assistance and poetry relating to a cancer experience.

Requests for articles were sent to highly recommended individuals and nearly everyone responded positively. In this age of cynicism, it is gratifying to interact with the remarkable people who have made this book possible. The articles are written by authors in the United States, Canada, Cambodia and Israel. Most of the authors have never met in person but some have been exchanging ideas over the Internet for the past three years, since the conception of this book. This collaboration is truly a product of the miracle of modern communication.

Each author presents a personal point of view. Occasionally opinions differ, but that should help the reader discover what questions to ask and in which direction to go. However, patients should always consult their own doctor or doctors for their most current recommendations.

Besides providing information, *Surviving Cancer* encourages early detection. While reading the survivors' stories, it becomes apparent that early detection makes a difference—when cancer is found at an early stage, a greater percentage of patients are cured.

Through the process of compiling this book, I could not help but notice how overcoming cancer has given many survivors a mission to do something to help others, whether it takes the shape of creating an organization, speaking to groups of patients, writing a narration, making sculptures to encourage early detection or collaborating to create a book.

All of the contributors hope that those who read this book will benefit from our joint effort.

Marion Behr

Acknowledgments

This book evolved as a result of the experiences of so many individuals who have been through, fought and won the battle against cancer in a variety of ways. As survivors they are sharing their stories with others to help make the road easier to travel. I thank all of the authors of the narrations for giving of themselves so generously and courageously; for sharing their lives, contributing their thoughts and often giving advice that can only come through life's experiences.

The doctors who contributed did so selflessly, offering their expertise in order to help win the fight against cancer. Equally important is their desire to assist every person who has been informed "you have cancer." Kathleen Toomey, M.D., thank you for suggesting the need for a "cancer team of doctors," as well as for your continuous support and advice. It seems a while ago since you first came to my studio to view the cancer sculptures and decided to show them at Steeplechase Cancer Center in Somerville, New Jersey. Look at what you started! *Surviving Cancer: Our Voices and Choices* came into existence as a direct result of interchanges that occurred during that show and others that followed.

Hanna Fox, you are not only an amazing editor, but a dear friend. We have known each other since childhood, and I am fortunate to have been able to work together with you now. It has been a privilege for me.

Amy Hick, thank you for continuously inspecting, detecting and orchestrating the book. Kelsey Blackwell, your comprehensive and beautiful design concept influences every page.

Tom Heller, I'm so grateful you shared your expertise with photography and your enthusiasm for this project for all to see. Yaritsa Arenas, your texture photographs, design sense and quietude have been invaluable. Ilana Ventura, endless gratitude for your sharp eyes. Many thanks go to Jeffrey Kostich, inventor of the Alpha® Cradles, for your ingenuity. To the Radiation Oncology Department at St. Barnabas Hospital, Livingston, New Jersey, thank you for donating the cradles used as armatures for the sculptures. Sara Angel, thank you for your wisdom and for sharing it. Frank Greenagle, we appreciate your valuable publication advice.

Dorothy Reed, thanks for not only contributing your knowledge, but also for being an original motivator when we began to dream about doing a book. Diane Carr, thank you for all your efforts to make that dream come true. Jane Tuvia, M.D., Anne Johnston, Ph.D., Wanda Diak and Virginia Bruner, you are appreciated for answering questions endlessly and never hanging up a phone or ignoring an e-mail. Dawn Behr-Ventura, M.D. and Steven Lev, M.D., we are grateful for your introductions to contributing colleagues. Michael Kurtz, your contact renewed our vitality. To you, Charulata Prasada, heartfelt gratitude for traveling into Cambodian villages to open our eyes to the plight of so many women we rarely hear about and for your enduring patience in gathering information that left an indelible mark on this collection.

Robyn Tromeur, you are not only a very special curator, but a person who is willing to step outside a circle and dance. Thank you for the show at The Center for Contemporary Art, Bedminster, New Jersey, and thank you, Ellen Rannells and Norma Rahn, for having the panel discussion on cancer one evening during the show. Three of the young women from that evening contributed to this collection and their stories have pushed me forward innumerable times.

My deep appreciation goes to my husband, Omri Marc Behr, Ph.D., J.D., and our children, Dawn, Darrin and Dana, and their spouses, David and Asha, for seeing me through my cancer and for always being there. Marc, this book could not have happened without all you do behind the scenes, so to you from me, all my love and appreciation. Carol Howard, a dear friend, you are still an inspiration for the pages that follow.

A Set of Questions to Help Define What You May Need to Know

To be active in one's healing process means participating in getting the best treatment and information possible. Therefore, in your fight against cancer it's very important to ask questions!

Our goal is to get you thinking about the myriad questions that will arise as you seek treatment, and to begin to answer many of them. The list below outlines some of these preliminary questions, and guides you to the articles in the following pages that will begin to offer answers. We have also provided lists of additional resources (p. 236). Of course, we echo the advice of many of our experts to write down any remaining questions that are directed to your particular doctor's area of expertise before going to your appointments.

1. Q – How do I find the best possible doctor?
   A – Kathleen Toomey, M.D., *p. 25*
       Barrie Raik, M.D., *p. 30–32*
       Richard Margolese, M.D., *p. 97, 100*

2. Q – What should I look for in a doctor? Are there professional designations I should check?
   A – Kathleen Toomey, M.D., *p. 25*
       Barrie Raik, M.D., *p. 30–31*
       Richard Margolese, M.D., *p. 97, 100*

3. Q – Does the doctor of your choice participate in a tumor board?
   A – See the definition of tumor board in the Glossary, *p. 259*

4. Q – How important is an early diagnosis? Why?
   A – Jane Tuvia, M.D., *p. 74*
       Lora Weiselberg, M.D., *p. 233*
       Christine Bonney, *p. 183*
       Nora Macdonald, *p. 61*
       Angela Lanfranchi, M.D., *p. 231*
       Naov Davin, *p. 92*
       Evie Hammerman, M.S.W., *p. 131*
       Sushma Prasada, *p. 43, 45*
       Kathi Edelson Wolder, *p. 203, 206*
       Marcy McCaw, B.Sc.P.T., *p. 114*
       Julie Ann Juliano, M.D., *p. 37*
       Dorothy Reed, *p. 199*

5. Q – What is cancer?
   A – Barrie Raik, M.D., *p. 31*

6. Q – What are cancer cells?
   A – Abnormal cells that divide without control and are able to invade other tissues. (National Cancer Institute)

7.   Q – What is:
     i. a *benign* tumor?
     A – Jane Tuvia, M.D., *p. 74*

     ii. a *malignant* tumor?
     A – Barrie Raik, M.D., *p. 31*

     iii. *metastasis*?
     A – Barrie Raik, M.D., *p. 31*
         Richard Margolese, M.D., *p. 97*

8.   Q – Why is compression necessary when having
         a mammogram?
     A – Sandra Scott, R.T.(R.)(M.), *p. 79*

9.   Q – What type of cancer do I have?
     A – Ask your oncologist.

10. Q – Are there different types of cancers?
     A – Christine Rizk, M.D., *p. 105*
         Myra Barginear, M.D., *p. 119*
         Susan McCoy, M.D., *p. 50*
         Kathleen Toomey, M.D., *p. 25*
         Ruth Oratz, M.D., *p. 59, 61*

11. Q – What are the various cancer stages?
     A – Myra Barginear, M.D., *p. 118–19*
         Christine Rizk, M.D., *p. 106–7*

12. Q – What stage of cancer do I have and how
         does that affect my treatment?
     A – Ask your radiologist, then your surgeon
         and medical oncologist.

13. Q – When should a patient ask for a second
         opinion? A third?
     A – Kathleen Toomey, M.D., *p. 25–26*
         Joyce Greenberg Lott, *p. 35, 37*
         Marion Behr, *p. 29*
         Barrie Raik, M.D., *p. 31*

William Scarlett, D.O., *p. 114*
Richard Margolese, M.D., *p. 222–23*

14. Q – Will your insurance cover the hospital/
         doctors you intend to see? You may also
         want to ask if your insurance covers second
         or third opinions.
     A – Check your insurance and talk with your
         insurance broker.
         Stuart Van Winkle, C.F.P., *p. 177–79*
     A – Ask a social worker to guide you
         to answers.
         Vilmarie Rodriguez, M.S.W., *p. 139*
         Megan McQuarrie, *p. 173, 175*
         Barrie Raik, M.D., *p. 30, 32*

15. Q – Is there more than one direction of treat-
         ment for any given cancer and if so, how
         can I decide which direction to take?
     A – Richard Margolese, M.D., *p. 97, 99–100*
         Joyce Greenberg Lott, *p. 35, 37*
         Barrie Raik, M.D., *p. 31–32*

16. Q – You will often be asked to bring a complete
         copy of your records to your doctor (pref-
         erably on CDs). What should these include?
     A – i. Medical reports that include consultation
         reports from all your physicians:
         – primary care physician
         – gynecologist
         – radiologist
         – oncologists: surgical, medical, radiation
     A – ii. Radiology reports and imaging include:
         a) X-rays
         b) mammograms
         c) ultrasound
         d) CAT (Computer Axial Tomography)
         e) MRI or MRT (Magnetic Resonance
            Imaging or Tomography)
         f) PET (Positron Emission Tomography)

g) DEXA scans (bone density)

h) MUGA (multigated acquisition scans for heart)

A – iii. Pathology reports and pathology slides. Get a copy of all pathology, X-ray, consultant and treatment studies and keep them always.

Kathleen Toomey, M.D., *p. 25*

Radiology images and pathology slides may not be held by your doctor(s) so it's important to know how to access them if necessary. Find out where these can be located.

They may be with the radiology office where they were made or the hospital lab where a biopsy was done. Always ask to have this information sent to your primary doctor so one doctor will have all the information together. Above all, make sure to have all the information yourself.

17. Q – What are the differences between mammogram, ultrasound and MRI?

A – Jane Tuvia, M.D., *p. 74–77*

18. Q – What does a biopsy involve?

A – Susan McCoy, M.D., *p. 49*
Jane Tuvia, M.D., *p. 77*
Sandra Scott, R.T.(R.)(M.), *p. 79–80*
Christine Rizk, M.D., *p. 105–6*
Barrie Raik, M.D., *p. 30–31*

19. Q – How can I alleviate the initial fear, depression and/or stress that often come along with a cancer diagnosis?

A – Ask a nurse navigator, nurse practitioner, social worker, psychologist or inquire at a support organization.
Vilmarie Rodriguez, M.S.W., *p. 139, 141*
Sherry Melinyshyn, R.N.(F.C.), *p. 143–44*
Ellen Levine, M.S.W., *p. 195–96*
Richard Dickens, L.C.S.W.-R., *p. 163–68*
Kerry Kay, *p. 168–70*

20. Q – How important is family history?

A – Ruth Oratz, M.D., *p. 58–59, 61*
Susan McCoy, M.D., *p. 47*

21. Q – What are BRCA mutations?

A – Ruth Oratz, M.D., *p. 59, 61*

22. Q – Can men get breast cancer?

A – Dawn Behr-Ventura, M.D., *p. 63–66*
Rich Loreti, *p. 66–67, 69–70*
Ruth Oratz, M.D., *p. 58*

23. Q – What determines the type of surgical procedure required?

A – Christine Rizk, M.D., *p. 107, 109*
Richard Margolese, M.D., *p. 97*

24. Q – When can reconstructive surgery be performed?

A – William Scarlett, D.O., *p. 111, 113*

25. Q – What causes lymphedema?

A – Marcy McCaw, B.Sc.P.T., *p. 114*

26. Q – What are the side effects of my planned chemotherapy regimen?

A – Myra Barginear, M.D., *p. 120–21*
Karen Connelly, R.D., *p. 149*
Susan McCoy, M.D., *p. 50–51*
Meryl Marger Picard, Ph.D., *p. 152*

27. Q – Can some side effects be controlled? If so, how and when?

A – Myra Barginear, M.D., *p. 120–21*
Susan McCoy, M.D., *p. 50*
Meryl Marger Picard, Ph.D., *p. 152*

28. Q – Usually, are side effects from chemotherapy temporary or permanent?

A – Myra Barginear, M.D., *p. 120–21*

29. Q – What is a port?

A – Myra Barginear, M.D., *p. 119*
Annelise DeCoursin, *p. 121*

30. Q – When hair is lost due to chemotherapy, does it come back? If so, how long does it take before it grows in again?
A – Yes, hair usually begins to regrow after about 6–12 months. Chemotherapy agents must first clear the system. (www.cancer.net)

31. Q – What is CRF (Cancer-Related Fatigue)?
A – Meryl Marger Picard, Ph.D., *p. 151–53, 155*

32. Q – Are any cancer treatments given as outpatient treatments?
A – Myra Barginear, M.D., *p. 119*
Debra Walz, R.N., *p. 41*

33. Q – What are the side effects from radiation? Can they be controlled? How?
A – Mitchell Karten, M.D., *p. 130–31*
Christine Rizk, M.D., *p. 110*

34. Q – How is radiation used in conservative therapy?
A – Mitchell Karten, M.D., *p. 130*

35. Q – Does external beam radiation therapy make you radioactive?
A – Mitchell Karten, M.D., *p. 130–31*

36. Q – What is HER2?
A – Richard Margolese, M.D., *p. 100*
Mariann Linfante Jacobson, *p. 193*
Glossary, *p. 255*

37. Q – What is Herceptin?
A – Richard Margolese, M.D., *p. 100*

38. Q – Is the prior use of HRT (hormone replacement therapy) related to getting breast cancer?
A – Anne Johnston, Ph.D., *p. 84*
A – Angela Lanfranchi, M.D., *p. 231*

39. Q – What is targeted therapy?
A – Karen Connelly, R.D., *p. 149*

40. Q – Can spiritual support help a cancer patient?
A – Dorothy Reed, *p. 199*
Lucinda Newsome, *p. 199*
Nomi Roth Elbert, *p. 159*

41. Q – What is complementary medicine and might it be useful in my case in conjunction with my current treatment?
A – Richard Dickens, L.C.S.W.-R., *p. 163*
Kerry Kay, *p. 169*

If you are considering any complementary treatments, ALWAYS ask your doctor which dietary supplements or over-the-counter vitamins can interact with your cancer medications in a negative way.

42. Q – What is a clinical trial? Can it benefit me? How do I find out about it?
A – Richard Margolese, M.D., *p. 99–100*
Andrew Schally, Ph.D., *p. 220*
Kathi Edelson Wolder, *p. 206*
Richard Dickens, L.C.S.W.-R., *p. 163*

See www.cancer.gov/clinicaltrials. If you are interested, ask if clinical trials are available where you are being treated.

43. Q – Are there programs that help patients find assistance with everyday chores?
A – Vilmarie Rodriguez, M.S.W., *p. 139, 142*
Megan McQuarrie, *p. 176*
Meryl Marger Picard, Ph.D., *p. 153*

44. Q – How can I find information regarding the most recent cancer research and treatments?
A – Go to the website of the National Cancer Institute of the National Institutes of Health: www.cancer.gov

For further questions, including "types of cancer," go to www.breastcancer.org/symptoms.

I

First Steps—
Facing a diagnosis and assembling your team

How to Find the Medical Team for You

Kathleen Toomey, M.D.

Any cancer diagnosis is frightening. Most women fear the diagnosis of breast cancer all their lives. It is important to have the right medical team when faced with a cancer diagnosis. The most important attribute of physicians is that they feel right to you. They must be able to communicate with you in language you understand. Board certification in their subspecialty is important as well. At Somerset Medical Center, where I practice, board certification is required for membership on the medical staff. Every hospital and facility has a website you can access to see how it is ranked against others. Today, breast centers are being certified by the American College of Surgeons. This is an important certification and means that the breast center meets certain strict criteria for standards and functions.

Important questions to ask your health care team are: What kind of cancer do I have? What is my stage? Remember to get a copy of all pathology, X-ray, consultant and treatment summaries and keep them always. Ask about the medications and therapies you will receive, their potential side effects and when you should call your physician. Ask about the type of tests needed for staging and monitoring. Ask what guidelines, such as the National Comprehensive Cancer Network (NCCN) or American Society of Clinical Oncology (ASCO) guidelines, will be used for treatment and follow-up. The websites for these organizations—nccn.org or cancer.net (ASCO)—are very helpful to the layperson. The American Cancer Society website, local hospital/cancer center websites and resource libraries in cancer centers are all places to go for information you can trust. Centers that participate in clinical trials are most likely to be on the cutting edge of new information. Get information that can help alleviate your anxiety at organizations such as the Cancer Support Community (CSC) and through local support groups.

CANCER SUPPORT
ORGANIZATIONS

breastcancer.org
cancer.gov
cancer.net
cancercenter.com
cancersupportcommunity.org
skincancer.about.com

A second opinion should never be a problem. There are new tests to determine if chemotherapy might be helpful in your case. In the case of breast cancer, know the estrogen and progesterone status of your tumor as well as the HER2 status. Go to see your physician with a list of questions. Write down the answers in a book or folder.

A team has multiple players. For a breast cancer patient this means a primary physician and/or gynecologist, a breast radiologist, a breast surgeon, a reconstruction surgeon, a medical oncologist and radiation oncologist. Oncology nurses, nurse practitioners/physician assistants, breast center technicians, social workers, dietitians and financial counselors can be useful sources of information as well. Support groups and organizations, family and friends (especially those who have had cancer) can also be helpful.

Remember treatment is urgent but not an emergency. You have time to make informed decisions. Don't let yourself be rushed; you must be comfortable with your team. If something doesn't seem right to you, get another opinion. It takes a team to care for a cancer patient and you want to be on the very best team you can get.

I Was Only Twenty-Seven
Pamela Adams

Being told that I would likely lose my hair and my breasts was quite a blow. I was young, out on my own, far from family, beginning my career and had yet to find that special someone. And this new predicament was certainly not going to help in that respect!

I felt the lump one morning while showering and thought to myself, this is impossible. I continued feeling it over the next few mornings, fearing the conversation I'd have with my doctor. I was certain he'd say, "you're too young, it has to do with your cycle, come back in a few months," but I made the appointment anyway. He and the other doctors proved me wrong and set to work examining my lump and eventually removed it. With that came the cancer diagnosis. I was only twenty-seven years old.

Over the next couple of months, cancer changed me in ways I never expected. There were the obvious changes: I lost my hair and had both breasts removed. However, if you ask anyone who knew me then, I was at my sexiest during those months—with no hair and tissue-expanding boobs—because I believed it was true. That was a change I never expected to gain from a cancer diagnosis. I made the decision not to let cancer slow me down. This was my life and I wasn't going to let this get in the way!

Besides, I was extremely proud of what I was doing—battling cancer—and I wanted everyone to know. Every morning, as I put on makeup, willing my remaining three eyelashes to hang in there, I believed that I was hot. I stepped back from the mirror and thought, "you look great!" You couldn't have convinced me otherwise. I went out to bars and knew that every man in the place was looking at me (mind you, they probably were, but not for the reasons I thought). I wasn't delusional. I knew that I was bald and that my low-cut, tight-fitting shirt didn't look quite right, but I also knew that if people looked at me and saw that I was willing to go out to a bar looking like I did, they'd see right through my physical imperfections and admire the woman who had the strength to go out, rather than hide.

It's been almost four years since my diagnosis and you could say I've been myself physically for about three years now. Once the physical effects wore off and I was no longer consumed with being a patient, some of the emotional effects of cancer began to sink in. I know how it feels to have my body turn against me and to wake up every morning wondering if it will turn against me again.

But I've also had the extreme pleasure of knowing what it's like to help other women who have been affected by the disease and to help guide them along their own journey. I am an advocate and fundraiser for a cause that I care passionately about. I truly appreciate every single day and take advantage of every opportunity. The humbling truth is that no matter how much chemo is in me, how bald I am or how funky my breasts are, it truly can always be worse. I have learned to accept what I cannot control.

Most importantly, I now know that my body didn't turn against me. My body met the challenge of cancer head-on—it got me through many surgeries, chemo and radiation—and I am stronger now because of it. I know just how far my body can go and find joy in pushing it harder every day. I know that whatever life hands me next, I will be both physically and emotionally strong enough to face it.

Life dealt me a tough blow, and I imagine it will deal me many more throughout the rest of my life. Life deals lots of people tough blows of varying degrees every day but what's important is how a person chooses to deal with those challenges. I will never forgive cancer for the things it took from me, but I will forever be grateful for the strength, wisdom and life it gave to me.

CHEMOTHERAPY

A drug treatment that uses powerful chemicals to kill fast-growing cells in your body. Many different chemotherapy drugs are available. They may be used alone or in combination to treat a wide variety of cancers.

Focusing Beyond the Cancer
Marion Behr

I was lying on the table, anchored in a blue plastic cradle, looking around—to the left, then to the right. The room's details were taking shape. There were voices in the background. Halfway up the right wall, stacks of blue cradles filled layers of shelves. There were so many cradles!

At other times, other individuals must have been lying in each of those cradles in similar positions to mine. What were they thinking and feeling lying here? Were they anxious or scared? In my mind, the plastic cradles took body-like forms. Then, overhead, a tiny red light switched on. The radiation process began.

At this point, my cancer journey was coming to a close. There were just six weeks of radiation treatments and a preventative medication to be taken. A friend, another cancer survivor, suggested taking this medication right after lunch. After trial and error, that worked for her. Her advice worked for me as well.

Shortly after the first radiation procedure, I asked and was given permission to bring several of the blue cradles home to my studio. They had been used for past radiation treatments and could not be recycled. During following office visits I listened to other patients carefully. Some were relieved, scared, religious or family conscious. Others were joyful to be finishing their sessions. All of us wanted to live! When I was home, I would reshape the cradles to represent people and their emotions as they fought for a healthy life.

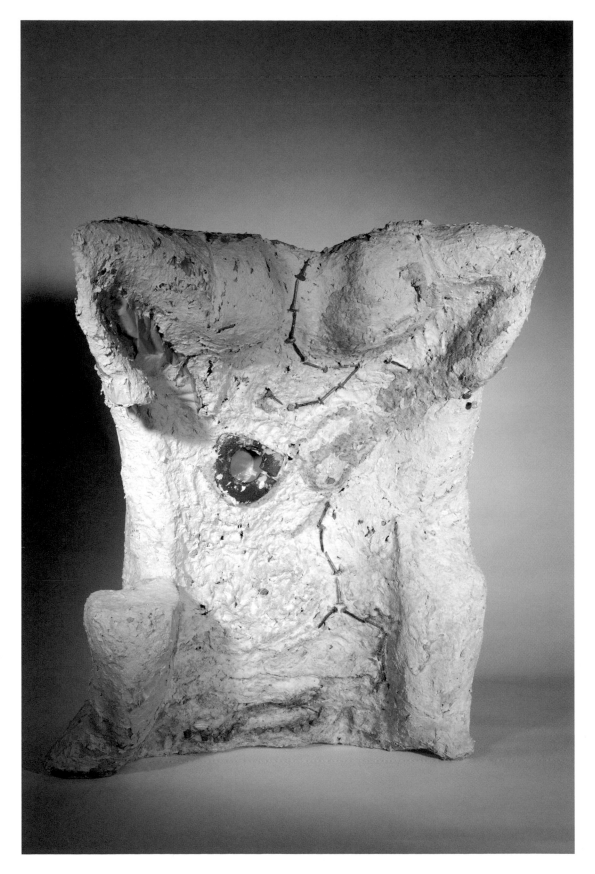

My kids had pushed me to get a mammogram approximately one year before. With busy schedules and a very full life, it's so easy to skip a year or two and not realize that so much time has gone by. Thank heaven for my kids! Waiting longer might have caused a considerable problem. Early mammograms can make a difference—it did for me. Since one good turn deserves another, the sculptures would become my way to encourage others to *Cancel Cancer* and *Image Early*.

Naturally, I went through all the fears and reactions a person has when told, "you have cancer." However, as a result of this experience, the sculptures were born. Four exhibits, aimed at encouraging women to get mammograms, came to life. This book evolved as a result of a panel presentation and numerous discussions.

My cancer was removed five months before the radiation treatment began and the removal was far less painful than the gripping fears that preceded the operation. These experiences were punctuated by statements that created unimaginable turmoil in my mind. "We see a calcium deposit on your mammogram." "There may be a cancer." "The radiologist has read your sonogram and will be right in to talk to you." "You have a small cancer." "You have to speak to a surgeon."

I had no idea where to look for the doctor who would be right for me. Where could I find the best advice? What professional would spend the necessary time to explain what route was best for me to take? There were certainly plenty of choices. My eldest daughter, a physician, researched with her team. My youngest daughter and son kept me talking about any possible concerns. My daughter-in-law investigated doctors' reputations. My kids and friends provided information and support. My husband and I got on the Internet to do some research of our own. Then the sifting began. Ultimately, the final choice had to be my own. A plan took shape.

During those months I learned a lot from my experiences. It's important that both the cancer patient and family members ask questions. For example, I am allergic to latex. At one point a technician taking blood was wearing latex gloves. My husband, who was with me, asked about the material of the technician's gloves. Under those circumstances, I would not have noticed nor bothered to ask. If possible, have a partner, relative or friend come along to your hospital and doctor visits. It is important to have an advocate, someone else to ask questions you might miss. Write down your questions before the appointment. Have your advocate take notes on the doctor's answers and any other important information, so you can discuss everything after leaving the doctor's office. Keeping written records of all doctors' responses will be helpful in making final decisions.

Don't be afraid to get second opinions or to have reports checked. During my surgery, three lymph nodes were removed. An extremely low cancer count was found in one node during a second testing. My original report stated the cluster size was under 2 mm. To be safe, the surgeon suggested a lymphectomy. My daughter's team asked for a very careful recount. The count was done once more and the cluster size was under 0.2 mm. As a result, no lymph nodes needed to be removed. Since I am left-handed and need my left arm to create art, it was a huge relief not to have to have more surgery under that arm.

"Yearly mammograms can lead to early detection of breast cancers when they are most curable and breast conservation therapies are available. The most recent recommendations are for getting annual mammograms starting at age 40."

— Jane Tuvia, M.D.

Along with the inevitable complications, some positive experiences evolved too. Life became more important than ever. My husband, Marc, and I worked to spend extra quality time together. Projects for the future solidified in my mind, and little memorable moments truly made my days.

The day after my operation all our children and grandchildren came to our house. I was in bed so Marc went out to get sushi for the family. Everyone was sitting on or near the bed eating when suddenly my then four-year-old grandson piped up, "Grammy, this is the best picnic I've ever been to!" That certainly put an interesting perspective on the whole situation.

The next morning it felt good to get back to work in the studio. Survival, for me, is focusing beyond the cancer and living life to its fullest, every day.

The Primary Care Doctor on the Cancer Team
Barrie L. Raik, M.D.

What is the role of the primary care doctor? What can a patient and his or her family expect from this person?

The primary care doctor should be a physician who knows the patient and the patient's medical history. He or she is responsible for guiding and counseling his or her patients in many aspects of their health care. This, of course, includes being a guide in the case of suspicion, diagnosis and treatment of cancer, especially when other medical specialists are involved.

If you don't have a primary care physician, it may be necessary or desirable to select one. Sometimes your insurance plan requires one physician who refers you to specialists and orders tests. Sometimes you may have been assigned a primary care physician by your insurer but don't like or feel comfortable with this person. If the treatment decisions are not urgent, you may have time to interview several doctors in your plan to find one you trust and can work with. Other resources for finding a good primary care physician include checking with medical organizations and hospitals, as well as recommendations from those in your community. If you need to begin your cancer treatment right away, focus on finding the cancer specialists first, and then search for a primary care physician.

An investigation of the possibility of cancer will commence when either a patient feels something strange, a routine blood test turns up an abnormality or through a routine mammogram.

Often the primary care physician is the doctor who begins the investigation of a problem, orders a test and then refers the patient to a specialist for an appropriate procedure. This may be non-invasive through a mammogram or a sonogram, or invasive through a biopsy.

A biopsy involves obtaining a small piece of tissue to analyze. This can be done in various ways. Sometimes a radiologist uses a needle to obtain tissue

"...I felt the lump one morning and thought, this is impossible."

— Pamela Adams

from the breast lesion seen on a mammogram or sonogram. Sometimes the surgeon does an excisional biopsy, taking a larger piece of the area of concern. Cancer is diagnosed by a pathologist examining the specially stained tissue under a microscope. The results from the pathologist help the other cancer specialists stage the cancer and plan the treatment.

It is often likely that the primary care physician is the first to give the cancer diagnosis. The manner of telling the patient that cancer has been found is important. If patients are told too abruptly they may not be able to absorb the information. If the message is too gently phrased, they may not really understand that they have cancer and need to make decisions about their treatment.

Cancer is defined as a condition in which the cells of an organ grow abnormally. Neoplasm means new growth. Malignant neoplasm means a new growth that continues to grow abnormally and sometimes spreads to other parts of the body. The spread is called metastasis. Many types of cancers need to be staged before a treatment can be recommended. This involves the size, location and the cellular type of the tumor.

Q — What is cancer?

All this information may be new and frightening to the patient. The patient needs time to absorb a large amount of information, deal with emotional responses and develop strength to proceed with treatment. Many doctors also provide patients and their families with information through text or video. Sometimes there are group sessions or classes where the most common anxieties and questions can be answered for several patients at once.

Some patients function better not knowing every detail of what is happening. One way to handle this is to identify a trusted family member or friend who will take on the task of managing all the information and details that may be overwhelming for the patient. If the patient just wants to trust the doctor to select the most appropriate course of treatment, the patient and doctor should have a clear understanding of what kind of information the patient wants to avoid hearing. For example, it would be hard to treat a patient who doesn't want to know about metastatic disease when the treatment involves chemotherapy.

The patient's next step after diagnosis is generally to meet with one or several specialists for treatment. It may be helpful if the primary care physician can refer the patient to colleagues. Sometimes the patient will be able to locate one specialist, who may then make a referral to the others. It is common for patients with breast cancer and other cancers to be treated by different specialists: the surgeon, the radiation oncologist who administers radiation therapy and the oncologist who manages the chemotherapy and often the overall care of the patient. Finding the right specialist or group of specialists is important because the patient will spend a lot of time interacting with these doctors, their nurses and office staff. It is sometimes appropriate to get a second opinion and even a third.

Q — How do I find the best possible doctor?

When recommendations are not well understood, primary care doctors can help explain them. While primary care doctors may not be experts in the management of cancers, they will be able to speak to the specialists and take the time to explain the patient's different choices, the possible side effects, as well as the risks and the benefits of particular treatments. Although primary care doctors won't make the choice for the patient, they can assist in decision making.

Once treatment choices are presented to the patient, the primary care physician may be able to help the patient make the decision about different treatment options based on personal values, medical history and family history. A doctor who knows the patient well will also be able to provide emotional support at a difficult time.

For all appointments with various specialists, it is a good idea to bring a list of questions and have a friend or family member present to take notes.

In an ideal world, the patient has medical insurance that covers these visits and ongoing treatment in and out of the hospital. Sometimes, however, the patient doesn't have a primary care physician or doesn't have insurance. Most teaching hospitals have programs to help patients without insurance. A breast cancer clinic will often have a social worker who can find out whether or not the patient is eligible for Medicaid or other low-cost insurances.

If the patient and family are overwhelmed with the diagnosis of cancer, the physician can outline in general terms what the next steps are likely to be. Most doctors who accept insurance work with nurse practitioners and physician assistants. These valuable clinicians are able to spend longer sessions with the patient, especially in the initial stages of diagnosis and treatment.

Usually, there is time to seek more than one opinion about treatment options. Occasionally, the cancer is first seen in an emergency setting and there is no time for a second opinion. In those cases, the primary care physician can and should reassure the patient that the team caring for him or her is providing the best possible care.

During the treatment phase, the patient (along with family and others helping) will be very busy with visits to the various specialists, a treatment center or a hospital. Often the patient won't be in contact with the primary care physician because other doctors will be providing the care. However, it is important to ensure that the specialists keep the primary care physician informed, either by electronic medical records or telephone communication. If there are complications, hospitalizations or other issues, the primary care physician should participate more actively in treatment.

If the patient goes into remission, the cancer specialists will likely continue to see the patient, but less frequently. When the patient returns to the care of the primary physician, as a cancer survivor, close monitoring will be needed to observe long-term effects of treatment, for recurrence and for secondary complications such as heart problems from Adriamycin (a chemotherapy drug). The primary care physician should be competent in this post-treatment phase and continue to collaborate with the oncologists.

If the patient's course does not lead to a cure, the patient could be advised that the pursuit of further aggressive treatment is not in her or his best interest. At that time, the patient may want to discuss palliative or hospice care. This is another area that the primary care physician should be able to discuss with the patient and loved ones.

Primary care physicians can make the cancer journey easier for the patient by being available and supportive because they are aware of the many psychological aspects of cancer. They can also offer treatment and referrals if the patient develops depression, anxiety, insomnia or other symptoms. Since the primary care physician will follow the patient after treatment has been completed, the physician also needs to be aware of the risks and concerns for cancer survivors.

Denial

Joyce Greenberg Lott

Twenty-seven years ago, after a divorce, I fell in love with and married my second husband, Gary. It didn't bother me that we had five children between us or that we were both high school teachers with limited incomes. We trained for a marathon together, planted a garden that covered almost an acre and put an addition on our house with beams and skylights. We felt strong and confident. All we craved together was time—time to do the things we enjoyed, which included his painting and my poetry.

Thirteen years after our wedding, Gary woke up one morning and discovered blood in his urine. Several weeks later, we took the train to the Memorial Sloan-Kettering Cancer Center, an hour away in New York City, and a surgeon removed a large portion of Gary's bladder. For five years after that, Gary taught and eventually retired, continued to add onto and improve our house, cooked delicious meals with food from our garden, painted watercolors and began to work in clay.

His cancer didn't metastasize (at least it wasn't evident to us or to the surgeon at Sloan whom he visited regularly) until six years after his operation. But when it did, it entered Gary's bones. In terrible pain, he still wanted to live. He was only sixty-eight and there was much he wanted to do.

He did live for seven months after his diagnosis, undergoing every awful treatment his doctor suggested. The night he died, Gary tried to fight off death with his last breaths.

Gary's prolonged suffering helped me accept his death. I vowed, deep in my heart, that I would accept my own death, not fight it, when the time came.

But of course death doesn't come just because you're ready for it. Loneliness came, along with the chore of cleaning out Gary's belongings. The following year, retirement came. Shortly after that, Joe came into my life—a widower twelve years older than I, who enjoyed skiing and tennis the way I do and who invited me to travel all over the world with him. As much as I enjoyed this new relationship, I feared that, because of Joe's age, he would get sick and die and I would be a caretaker and grief-stricken all over again.

When Joe and I weren't traveling, we spent weekends together. We lived alone during the week, an hour and a half apart, he in an apartment and I in the house Gary and I had lived in.

Two and a half years after I met Joe, I returned from a trip to Egypt with a cough and sore throat that I couldn't get rid of. I lost my appetite, experienced night sweats and felt tired. I thought maybe I had picked up some weird germ along the Nile. For more than a year, I knew I had a swelling in my right groin. I didn't tell anyone about it and I didn't connect it with my malaise. When I thought about the swelling, I told myself that I probably pulled something playing tennis. Denial has always been one of my strong suits.

Two months after we returned from Egypt, Joe took me out to dinner with friends in New York City. It was a more expensive meal than I was used to and as much as I wanted to eat it, I could hardly swallow. When we got back to his apartment, I lay on his bed and cried and cried. "I'm so tired and I can't eat," I said. And then I showed him. "I have this swelling in my groin."

Joe acted immediately, dragging me out of my passivity and denial. He telephoned his best friend, a doctor, that night and brought me right over to see him. Another friend of Joe's, a surgeon, performed a biopsy the next day. Ironically, Joe, the man twelve years older than I, was taking care of me, not the other way around.

When I got my diagnosis—stage 1 B-cell non-Hodgkin's lymphoma—I knew little about my disease. I hadn't yet spoken to an oncologist nor had I been on the Internet to read about my condition. All I knew was that I had vowed to myself that when my time came, I would accept my death.

I spent the next week doing just that. To begin, I told myself I didn't want to grow old anyway. Seventy-one was old enough. I could still run around the tennis court and look halfway decent. Did I really need wrinkles and dementia and a cane? My children would be fine. They no longer needed me in basic ways.

More importantly, I reviewed my life and realized that I had really lived. I had no big regrets. Oh sure, I'd done some dumb things, even some nasty ones, but I'd learned from them and grown as a person. Someone once told me we only regret what we haven't done. That person was right. I did have one regret: I wanted to take all my children and grandchildren on a vacation together. Every time I started to plan it, I ended up thinking it would be too expensive. "If I get better, I'm going to take that vacation," I vowed.

When I discussed my condition with my oncologist, I learned that with strong chemo, the kind you lose your hair from, stage 1 non-Hodgkin's lymphoma is treatable. Even though I had succumbed to one of the world's worst cases of denial, I had lucked out. I might not have to accept my death after all. If I turned out to be one of the lucky ones, I could go into remission.

I opted to do my chemo in Princeton instead of traveling to New York. I learned that the protocol (R-CHOP) would be the same no matter who treated me; and as a result of my disease, I was pretty tired out. I had friends in Princeton and my older daughter and son lived within driving distance. I wanted to spare Joe the primary caretaking role I had performed for Gary. I knew just how draining that job can be.

My oncologist, Dr. Yi, arranged for my first transfusion at University Medical Center at Princeton. I am most grateful to him for this because I had an allergic reaction to Rituxan, the first drug in my infusion and the most important in fighting my condition. I received emergency care in the hospital and Dr. Yi monitored me, giving me the drug overnight in an extremely slow drip.

Although I was able to continue the chemotherapy, I did not have a good reaction to it. I suffered from nausea and diarrhea, developed fevers and lay around the house pretty much exhausted. The telephone turned out to be my nemesis. Every time I lay down to take a nap or boiled water for tea, it rang—making me aware for the first time how I had taken over the responsibility of communication during my husband's illness.

One of the things I had to decide, without a live-in support person, was how to communicate with friends and family. I chose not to pick up the phone unless I wanted to talk. Instead, I left a message thanking callers, saying I really appreciated their calls and would get back to them when I could. I also sent my daughter an e-mail list of concerned friends and family. She communicated to them in a mass e-mail on a regular basis.

I answered my friends honestly when they asked what they could do. My friend Barbara brought me nutritious food from Whole Foods and my friend Betty brought me soups she made with farm stand vegetables. Joe continued to stay with me every weekend and sometimes during the week when I needed him. He was a miracle. Here I was, a bald, skinny and sick seventy-one-year-old, who spent most of her time on the toilet. And I had a boyfriend who loved me.

Much to my surprise, I found I didn't mind being bald. People complimented me on the shape of my head. "Your mother must have made you sleep on your stomach," one woman said. I dismissed wigs and fell in love with earrings and hats when I felt well enough to dress. I remember washing my hands in the bathroom at the Infusion Room for the first time and feeling liberated. I no longer needed to look in the mirror and rearrange my hair.

Approximately once a month, I went to the Infusion Room at the hospital in Princeton with either one of my daughters or Joe. I did this three times, after which Dr. Yi ordered another PET scan. The chemo had been successful—no indication of cancer!

However, when I met with Dr. Yi, he informed me that, even though I was cancer free, I must have three more infusions. In tears, I asked why. He produced statistics and graphs that, after measuring my age and the size of the swelling in the lymph node in my right groin, came up with the result: a minimum of three additional treatments.

I knew the side effects of the drugs I had been taking, including a weakened heart later in life. I also knew their immediate effects on my own body. I talked with my older daughter, Elizabeth Greenberg, and we both agreed I needed a

"Fatigue is the great disrupter of life roles, habits and routines. It is debilitating and is often described as the most stressful symptom cancer patients identify."

— Meryl Marger Picard, Ph.D.

SIDE EFFECTS

Side effects are undesirable and possibly harmful and unintended effects of medications.

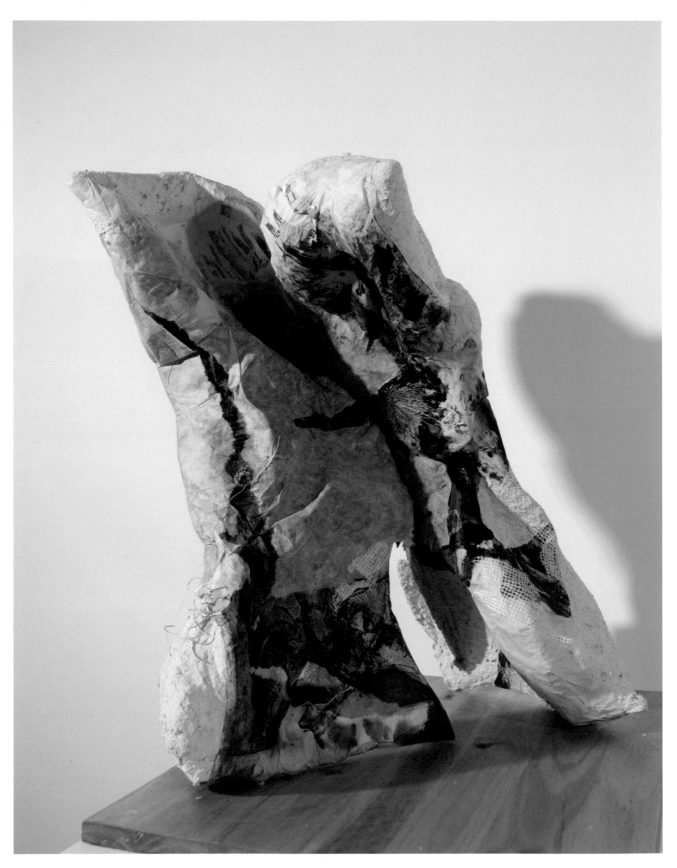

CONDUCTING

second opinion. Elizabeth did the research and found Dr. John P. Leonard, Professor of Hematology and Medical Oncology at Weill Cornell Medical College/New York-Presbyterian Hospital and clinical director of the New York-Cornell Center for Lymphoma and Myeloma. Even more difficult than finding Dr. Leonard was getting a chance to see him. It took Elizabeth over a week to schedule an appointment.

I shipped all my pathology reports to Dr. Leonard and Elizabeth, Joe and I traveled to New York. The best I could hope for, I thought, was reducing my chemotherapy by one round. Instead, after examining me thoroughly, Dr. Leonard told me that the latest research on stage 1 B-cell non-Hodgkin's lymphoma showed that I had already had sufficient chemo.

Dr. Leonard, however, recommended radiation every day for a month. It was not proven it would help, he said, but all the studies included it. Dr. Leonard called Dr. Yi to inform him about my treatment. The radiation oncologist—a former student of Gary's—gave me the smallest dose possible.

For the past two years, I have lived life cancer free. I play tennis regularly and get my hair cut every couple of months. Joe and I traveled to Italy the fall after Dr. Leonard's good news. I ate so much pasta there, I began to think I might even have to watch my weight. Last fall Joe and I took a trip to Spain and Portugal.

I splurged and took all fourteen of my children and grandchildren on a wonderful vacation at the Mohonk Mountain Resort in New York State. They continue to ask me when we're going to do it again.

I have been one of the fortunate ones. Unlike my husband Gary, I have not had to accept my death. I am, however, constantly aware of my mortality and of the preciousness of life.

Concerns of a Family Physician
Julie Ann Juliano, M.D.

Family physicians have a long-term and caring relationship with patients and their families. This is an extraordinary relationship with two sides; we get to share the joys of our patients' lives as well as help them through difficult times. We make sure that our patients and their families get the routine preventive care needed to not only keep them healthy but also to detect diseases early in their course for the best possible outcomes. Most patients avoid routine care because they are fearful that something will be found. That is why breaking the news after a routine exam is the most difficult conversation for both the patient and the family physician. We don't want to tell patients difficult news on the phone, because they could be alone, at work or out in public on a cell phone. We want to be able to monitor and control the situation to make sure our patient takes the news in the best possible way. However, in order to tell patients in person they must be invited into the office without knowing the reason and are advised to come with a family member or close friend.

Patients need to have the support of someone with them for three reasons. The first and most pressing is to take over transportation home, which may be overwhelming or unsafe if the patient is very upset, the second is to be supportive and the third is to listen to all of the information. The last is the most important, since once a doctor says the words, "I think you might have cancer," patients often shut down due to distress and they find it difficult to follow or later recall the conversation. Doctors see the terror, disbelief and confusion in their patients' eyes. We have to wait for the information just stated to sink in and process in our patients' minds. Then, I usually repeat the information and begin to answer the difficult questions that come next. As doctors, we've known our patients for years, we have a long-standing relationship and we want to comfort, address their concerns and reassure them that they are not alone.

That first conversation is vital to how patients will deal with the long process that follows. The conversation must proceed slowly. After the initial shock sinks in, the conversation must deal with all the stages of grief in a very brief period of time. Patients are taken through: "not me," "why me," "what will my family do without me," "this is not fair," crying and then, finally, "now what do I do?" Once we get there, questions are asked that we, as family physicians, usually cannot answer. "How far along is the cancer," "will I lose my hair," "how long will I live," "what will the treatment be and for how long?" This part of the conversation is extremely difficult. It is not necessary to paint either the worst picture or the best picture; we have to give a range of possibilities while restating that a tissue diagnosis and staging are the next steps, and only then can we really know the answers to any questions.

The next part of the conversation involves the family member or friend. We need to ask if he or she has any questions for us and address any questions or fears. Then we ask patients again if they have any questions they would like to ask. The questions can be scattered and sometimes irrelevant to the issues at hand, but nevertheless they are important—patients are vulnerable and often feel violated.

Then we address the testing needed to confirm or disprove the diagnosis of cancer. This is where a caring office staff becomes vital to the smooth transition to the upcoming care. If further testing is needed, it must be scheduled and the paperwork must be prepared at the end of the visit. If appointments are needed, referrals have to be arranged in advance and the consultant doctors' contact information must be given to the patient. This is all prepared in a packet, which is then handed to the patient with verbal instructions.

Follow-up is another important step. Office staff makes a phone call to the patient the next day to be sure that everything is going well and to answer any further questions. Frequently, questions will come to light because it is common for people to go home and research online the worst-case outcomes, which make them scared and upset. We try to reassure patients that until there is a

"When I got my diagnosis—stage 1 B-cell non-Hodgkin's lymphoma—I knew little about my disease."

— Joyce Greenberg Lott

A — Always ask to have all information sent to your primary doctor so one doctor will have the information together. Make sure to have all the information yourself.

tissue diagnosis and staging, they should stay off the Internet because they are reading things that probably do not pertain to them, and which could increase their distress.

After the diagnosis comes in, the family physician is there to support and appropriately transition the patient to the other doctors who take over the patient's care. Medical oncologists, surgeons, radiation oncologists, plastic surgeons and others all become the center of the patient's care. Trying to keep track of all the events happening can be challenging for the family physician. The patient will return to the family physician for comfort and to review the diagnosis and the care plan. At this point, when the patient has a grasp of the diagnosis and what he or she is facing, we then become a team that fights the cancer together.

II

Hand in Hand—
Additional partners on the road to wellness

Your Oncology Nurse Practitioner

Debra A. Walz, R.N., M.S., W.H.N.P.-B.C., A.O.C.N.P., STAR/C

You may find along the path of your cancer journey that your physician brings in a team of specially trained people who will play a part in your treatment and care. One member of the team could be a nurse practitioner, who quite possibly may be the first oncology team member you meet. Your oncology nurse practitioner has been educated and trained to perform the following: document your health history, perform your physical exam, order tests, evaluate your symptoms and test results, and in consultation with your oncologist develop your cancer treatment plan and perform specific treatments.

Oncology nurse practitioners can fulfill many roles in a patient's cancer journey. They can function as clinicians, consultants, educators, navigators, researchers, coordinators and case managers. Their specific role or roles depend upon the structure of the organization for which they work and the settings in which they work. The roles vary greatly between the nurse practitioner who works in a community hospital, a teaching hospital, an outpatient specialty clinic, or private practice, and one who works in the patient's home. The roles also vary depending upon the needs of those with whom they work and the needs of the patients, as well as their own areas of specialty and goals.

Each state has its own nursing guidelines that nurse practitioners are required to follow. All nurse practitioners must practice within the guidelines that have been established by their state Board of Nursing and its Nursing Practice Acts. For instance, in some states nurse practitioners have no restrictions when writing prescriptions; in other states they are not allowed to prescribe narcotics; and in others they are not allowed to prescribe any medications or treatments. In some states nurse practitioners are allowed to work independently; other states require that nurse practitioners have a collaborative agreement with a doctor; and in other states they must work with a doctor. When nurse practitioners are required to work in collaboration with a physician, it means the physician has agreed to be available to consult with the nurse practitioner on difficult cases or if she or he requires assistance in caring for the patient. The physician agrees to be available by telephone for consultation and is required to review a certain number of the nurse practitioner's cases and patient charts during a specified time frame.

The difference between a nurse and a nurse practitioner is that a nurse cares for patients and may administer medications and procedures that have been prescribed by a doctor or a nurse practitioner. The nurse practitioner has received advanced education and training and has been licensed to examine, diagnose and treat patients and their illnesses, prescribe medications and order procedures and tests, in addition to providing patient care and administering medications.

"Most doctors who accept insurance work with nurse practitioners and physician assistants. These valuable clinicians are able to spend longer sessions with the patient, especially in the initial stages of diagnosis and treatment."

— Barrie Raik, M.D.

In 1965, due to a lack of physicians and with the hope of meeting the health care needs of underserved areas in rural North America, the first nurse practitioner training program was founded at the University of Colorado by Loretta Ford, R.N., and Henry Silver, M.D. The first nurses who completed this program were highly scrutinized by physicians and critics. They met them head-on with the highest of nursing skills combined with strong competence in assessment and diagnostic skills.

Today, nurse practitioners have, at a minimum, acquired a master's level education and obtained National Board Certification as an Adult N.P., Family N.P., Women's Health N.P., Pediatric N.P. or Geriatric N.P. Some have also obtained further specialized education and training and have received National Board Certification in other areas such as an Advanced Oncology Certified Nurse Practitioner (A.O.C.N.P.).

As your treatment starts, your nurse practitioner may see you along with your physician or independently. The nurse practitioner can examine you and assess your response to treatment as well as your side effects from treatment. She or he might prescribe medications that work in conjunction with your cancer treatments and help with the side effects of your treatment. The nurse practitioner will provide education to you and your family about your diagnosis, recommended treatment and the expected side effects, as well as giving you and your family support throughout your journey and making referrals specific to your needs. One of the most important roles of the oncology nurse practitioner is to provide continuity of care throughout your journey. The Oncology Nurses Society (ONS) reports that studies have found that Advanced Oncology Certified Nurse Practitioners provide better patient education, which results in greater access to care, greater patient adherence to the prescribed procedures, improved quality of life and increased patient satisfaction.

So you may ask, what is the actual difference between my nurse practitioner and my doctor? Again, this does depend upon where you are being treated and in what state you live. Like doctors, nurse practitioners have been trained to diagnose and treat the patient's illness, but nurse practitioners also evaluate and manage the effects of the illness on both the patient and the patient's family. Nurse practitioners have been trained in the theory and practice of nursing, which encompasses the care of the whole patient. In the oncology setting the nurse practitioner works with the physician to develop the treatment plan and cares for you while you are receiving treatment.

You may find along your journey that you have unanswered questions or concerns or are experiencing difficulties making decisions regarding your treatment. Your nurse practitioner may be able to answer some of your questions and will work to help you discuss with your doctors some of the concerns you might have about your treatment options.

If your nurse practitioner remains part of your care team after your treatment is finished, your oncologist and nurse practitioner could share your follow-up visits and exams and the ordering of specific tests and/or therapies.

TUMOR BOARD

A tumor board is a treatment planning approach in which a number of doctors who are experts in different specialties (disciplines) review and discuss the medical condition and treatment options of a patient.

She or he will continue to assess and help manage the effects of your cancer and its treatment on you and your loved ones.

The most important thing to remember is that your nurse practitioner is there to help you get the best care and treatment for your cancer, help you to have open communication with your doctors and to help support you and your family through a time that can be very emotional and stressful.

References

Office of the Professions, New York State Education Department. July, 2003. Nursing Guide to Practice. Albany, NY.

Pearce, C. The History of Nurse Practitioners. Accessed May 31, 2012, at www.ehow.com/facts_6805736_history-nurse-practitioners.html.

Nurse Practitioner. Accessed May 31, 2012, at www.en.m.wikipedia.org/ wiki/Nurse_practitioner.

Gobelin, B.H., Triest-Robertson, S., & Vogel, W.H. (2009). Advanced Oncology Nursing Certification: Review and Resource Manual. Pittsburgh, PA.

My Experience as a Cancer Study Participant
Sushma Prasada

My father battled cancer for three years before he succumbed to it in 1967, at the age of fifty-four, in India. I was not aware of his illness for two and a half of these three years because, at that time, I was living in the U.S.—my father tried to protect me by not informing me. The death of a parent is hard to accept at any time. Under the unusual circumstances in my case, it left me devastated. My only consolation was that we had returned to India a few months before his death. He was able to see and play with his first grandchild and I was able to support my family emotionally during this time of crisis.

My husband, Biren, and I with our son, Sandeep, and daughter, Charu, immigrated to Canada in 1976. When we moved to Montreal, we did not know anyone there and were unable to make friends for several years. Biren was busy with his work. Sandeep and Charu went to school. I took several courses at McGill and Concordia universities and did volunteer work in a local school in order to enhance my earlier degrees: B.Ed. from India and M.S. in Educational Psychology from the U.S. In 1978, I accepted a position as an assistant teacher. A month later, I was offered the position of teacher. I started teaching developmentally delayed and emotionally disturbed children.

In 1981, I heard of a study being conducted by some doctors in Montreal hospitals about early diagnosis of breast cancer. I wanted to help in this research and volunteered as a subject. It involved going to the hospital once a year for a

"In the clinical trial process…the old treatment is compared against the new and if the new treatment is found to be superior, this treatment becomes the new standard."

— Richard Margolese, M.D.

mammogram for a period of five years. In 1986, I went for my last appointment with a great feeling of relief that all was well and I would not have to go again. It was not to be so.

They had spotted something in the mammogram and a follow-up was recommended. As my knowledge of French was minimal, I requested a referral to a doctor in the English stream. I had gone alone for my appointment. I was in a daze. I could not comprehend the situation or grasp its meaning. The nurse mentioned the name of Dr. Margolese at the Jewish General Hospital and gave me his telephone number. I told her that I felt lost and requested that she make the call for me. She was kind and understanding and made an appointment for me—the earliest available one—almost two months later.

It was a long bus ride home and it gave me time to assess the situation. I decided to break the news as gently as I could to Biren. But panic gripped both of us. We tried to comfort each other. No one had used the word cancer yet, but the possibility took possession of our minds. It became all pervasive. We knew nothing about breast cancer. We felt the urgent need for diagnosis and treatment. We decided to consult our family physician, who picked up the phone and made an appointment with a general surgeon in his hospital. The surgeon recommended surgery and was prepared to schedule it within a week. I just did not know what to do or who to ask. Finally we decided to wait for the appointment with Dr. Margolese. We also decided to tell everything to Sandeep and Charu.

Despite the fact that cancer had claimed my father's life, it had never occurred to me that I could also be a victim. I was forty-six years old and my life was falling apart. Our lives had been turned upside down. The stress in the home was devastating, each of us trying to cope in our own way. Charu was crying in her sleep, Sandeep was suffering quietly and stoically and Biren was tossing and turning and talking in his sleep. We did not have extended family in Montreal for sharing and emotional support. We tried to lead our lives in as normal a way as possible, going to school and our respective jobs. However, all the time, I kept thinking of my children and my husband and how it would affect their lives. My heart was breaking. Unable to face my own mortality, I was falling apart.

Why? Why? Why?
Been a good person
Lived a healthy life
Ate balanced, nutritious food
Exercised and meditated
Have loved and been loved
Am strong and giving.

Why? Why? Why?
Desperation
Anger
Depression

Be strong
Succumb not
Patience
Optimism
Faith
Hope

So much love to give
Done a lot
So much more to do
So little time left
Dreams unfulfilled
A little more time
Watch children grow up
See grandchildren dance in the rain
Grow old with my husband
A little more time
May be four years, ten, twenty
Or with great luck thirty
Hope

Since 1987, throughout the difficult and good times I have been treated and followed by Dr. Margolese at the Jewish General Hospital. No amount of praise is enough for the excellent medical attention, treatment and support that I have received.

I remained fine for twelve years and then the cancer returned. I had to undergo treatment again. It is almost twelve years since the second episode and I am very grateful to be alive.

After the first episode of cancer, I suffered from a severe case of Hashimoto's disease (hypothyroidism) and then after the second episode I had sarcoidosis (a disease of unknown cause, in which inflammation occurs in the lymph nodes, lungs, liver, eyes, skin or other tissues). In my case, it attacked my liver and eyes. By God's grace, I have reached the age of seventy-one. I am ever thankful that I am alive and well, enjoying my two grandchildren and eagerly looking forward to the arrival of the third. I am very lucky indeed.

In retrospect, what has helped me?

I felt that I did not have time to prove or disprove theories, so I followed a multifaceted holistic approach. Perhaps the following helped me:

– Early diagnosis
– Excellent medical treatment and follow-up
– Unflinching support of my husband, son, daughter and close
  family members

"...have the right medical team when faced with a diagnosis of breast cancer."

— Kathleen Toomey, M.D.

– After the initial shock, panic, anger, tears and sadness, the realization that negativity was only going to hurt me
– Acceptance of the disease
– Positive attitude
– Focus on everything that I had and counting my blessings
– Awareness that lots of people are much worse off than me
– Prayers
– Living a well-balanced lifestyle that included:
  • Good nutrition and exercise
  • Balance of rest and activity
  • Transcendental Meditation
  • Tai Chi
  • Setting up goals that helped in feeling fulfilled
  • Cherishing family and friends
  • Welcoming the beginning of a new day with joy
  • Going to bed thankful.

Will I Live?
Peggy S.

"We (oncology social workers)… can help navigate the health care system and intervene with day to day challenges that accompany a cancer diagnosis."

— Vilmarie Rodriguez, M.S.W.

We all pursue different paths throughout our journeys in life. It is the ones we don't choose and are forced to travel that mold us into who we are today. At thirty-four, with two wonderful children who were seven and four at that time, a devoted husband, good health and a happy life, I never expected to hear the words, "The lump is malignant." I looked at my husband and burst into tears, literally nauseated, feeling as if I had walked head-first into a brick wall. I have cancer! Will I live? Am I being punished? How do I tell my children and the rest of the family? These questions overwhelmed me. Once the shock subsided I knew I needed to face the reality of the situation. My husband immediately comforted me and said we would get through this together. True, he would be there, but what needed to be done to conquer this, and did I have what it would take to do so? Looking into the eyes of my husband and children reassured me that the answer was an emphatic yes. I would need to be strong for my family and myself.

June 1990 was the beginning of a journey I never thought I would take. A mastectomy was followed by six months of chemotherapy. Just when it seemed impossible to handle anything more, I was faced with a new obstacle. The day before starting my first chemo treatment, my father suffered a massive stroke and was in a coma. God works in mysterious ways. My father's illness became my major concern and I was extremely worried about my mom. Our family ties were strong and my sisters were all close by. Faith is an important part of my life. The love and support of my family, friends and church got me through this emotional roller coaster. I honestly believe God was working through my father. His illness preoccupied me so much that I didn't have time to feel sorry for myself and simply went through the motions of chemotherapy, then raced to be with my parents, husband and children. A year later, despite my initial hesitancy, I had reconstructive surgery, which turned out to be a good choice. At thirty-five, it boosted my self-esteem and morale.

While this was definitely the worst time in my life, much good evolved from the bad. I learned to appreciate each day and try not to take things for granted. There are the wonderful people I've met who have struggled with the same issues and I've greatly appreciated the special bond with other breast cancer survivors.

God gave me a second chance at life. I am a twenty-year breast cancer survivor—extremely thankful for that—and am a stronger, more confident person than twenty years ago, defined not by the scars on my body but rather by the person deep inside. I am grateful for the excellent, caring medical staff that treated me and the unconditional love and support of family and friends. My husband was my rock and loved me unconditionally through all this and still does. Although I did not choose this path, it took me to places I needed to go and provided me with the strength and maturity to face the unknown.

"It is important to listen effectively while providing a spiritual care plan that can utilize religious and spiritual resources while considering cultural and socio-economic factors."

— Nomi Roth Elbert, M.Ed.,
Spiritual Care Provider

The Role of the Gynecologist in Breast Cancer
Susan N. McCoy, M.D.

It is imperative to have a partnership with your doctor so you can help each other. There is no one-size-fits-all. Many women of childbearing age, or older women without medical problems, often use the ob-gyn as their primary care doctor. Other women have an internist as their primary care physician but are more comfortable having the gynecologist do the breast and pelvic exams. Whatever the situation, the doctor in charge of the breasts should be the one helping to guide the patient through the increasingly confusing maze of breast health.

Each woman needs to know what her risk factors are for breast cancer and what she can do to modify them, such as weight management, diet, alcohol use and exercise. If she has a family history that might be suspicious for a genetically inherited risk of breast cancer, some doctors offer the testing in their office and some refer the patient for genetic counseling. It is important to update and review your family history annually. If breast cancer has occurred in family members younger than fifty, or in multiple relatives on the same side of the family, or ovarian cancer at any age, you should make an effort to determine if that relative had genetic testing and convey that information to your doctor.

After determining your risks, you and your doctor can decide on the frequency of mammography and breast exams. There is conflicting advice

"I feel very lucky to have been examined here (in the States) by a gynecological specialist…"

— Pam Cooper

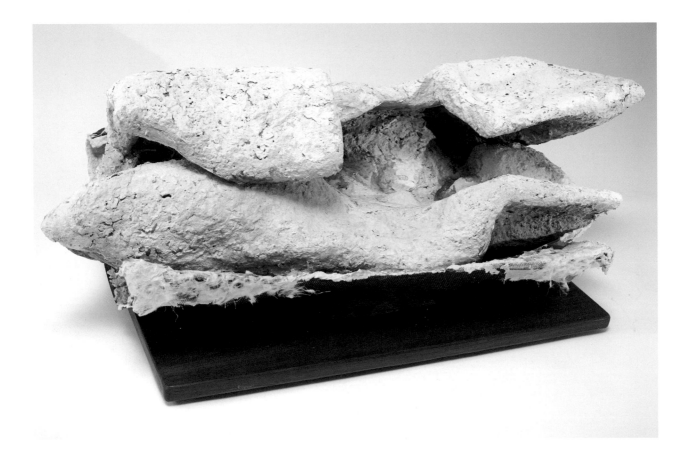

about hormones, the advisability and frequency of mammography screening and even whether or not to do self breast exams. It can be daunting both for physicians and patients to figure out what to do. In the current medical climate where doctors are increasingly pressed for time, complex explanations are difficult to convey and difficult for patients to understand.

I am amazed how often women assume that a yearly mammogram is sufficient for screening and are unaware that mammography may miss 10–15% of breast cancers, and not because they were overlooked. Some cancers just don't show up on a mammogram but may be felt by you or your doctor. When you go for your breast exam you should let your doctor know if you have noticed any change in your breast such as unusual pain (not related to the menstrual cycle) or nipple discharge. If you notice any of these symptoms or think you feel a lump in your breast, call and schedule an appointment for an exam. If you or the doctor has concerns, a diagnostic mammogram (rather than a routine screening study) will be ordered. The radiologist may then focus additional attention to a particular area of the breast or include an ultrasound or other studies if indicated.

Many women have had the heart-stopping experience of being called back for more testing after their mammogram. Fortunately, most of the time, this turns out to be a false alarm and with other views of the breast, the radiologist is able to determine that either no further testing is needed or that the finding is very likely benign. In some cases the radiologist recommends a six-month follow-up to ensure that there are no further changes that might warrant a biopsy. Many radiology offices and breast centers are responding to the anxiety caused by these callbacks and make an effort to bring the patient back as soon as possible and have the radiologist give the patient the result and recommendation immediately after the additional testing is completed. If a biopsy is recommended, the radiologist will most likely also call the referring doctor and speak to him or her directly.

If the mammography finding is more worrisome or suggestive of breast cancer, the radiologist will recommend a biopsy. The one-size-doesn't-fit-all rule applies here as well. Depending on the size, characteristics and location of the lesion, the biopsy may be done by the radiologist with the aid of a computer (stereotactic biopsy), by the radiologist or the surgeon using ultrasound guidance or directly by the surgeon in the office or the operating room. For instance, examination of a small area of suspicious calcifications that cannot be felt would most likely be done stereotactically, whereas a small lesion that is close to the surface of the breast and is easily felt by the surgeon might be biopsied in the office.

After a mammogram some doctors will choose to refer the patient to a general surgeon or breast surgeon prior to the biopsy; but because many of these biopsies will not show cancer, some doctors will wait until the biopsy result is back before a referral is made. The chosen course would also depend on the patient's preference and how suspicious the mammography or physical findings are. In the not too distant past, there were not many "breast" surgeons and most of the breast surgery was done by general surgeons. Now, especially in metropolitan areas and larger cities, there are likely to be breast centers and surgeons with advanced training in management of and surgery for breast cancer. However, where such specialists are not conveniently available there are still many excellent general surgeons who perform biopsies and breast surgery. Your primary doctor should be able to refer you to a surgeon, when appropriate.

If you are referred to a surgeon or diagnosed with breast cancer, it is important to keep your referring doctor in the loop. Most specialists are good about that, but it doesn't hurt to tell the surgeon, and other doctors involved in your care, who you would like to receive your information and updates. After a diagnosis of breast cancer, it is important to maintain your regular visits for gynecological care. Some of the side effects of cancer treatment or chemotherapy might be vaginal dryness, hot flashes or issues with sexual function, which your gynecologist may be able to help you manage or alleviate. Patients should always ask questions if anything seems to cause a concern or is not clear.

Women who have been diagnosed with certain BRCA gene mutations are also at increased risk for ovarian cancer. Younger women with these mutations, but without cancer, may be advised of the protective effect of oral contraceptives for the ovaries. Women who have completed childbearing may choose to have the fallopian tubes and ovaries surgically removed. This can be done with a laparoscope, often referred to as minimally invasive surgery. If there are other gynecologic issues, such as large fibroids or heavy bleeding, other options might include a complete hysterectomy. Fortunately, most breast cancer is NOT associated with the BRCA mutations and most women do not have to make these decisions, which can be life-altering especially for younger, pre-menopausal women.

There will continue to be new developments that may alter our recommendations for screening and health care in the future. For instance, did you ever think you would see the day when a yearly Pap smear is a relic of the past? For women with risk factors, the answers are clearer and regular mammography screening is indicated. For low-risk women, the answers are not so clear and are worthy of a discussion with the doctor to determine how frequently to have, and at what age to start, mammography screening. We still don't know how much of the decline in breast cancer death rates is due to early detection and how much is due to improvement in treatment.

Q — Are there different types of cancers?

Just as one size doesn't fit all for screening, not all breast cancers are alike. There is much to be learned about the behavior of different breast cancers. It is not inconceivable that in the future, we may be able to predict by molecular or genetic testing whether a cancer may be "indolent" and so slow growing that it may need minimal or no treatment at all. We are not there yet, but we do know that some cancers behave very aggressively, some are of the indolent variety and some are in between, but at this point, doctors are often unable to predict how a cancer will behave.

It seems the fear of breast cancer lurks in the back of every woman's mind, and that fear is often stoked by misinformation. If you look back just one generation, there has been a long list of hopeful changes. Long gone are the disfiguring radical surgeries that were once the norm, and the side effects from chemotherapy and radiation are better prevented and ameliorated. We should be cognizant that many of these advances have come through clinical trials and should be grateful for the thousands of women who have participated in these studies. We also know that a healthy lifestyle and positive attitude not only help prevent cancer but can decrease the chance of recurrence in women who have been diagnosed with breast cancer. As a plus, this lifestyle also helps prevent heart disease, which kills more women each year than breast cancer. So, in closing, know your body and take care of it, know your risk factors and how to manage them and know your doctor and be a proactive partner in your health care.

Experiencing Ovarian Cancer
Pam Cooper

I knew something was not quite right, but in my senior year at Pratt Institute, studying fine art and with my final exams and exhibit imminent, I didn't have time to worry about my health.

My family had moved to the U.S. four years previously for my husband's job. My two teenage children were none too happy about the move away from all their friends, especially my daughter. As I was unable to work, I decided to apply to art school; the previous year I attended Southampton College of Art part-time in the U.K. I applied and was accepted by Pratt Institute for a four-year fine arts degree course. This entailed traveling four days a week from Northern New Jersey to the Brooklyn Campus, starting just six weeks after arriving in the U.S. and only one week after moving into our house. It was a tough but manageable schedule, made possible by switching my thoughts from home to college, or vice versa, as I crossed the George Washington Bridge.

It was a very stressful four years, but I wouldn't have had it any other way. Maybe the upheaval and stress contributed to my upcoming experience— who knows.

I hadn't had a gynecological checkup since I left the U.K. so when school was finished in the summer of 1994, I rectified that. My periods were becoming more frequent. I was forty-five years old and was possibly starting menopause.

The doctor felt a lump on my ovary and sent me for an ultrasound. I had a sizeable mass on my ovary and needed to have a CA 125 test to see if it was cancerous. As I left the office the ultrasound technician patted me on the shoulder and wished me good luck. At that moment it all came home to me, and when I reached the car I just sat and cried.

CA 125

A CA 125 test is primarily used to monitor therapy during treatment for ovarian cancer.

A series of CA 125 tests that shows rising or falling concentrations is often more useful than a single result.

The CA 125 test turned out to be normal; there was no rush to schedule an operation as it was deemed to be a cyst. Now, seventeen years later, we know not to take the results of that test as definitive. I was scheduled for a half-hour operation on November 15. My doctor, also a gynecological surgeon, performed the operation. Five hours later my husband was informed I had cancer in both ovaries. Luckily the ovaries had not ruptured.

When I was told, apparently all I said was, "okay." I was dealing with pain medications and a tube down my throat—difficult to say anything at all. Thinking about it, what else can you say? Nothing is going to change; you just have to deal with the situation.

Six weeks later I started chemotherapy. I was given the choice to say no but decided to take all the precautions I could against a recurrence. Having been through the experience once I don't know if I could make the same decision today.

In 1994 chemotherapy for ovarian cancer was given by continuous drip over three days as an in-patient. Mine consisted of steroids, Taxol and Cisplatin, the last two guaranteed to make you lose your hair and make you nauseated. My hair started to fall out two weeks later. I had already selected a wig and decided to have my hair buzz cut when it started to fall out. This made me feel that I was in control of what was happening to me.

I rarely wore my wig. My hair is very fine and wigs are not made of fine hair. Each time I passed a mirror I frightened myself with my Tina Turner hairstyle. I wore hats in the winter and was bare headed in the summer. This is where my time in art school really paid off. I had a lot of young friends with shaved heads and just joined in. Eventually I even lost my facial hair. It is a very strange look without eyelashes and eyebrows, much more disturbing.

When you have been diagnosed with cancer, people have great difficulty knowing how to deal with you and will try to avoid the situation if at all possible. I found the easiest way of making people feel comfortable was just talking to them about the cancer or making jokes about having lost my hair. I have had people laugh at me because they thought I had shaved my head to join in with the other artists. Others looked at the floor so as not to engage with me. In one instance a woman rushed up and hugged me saying, "Hang in there." Obviously she had been through this ordeal herself. That brought a few tears. In a store with my daughter choosing hair clips, I could see the young shop assistant was very uncomfortable. I just looked at her and said, "Bad hair day." She couldn't help but laugh.

I endured five courses of treatment—the side effects from each were progressively worse. My oncologist tried everything to stop the nausea, to no avail.

Unfortunately, after finishing treatment, I developed a couple of other side effects that are with me to this day: neuropathy and tinnitus. That's now seventeen years. I'm not complaining; I can live with it.

I was lucky to have been diagnosed at such an early stage of the disease and I have no regrets that I chose chemotherapy. In the past seventeen years I have seen both my children married and have four small grandsons and another grandchild on the way. I don't think I could feel as relaxed as I do today if I hadn't had chemotherapy. I have a checkup every couple of years but the cancer does not define me. I am cancer free.

There are a lot of things wrong with health care in this country, but I feel very lucky to have been examined here by a gynecological specialist during those years and fortunate that my husband had health coverage. In the U.K. a woman does not see a gynecological doctor for her annual exam, but rather a general practice doctor. If my cancer had not been caught so early, the outcome could have been very different.

III

The Diagnostic Process—
Defining the condition

My Daughter Was Only Two and a Half
Meera Bagle

I love taking showers. They are comforting and relaxing. Sometimes I do my best thinking while taking them. That is exactly what I thought walking into one on a cold winter's day in February of 2001. But by the time I walked out, I had felt something I never felt before. Not in my mind, but rather in my body. There it was. A lump. No, it couldn't be.

I ignored the feeling for a while, thinking surely it would go away, but it didn't. So I saw my doctor, who concurred with my initial feeling. He said it should go away with my next menstrual cycle. It didn't. It was a mass, not liquid. He sent me to a surgeon to have it removed. The surgeons said it was probably nothing, a standard fibroadenoma, but why keep it in my body?

On May 11, 2001, at the age of thirty-one, I awoke in a hospital bed to the comforting faces of my loved ones by my side. What a relief. The anesthesia was wearing off. I could go home now to be with my daughter, Evani. The procedure was over and they took the growth out of my body. The worst was over, right? We were 99% sure, right?

Then the doctor came in. The words were spoken. "It's cancer." All I thought was: it can't be. It only happens when you are much older, if at all. I spent the next several days wondering why me, feeling as if my life were being stolen. Would I ever see my daughter come home from her first day of kindergarten? Would I see her dance in a recital, be able to help her with her homework, be there when she needed a dress for the prom or a ride home from college? Life was already tough enough. I was going through a divorce, and just one year earlier had lost my mother at the young age of fifty-six. I was thirty-one and still needed her, especially now. My daughter was only two and a half. I knew what it was like to live without a mother and could not let my daughter live without me.

I began to ask questions and educate myself. I learned that my cancer was caught early; it was stage 1. My lymph nodes were negative and the chances of it spreading were, hopefully, low. They could try to save most of my right breast by doing a lumpectomy. I do not carry the breast cancer gene. I would need to go through chemotherapy for the next four months, radiation thereafter and then take a tiny little pill called Tamoxifen—for the next five years. I learned that I would often feel weak, nauseated and maybe depressed, would lose my hair and may never have more children. Most importantly, I learned it wasn't a death sentence. Rather, I was being given another chance—at LIFE.

To this day, one of my most comforting memories of that time comes from the moment I decided to shave all the hair off my head. The chemotherapy was already causing clumps to fall out. It was just too hard to endure. There was only so much the scarf on my head could hold in place. It was time to let it go.

> "The family history should include all cases of cancer from both the mother's and the father's family ... cancer can be inherited from either parent."
>
> — Ruth Oratz, M.D.

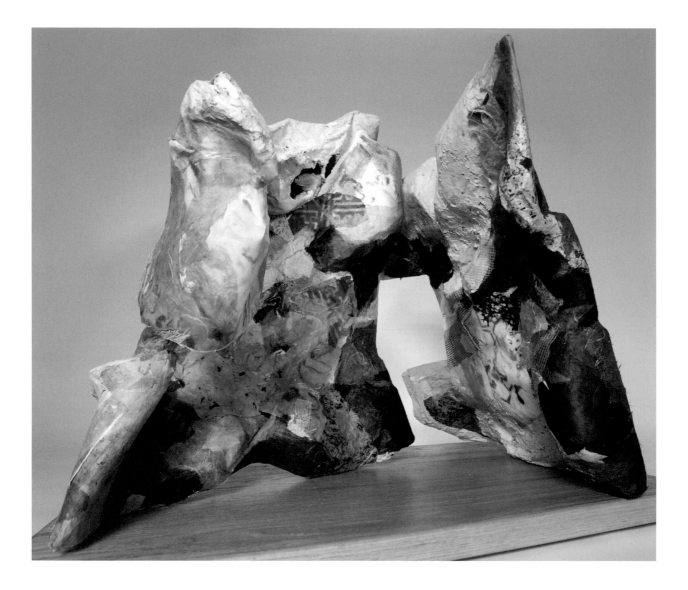

FRIENDSHIP

I went to my neighbor's house and she shaved it all off for me. My greatest fears were comforted when my baby girl ran into the room and right into her bald mommy's arms! She wasn't scared of me. It didn't matter what I looked like. I was still her beautiful mommy. I was going to be okay.

Rather than concentrate on what I could not control, I turned all my efforts towards the things I could and decided to stay positive no matter what. Sure, I was battling cancer and some days would feel weak. But that did not mean I could not live my life and provide a normal environment for my daughter. With the encouragement of my doctors, I decided to continue to work, keep up my exercising, enjoy concerts, take day trips, attend parties and dance at weddings. Sometimes I showed up all decked out—makeup, wig, hot flashes and all! Other days, my scarf would have to suffice. It didn't matter to me and, surprisingly, it didn't matter to others. If anything, I inspired them just by showing up! Life was more precious to me than ever. I was going to be really good at living it!

It has been eleven years since my diagnosis. I have since married an extremely kind and loving man, whose relentless support has been an instrumental element in my recovery from this disease. I have been blessed with two more children, Monika and Nikhil; though not born of my body, they are born of my heart. My daughter, Evani, is now fourteen years old and proudly supports me. By the way, she looked adorable on her first day of kindergarten and I've had many chances to help her with homework.

With each passing year, recollections of the details of my illness, medications and treatments are dimmer. Rather, my memories are those of trips to Paris, Greece and Italy, of taking my children to Disney to meet Cinderella, The Little Mermaid and Buzz Lightyear! And years later, of zip-lining with those same beautiful children through the rainforest in Costa Rica, memories of learning how to plant flowers in my garden, of meeting beautiful people with whom I have become the best of friends, of meeting special girlfriends who have become like sisters to me, memories of sipping wine and laughing until it hurts, of walking in marathons to raise money and awareness, of having a full head of hair again and choosing to donate over eleven inches of it, and memories of watching my daughter dance. I turned forty years old recently. There was a time I didn't believe I would make it to forty. But that was because I did not know better. Once I opened my mind to educate myself, I was able to change the outcome of my life's circumstances.

In the years since my diagnosis I have been blessed with the ability to share my story and hopefully to be an inspiration to many women who face similar battles. The way I see it is this: my survivorship has enabled me to help others understand this disease. Through early detection and aggressive intervention, breast cancer can be overcome.

Cancer does not define me. It was part of my life. The fear of it coming back will always remain on the edge of my thoughts. However, I have chosen not to let that distant fear cripple me. Rather, it is a tool to empower me to live a better life. The surgeries scarred me, the cancer did not—it transformed me. Now, I am stronger and more determined. Some things have not changed: I still love showers and appreciate them more than ever with each passing day.

Family History and Genetic Susceptibility
Ruth Oratz, M.D., F.A.C.P.

"I knew nothing about the possibility of survival, only that my mother had died of breast cancer at forty-two."

— Nora Macdonald

Q — Can men get breast cancer?

After the initial shock of a breast cancer diagnosis, many women ask, "How did this happen to me?" There are many risk factors for developing this disease; the two most important of which are being female and living long enough to develop cancer. Other risk factors include issues related to a woman's hormonal history—facts about age at first menstrual period, age at first full-term pregnancy, number of pregnancies, age at menopause and use of exogenous hormones such as oral contraceptives (birth control pills) or hormone replacement therapy. Lifestyle factors such as obesity, physical activity and exercise, alcohol intake and smoking may also affect a woman's risk. For women who have very dense breast tissue, have had a previously abnormal breast biopsy or prior radiation therapy to the chest area, the risk may also be increased. Women who have a family history have a higher rate of developing the disease themselves. How important is family history?

Breast cancer risk is higher among women whose close relatives have the disease. There is a family history of breast cancer in twenty to thirty percent of women who have the disease. Having one affected first-degree relative (parent, sibling or child) doubles the risk, having two first-degree relatives with this condition leads to a fivefold increase in risk. Men with breast cancer are an important aspect of family history because it may indicate a genetic propensity in a family.

Another important sign that genetic factors may play a role in increasing the predisposition for breast cancer is the age at which this condition develops. If there is an early onset in the family (prior to age fifty), the probability is higher that genetic susceptibility is a prominent risk factor. There is a link between breast and ovarian cancer in genetic syndromes, so that if ovarian cancer is also present in the family, the likelihood of a heritable risk for breast cancer is increased. Sometimes other malignancies may cluster in families that have a high incidence of breast cancer. These may include pancreatic, prostate, endometrial (uterine), thyroid or colon cancer.

It is very important that your physician take a complete family history. The family history should include all cases of cancer from both the mother's and the father's family, as the genes that might be implicated in causing breast cancer can be inherited from either parent and are not limited to the mother's family or only to female relatives.

A number of different genetic syndromes have been identified that increase the risk of developing cancer in the breast. The most important and prominent genes are BRCA1 and BRCA2. Both of these genes are located on chromosomes that we inherit from our parents, one copy from the mother and one copy from the father. This means that the genes are not sex-linked and are not connected only to female relations. We believe that the normal function of these genes is to suppress the development of cancer. If a mutation or abnormality in the gene occurs, then the normal tumor suppressor function is not working and the individual is at increased risk for developing cancer.

Mutations in BRCA1 or BRCA2 are associated with a very high lifetime risk of breast or ovarian cancer.

Breast and Ovarian Cancer Risk Associated with BRCA1 or BRCA2 Mutations

	BRCA1 Mutation	BRCA2 Mutation	General Population
Breast Cancer Lifetime Risk	36–85%	36–85%	12.8%
Ovarian Cancer Lifetime Risk	40–60%	16–27%	1–2%
2nd Breast Cancer Following 1st Diagnosis	40–50%	30–50%	11%
Ovarian Cancer Following 1st Breast Cancer	Tenfold increase	16%	2–6%

"There were four tests to check whether I was a carrier and whether the cancer could somehow be a result of heredity. The BRCA test is the genetic test… I took all of the basic tests because of my girls. There was always the thought: 'What if I'm a carrier?'"
— Rich Loreti

Does everyone with a mutation in BRCA1 or BRCA2 develop cancer? No. Some individuals with BRCA mutations never develop cancer. This can make the cancer appear to skip generations. However, individuals with a mutation, regardless of whether or not they develop cancer, have a 50/50 chance of passing the mutation on to the next generation. Also, since these mutations can pass via men, who do not often develop breast cancer (and never develop ovarian cancer), the pattern of inheritance may seem spotty in a particular family. This is why a very careful family history should be obtained. If there is any suggestion that a heritable susceptibility for cancer is present, genetic counseling and testing should be part of the treatment plan.

There are some differences in the types of breast cancer that arise in individuals with BRCA mutations, compared with those who do not have BRCA mutations. Those that develop in women with mutations in BRCA1 or BRCA2 may arise at a younger age and may be more aggressive. These

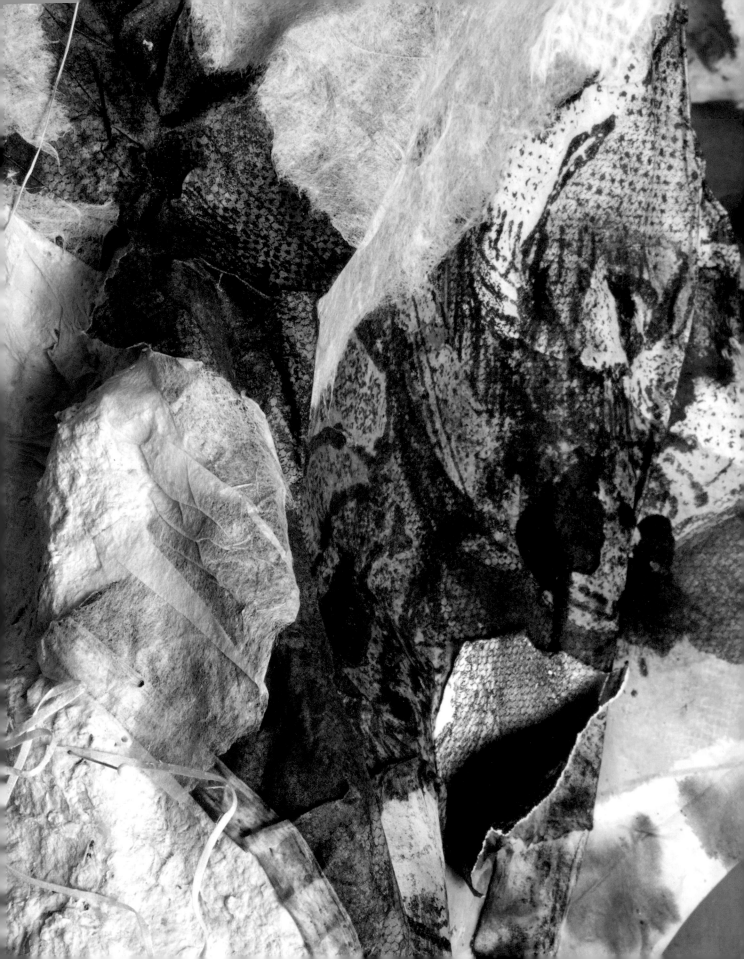

The Diagnostic Process   61

tumors are more likely to require treatment with chemotherapy and may not be responsive to hormonal therapies. Treatment options and decisions about follow-up and surveillance following treatment are different for BRCA mutation carriers than for non-carriers. Counseling for family members who may also be at increased risk (brothers and sisters, children and others) is also a serious consideration.

Family history and genetic susceptibility is an important issue. Although only a small percentage of affected women will carry a mutation in BRCA1 or BRCA2 (10–15% of all breast cancer patients), this information is vitally important for those individuals and families who do harbor these mutations.

Once a diagnosis is made, be sure that a complete family history is obtained. Further, if genetic susceptibility for cancer is a possibility, appropriate counseling and testing ought to be undertaken. Knowledge is power. Identifying individuals at risk before cancer develops may help save lives. Do not be afraid to investigate this issue and share the information with appropriate family members. New screening and surveillance technologies, as well as risk-reducing interventions, may significantly decrease the risk in close relatives. Research to find treatments and prevention specific to BRCA-related breast cancers is also underway. We are confident that identifying individuals at risk, before they develop cancer, will make a difference!

"BRCA1 and 2 are tumor suppressor genes that play an important role in repairing errors in DNA. If there is a mutation or error in these genes they do not function properly."

— Dawn Behr-Ventura, M.D.

My Mother Died of Breast Cancer at Forty-Two
Nora Macdonald

I'm telling my story to encourage women to be vigilant. Early detection of breast cancer, while scary, is life-saving. If there is a history of breast or ovarian cancer in your family, talk to your doctor about being screened for the BRCA1 and 2 genes. Knowing that you carry the gene will give you choices you may not have once cancer is diagnosed.

One December evening in 1986 I put my seven-year-old daughter to bed and then took a bath. As I splashed warm water over myself I felt something near my left nipple. It felt abnormal. I touched it again. It would go away during the night, I hoped. A few weeks previously I had had my first mammogram and the radiologist had said that everything seemed normal.

The lump didn't go away the next day, or the day after. I called my internist. After the examination he said that I should go for a biopsy. Next on the agenda was a needle biopsy followed two weeks later by an outpatient lump biopsy. Waiting for results was the worst. During those weeks my anxiety level went through the roof. I was turning forty-two, widowed and alone with my little daughter. I knew nothing about the possibility of survival—only that my mother had died of breast cancer at forty-two.

"Diagnosis starts with a suspicion either on examination or on a mammogram. … The most important advice I can give to women is to have an awareness of your body and know if anything has changed."

— Christine Rizk, M.D.

The lab results were positive and the perimeter of the removed lump was not clear. I was fortunate to have had a wonderful surgeon. I'll never forget the doodle he drew on a sheet of paper explaining a mastectomy! The panic that gripped me was paralyzing. As I drove home after the diagnosis, my mind was racing. What would happen to my daughter? How could I possibly tell her, "Mommy is going to die"? It made me think about my own experience of losing my mother at such a young age. I needed information badly, but there was very little available at that time. The Internet, a great source of helpful information, did not exist back then, and breast cancer was not a topic people discussed.

After the surgery, an oncologist came into my room at the hospital to say that I had affected nodes and should start chemotherapy in three weeks. Oh my God—I had lost a breast (simultaneous reconstruction was not an option back then), was going to lose my hair and had to face my seven year old! While the doctors tried to give me positive reassurance, I was convinced that the end was in sight.

We got through the next six months of chemo, hair loss and fatigue. My daughter's teacher, who had lost a son in a skiing accident, was our savior. She took care of my daughter when I was feeling sick, giving us both love and reassurance. I also joined a support group. While family and friends were a source of strength, discussing feelings and fears with other breast cancer survivors was invaluable. Thinking back on that time, I realize I could have made life easier. I felt I had to make everything all right, trying to be super mom and pushing myself to prove that I was okay.

Five years later I was alive and well—cancer free. It was eleven years later during a routine mammogram on the other breast that the radiologist discovered another abnormality. A different type of cancer was diagnosed this time. Given my history, my internist suggested another mastectomy, which turned out to be the right decision; the subsequent pathology report showed another cancerous spot.

Twenty-five years after my first diagnosis, I am happy to be alive, proud of my daughter who is an M.D. and am privileged to share my experience and gratitude with other women, knowing that many of us survive to live healthy, grateful and productive lives. As a cancer survivor I have a greater appreciation of life, an understanding of what is truly important to me and a deep empathy for others who are battling the disease.

"Don't be afraid to go to a support group, a private psychologist or psychiatrist, or now with the Internet, an online site."

— Monica Becker

Lumps and Bumps in the Male Breast: Men Can Get Breast Cancer Too

Dawn Behr-Ventura, M.D., M.P.H.

Men do get breast cancer. Survival rates for breast cancer in men are stage for stage the same as women. However, men typically first seek medical evaluation with higher stages of breast cancer. Men with the BRCA2 gene mutation, Li-Fraumeni syndrome, Klinefelter syndrome, Cowden syndrome or a family history of breast cancer are at an increased risk for breast cancer. Reasons to obtain mammography in the male population include: a palpable mass, recent onset of breast enlargement or tenderness, changes in the skin related to the nipple-areola complex, nipple discharge or a history of previous breast cancer.

When people think about breast cancer, they envision it to be a disease that only affects the female population. However, men can get breast cancer too! In 2013, there will be approximately 2,240 new cases of male breast cancer and 410 deaths from male breast cancer in the United States.[1]

In order to understand where breast cancer occurs, it is helpful to have a basic understanding of breast anatomy, which is not the same in men and women. Breast tissue in an adult woman has lactiferous (milk) ducts, lobules and acini, along with supporting tissue, such as Cooper's ligaments, which extend from the deep tissue of the breast to the skin.

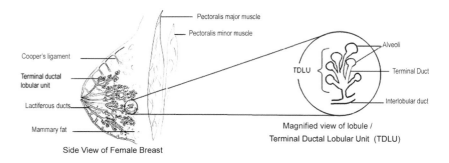

The purpose of the fully developed female breast is to produce milk. Milk production occurs in cellular components (termed acini or alveoli) located within sac-like branching portions of the breast (lobule or terminal ductal lobular unit) and then travels down more prominent ducts toward the nipple where a baby nurses. Of all mammals, only in humans do mature breasts develop prior to pregnancy.

In the prepubescent patient, male and female breast tissue is similar in appearance. For women, hormonal surges during puberty stimulate further growth of ductal and stromal elements, alveolar budding and lobular growth.[2] For men, hormonal surges may stimulate ductal and stromal elements, but not growth of alveoli or lobules. This makes sense as the male breast is not meant to produce milk. Men typically only get ductal, and not lobular, forms of breast cancer. The reason for this fact is not clearly understood, as both lobular and ductal carcinomas seem to originate from the same stem cells. Women can get both forms of breast cancer.

However, it is important to remember that not all "lumps" in the male breast signify cancer. Newborns may demonstrate breast tissue prominence due to transplacental exposure to estrogens (female hormones). This usually subsides in days to weeks after birth, but may last several months in breastfed infants. Furthermore, it is common for adolescent boys to experience intermittent breast tissue prominence as a result of increased hormonal activity. This is referred to as pubertal gynecomastia (breast tissue prominence in the pubertal male), which occurs in up to 64% of adolescent boys, with a peak incidence between thirteen and fourteen years of age.[3] Pubertal gynecomastia can last for one to two years and is often associated with breast tenderness. Though the prominent tissue is typically relatively similar in both breasts, it may be asymmetric in distribution. Nonetheless, this typically resolves on its own, usually by age twenty, and should not be of great concern. Young male patients should be counseled that this finding is part of normal development and does not usually require any intervention.

No one knows exactly what stimulates breast tissue prominence in adolescent boys. However, it is believed that breast tissue prominence is related to relatively high estradiol levels.[4] Testosterone (male hormone) and estradiol (a precursor of estrogen, a female hormone) are two molecules that are very similar to one another in appearance. It is not unusual, during adolescence, for there to be an overabundance of testosterone in the male body. When this happens, some molecules of testosterone can be converted to estradiol.

"At age sixty-eight while taking a shower, I noticed my left nipple seemed to be sticking out. I followed it for a week or two, and noticed an underlying hemispherical lump, growing right under the nipple, had become the size of a golf ball cut in half."

— Wilbur Dexter Johnston, Ph.D.

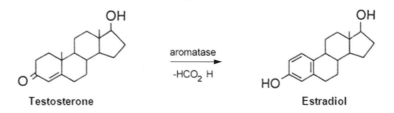

There may also be an association between pubertal gynecomastia and high levels of growth hormones (which are different from the sex hormones testosterone and estrogen).

Prominent breast tissue (gynecomastia) also occurs in adult men and can be stimulated by hormonal imbalance, related to certain medications or medical conditions. Examples of medications which may be associated with this condition include anabolic steroids, digitalis, cimetidine, diazepam and furosemide. Marijuana and heroin may also have this effect. Gynecomastia can also be seen as a side effect in patients with medical conditions such as renal failure, non-alcoholic and alcoholic cirrhosis (damage to the liver with resultant scarring), and malnutrition. Most often, it is the result of a benign process. However, prominence of breast tissue can also be seen in patients with testicular cancer.

Who are the male populations at risk for breast cancer and when should one worry? Typically men with gynecomastia will have easily moveable soft tissue below the level of the nipple in both breasts, which can be distinguished from the skin and subareolar disc (well-defined round tissue below the nipple). Prominent male breast tissue is much more common than cancer. However, any eccentric breast mass should be considered suspicious! Along these lines, indications for mammography in the male population include the following: presence of a mass, recent onset of breast enlargement or tenderness, changes in the skin related to the nipple-areola complex, nipple discharge or a history of previous breast cancer. While men can carry the BRCA1 gene mutation, it is extremely rare that this gene is expressed as male breast cancer; however, these men do have an increased risk of developing prostate cancer. BRCA2-positive men, which means they do have the gene mutation, do have an increased risk of breast cancer and are also at increased risk for other cancers such as prostate cancer, testicular cancer, pancreatic cancer, stomach cancer and melanoma. Men who have a BRCA gene mutation should have a discussion with their primary care physicians regarding how to appropriately screen for these potential cancers. Men with Li-Fraumeni syndrome, Klinefelter syndrome, Cowden syndrome or a family history of breast cancer also have an increased risk of breast cancer.[5]

As mentioned earlier, the proliferation of breast tissue in men is limited to the growth of ductal and stromal tissue. Furthermore, approximately 85% of breast cancers in the male population are the result of ductal cancer. However, men can also have cancerous lesions in breast tissue, which are not the result of breast cancer, but rather metastasized masses from other cancers, such as melanoma, renal cell carcinoma, lung carcinoma and prostate carcinoma. In addition, a patient may have neoplastic lesions in the breast related to lymphoma or leukemia. Survival rates for breast cancer in men are stage for stage the same as women. The problem, however, is that men typically first seek medical evaluation with higher stages of breast cancer. Many men already have metastatic axillary (underarm region) lymph node involvement at the time that their cancer is first diagnosed. The mean age of men with breast cancer is fifty-nine years old.[6] This is older than the mean age of women with breast cancer, which is between forty-eight and fifty-three years old. As young men more commonly present with gynecomastia, and the incidence

"The hard spot was of particular concern to him (my doctor) because it was located directly underneath my nipple. That's typical for male breast cancer."

— Rich Loreti

of breast cancer in men younger than thirty is extremely rare, typically mammography is not performed for men under forty-five years old unless they demonstrate the symptoms or possess the risk factors described above.

While the overall incidence of breast cancer in the male population is much lower than in the female population, men can still get breast cancer, as well as metastatic disease within the breast. Therefore, any man who notices lumps or other symptoms related to the breast should be appropriately evaluated. At the very least, he should receive a physical breast examination, along with additional testing as deemed necessary by his physician.

1. www.cancer.gov/cancertopics/types/breast
2. McFate, J. et al. Congenital and Acquired Disorders of the Breast in Advanced Therapy of Breast Disease. 2012, p 255.
3. Braunstein G. Gynecomastia, *N Engl J Med*. 1993; 328: 490–95.
4. Moore D., et.al. Hormonal changes during puberty: V. Transient X pubertal gynecomastia: abnormal androgen-estrogen ratios. *J Clin Endocrinol Metab*. 1984; 58: 492–499.
5. Weis, J.R. et al. Epidemiology of Male Breast Cancer. *Cancer Epidemiology, Biomarkers & Prevention*. Jan 2005 14; 20.
6. So G.J. et al. The Male Breast. Bassett, L.W. et al. Eds. in Diagnosis of Diseases of the Breast. W.B. Saunders Co., 1997. p 504.

Male Breast Cancer Is Real

Rich Loreti

Forty-three is a young age to find out you have cancer. That's how old I was this past summer, less than a year ago.

My wife, Sandy, was putting suntan lotion on my chest and felt the lump for the second time. Her face showed concern. Several days before, she had noticed a small lump under my nipple. It felt hard, almost like a marble. We talked about it a little and let the subject go. We didn't read much into it. This time, however, Sandy insisted it was time to make an appointment with our doctor— but I couldn't. We were on vacation. The kids needed me around! I promised to call the doctor right after Labor Day and did. Did I think it was cancer? Absolutely not, I didn't think that at all.

My wife and kids stay near the ocean most of the summer. I take off every weekend and Mondays and on Tuesdays go back to work. We own a garbage company and also a landscaping company. That Tuesday, one of the first things I did at work was to go online to Google: lumps, a hard place under my nipple and anything else that could describe what we felt in my chest. Everything started coming back to women's breast cancer. Then I tried male, because nobody really hears of male breast cancer. Momentarily I thought, "okay, I'm looking for the wrong thing." It was weird because male breast cancer didn't surface right away.

All the information on the screen addressed women's concerns regarding the disease. However, eventually male breast cancer did appear.

On the screen there was the description of a lumpectomy, then information stating that male breast cancer usually strikes men over the age of sixty. Ultimately all sorts of information came to the surface that made me nervous. It was time to take a break. I went online again a little bit later. After reading more articles, there was no panic—yet—just a definite concern about the unknown.

The next day, while speaking to my wife, she insisted in no uncertain terms that it was time to call the doctor. My response was: "Don't worry, I'll call tomorrow." But I didn't. I just kept procrastinating. Because of the scariness, the fear of the unknown, everything that goes through one's head, one just doesn't know how to react. On the weekend, when we were together, it was the right time to reveal all the pertinent information to Sandy. Everything found on the Internet indicated that cancer was a possibility. She responded, "I've heard of male breast cancer but one never hears of a real incident." It was at that point we decided to finish out our summer vacation. So, I promised to call the doctor around Labor Day, but I still wasn't mentally prepared to receive bad news.

Summer was over. I called my family doctor of twenty years right away and was able to get an appointment the day after Labor Day. Once in the office my vitals were checked, then the doctor entered the examining room and started asking questions. Almost immediately he began to examine my chest and felt the lump right away. He stopped the exam, sat down and began to write. "What's up?" I asked. He proceeded to explain: "It's definitely not fat cells, it's too hard. I'm sending you for imaging. You need a mammogram and a sonogram."

Since he had been my doctor for such a long time, I simply asked, "What is it?" His response: "I can't tell you because I don't know. What is clear is the lump has to be surgically removed."

The hard spot was of particular concern to him because it was located directly underneath my nipple. That's typical for male breast cancer. Lumps can be found in various places in a man's chest, just as they are located in different areas of a woman's breast, but this spot was typical for male breast cancer.

Two days later a mammogram and a sonogram were done at a local imaging center. Everything was moving fast now. The radiologist pointed out a 2.2-centimeter mass and asked if an appointment had already been made with a surgeon. It had been, with the assistance of our family physician. The appointment was already set for Friday.

Friday came. Sandy and I went to the surgeon. All my films came along with us. The surgeon went over everything again—pointing out the mass, exactly where it was, its diameter, all the details. He seemed very intelligent. I was on the examining table and my wife was sitting close by. He sat next to her facing me. We began talking and then he just told me to listen and to ask questions when he was finished. He brought up the sort of questions that must be on every patient's mind at a time like this. Why me? Do I have cancer? If so, what stage is it at? What do I do next? Which doctors will give me the best attention?

"I thought if it was a 'male menopause' thing it would be symmetrical. (Not true—gynecomastia, which is what it turned out to be, is typically asymmetrical and related to hormonal imbalance, either at puberty or at about age sixty.)"

— Wilbur Dexter Johnston, Ph.D.

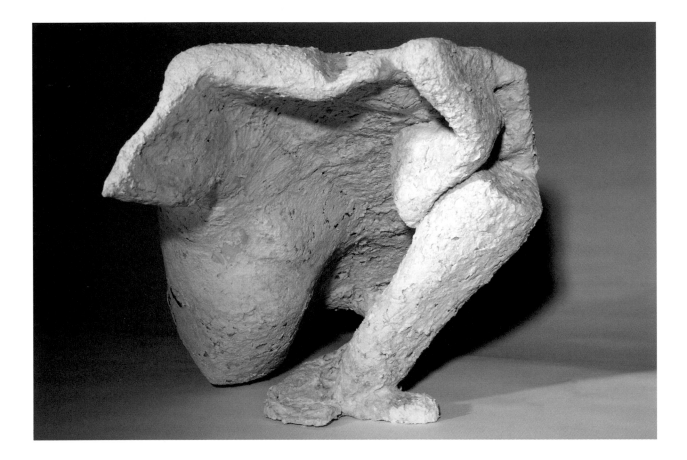

CONTEMPLATION

He immediately responded to each question after he asked it. Many of these questions had been going through my head. He went through about ten or twelve, at which point my wife asked, "Is it cancer?" Without doing a biopsy, he couldn't know. However, it was definitely a mass, and he proceeded to give us specifics regarding male breast cancer. He sees a man with breast cancer approximately every six to twelve months. I was his second patient during the year. He explained that if it were cancer I would require a mastectomy, and went on to describe what might need to be done, how things are attached, about lesions and everything else that could inform me of what might lie ahead.

The biopsy was done the following Monday. The surgeon clearly realized we were anxious to hear the results. On Wednesday we returned to the surgeon's office and were told it is definitely cancerous. It's malignant. It is stage 2 cancer. I was stunned and crying. My wife was crying like a baby. We have two kids. Cancer does not run in my family. People say you need an extra person to come along to the doctor's office to hear what is being said—I think two extra people is more like it. After this news, I didn't hear or remember a word the doctor said. My wife wasn't much better off. Fear was all over her face! The doctor, on the other hand, had been faced by cancer patients before.

Again, he explained it was necessary to have a mastectomy. I didn't know anything about surgery. My knowledge about male breast cancer went from nothing to an overwhelming amount within one month. My family and close friends all wanted me to get a second opinion from a doctor in a large New York City hospital. That was not what I wanted. Rather, my intent was to stay close to home with a doctor I knew and trusted.

If the operation was done locally, family and friends would be near, could help and be there emotionally for my wife and kids. Since my children are young (fourteen and ten) it was important for me to know I was close by. Different things are important to different people.

The mastectomy was performed by a surgeon our family knows. He is someone I trust and with whom I feel comfortable. I liked the other doctor a lot, but this is a person who comes to our school gatherings. This kind of comfort was important to me. He wasn't afraid to be emotional and supportive. The surgery took place on October 8. Not much time elapsed between the diagnosis and the surgery.

There were four tests to check whether I was a carrier and whether the cancer could somehow be a result of heredity. The BRCA test is the genetic test and the Oncotype DX test determines what type of treatment, if any, will be needed. I took all of the basic tests because of my girls. There was always the thought: "What if I'm a carrier?" There are three levels of the Oncotype DX test: low, medium and high. I'm just over the medium line. There is a 78% chance that I'm clean, a 22% chance of something coming back. That news was enough to get me to the oncologist's office.

Following the mastectomy, both my surgeon and oncologist recommended that I do four rounds of chemotherapy. The first two days weren't bad. The

"If there is early onset of breast cancer in the family (less than age fifty), the probability is higher that genetic susceptibility is a prominent risk factor."

— Ruth Oratz, M.D.

third day felt like I had hit a wall. The exhaustion was like nothing I had ever experienced. My hair started to fall out and the kids were clearly worried so we sat them down and explained exactly what was happening. I was scared, yet wanted to be well for my wife and children. They keep me going.

According to a doctor, the cancer could have started years ago, and it just escalated recently. We don't know why or what made that happen. Now I'm concerned with the present and the future. I'm going to a plastic surgeon next; at least I want my nipple back! In our society, women usually wear tops at the beach, men often don't. I have my health and am grateful to be alive, but men are seen in a certain way and there's no reason not to look and feel as well as possible.

I finished my fourth round of chemo three weeks ago and just went to the doctor today. I'm all done. To me, having chemotherapy was like an insurance policy because the percentage of something coming back went from 22% to approximately 5% to 7%. That move was a no-brainer. Today I also start taking a defensive drug called Tamoxifen.

Before the cancer, work and earning money were my main focus. Now I live for my wife and children. At 4:30 p.m., it's time to end the workday. There is tomorrow. Before the cancer it seemed that everything had to be finished today.

So many men don't discover their cancer until they hit stage 4. That's definitely too late. I was lucky. The cancer was still at stage 2 because we felt the lump early on. It doesn't occur to most guys to do a self-exam. I use a bar of soap to wash, so how many times do I touch my chest? Women do a self-exam, that's something that doesn't occur to most men. Be smart, most men don't get breast cancer, but if you do, it's good to catch it early. It can make the difference between life and death. At least once a month, check your chest. That's my advice. If you feel a lump, get to a doctor right away.

"Survival rates for breast cancer in men are stage for stage the same as women. However, men typically first seek medical evaluation with higher stages of breast cancer."

— Dawn Behr-Ventura, M.D.

Scars of Life and Love

Dawn Meade

It was an ordinary day at work as I picked up the phone to an unfamiliar number. The radiology center was calling to tell me I needed to come in for another mammography. I didn't think much of it and went about my day. Although I had felt a lump in my left breast, when I mentioned it to my doctor she didn't seem very concerned. My husband and I had been through our fair share of pain and suffering and had no idea one of our greatest challenges was about to occur. We had lived through 9/11 and had mourned the loss of our beloved brother-in-law. Four months later, I gave birth to premature twin boys who had a combined weight of a little over 5 lbs. To say our life was a bit hectic is an understatement. With my busy life and my job as a speech pathologist, I didn't have much time to worry about that call.

The following day, on November 14, 2006, I left my boys with my husband and went to the radiology center. While sitting in the waiting area, my mom appeared. Why was she there? Did she sense something? She would later admit that she had sensed something wasn't right and needed to be there with me. When they told me the word "cancer," I just didn't get it. How were they so certain? I'm a healthy thirty-eight-year-old woman with my entire life ahead of me. I feel great, how could I possibly have something that never even occurred to me? I couldn't even utter the words to my mom because I knew the pain I was about to inflict on her. I struggled with my emotions, stuck between fear of what I was about to put my family through, anger at how I might have prevented this, and the pure will and determination to beat this beast that I was burdened with. It wasn't the fact that I wanted to live, but needed to live. I wanted to be here for my family. It wasn't an option.

December 14, 2006, I had a lumpectomy and an axillary lymph node reduction. I recovered well and really didn't experience too much pain. My husband and I were about to celebrate our seven-year anniversary on December 18. I was still recovering from surgery and was held up at my mom's house because one of my twins had a stomach virus. My husband, Pat, was absolutely amazing and came to every appointment with a list of questions, as my sister took notes. He had a recorder in case he missed something. Pat challenged the doctors to ensure that they didn't miss a point. He listened to my fears and made promises to me that no husband should ever have to make to his wife. Our love for each other was always special; he is truly my best friend. Although I wasn't looking forward to our anniversary, I agreed to a quiet dinner at my mom's.

I saw something on his face when he arrived at my mom's. Excitement, yes, he was excited. I told myself that I would make a fuss over the present he was about to hand me. In my heart, I felt there wasn't a present he could give me that would lift my spirits. No piece of jewelry, no designer handbag or shoes could bring any happiness to my life at that point. As he lifted his shirt I wasn't sure what to make of the white bandage on his left breast. What had he done? As he removed the bandage my eyes welled with tears and my heart was completely filled with joy. A beautiful pink ribbon was tattooed in the exact spot I had my surgery. The words he said next will be with me forever, "If you are scarred, then I will be scarred with you." In that moment, I knew that my cancer journey was not mine alone. I shared it with all those around me. Especially my husband. Six years later, after eight rounds of chemotherapy, thirty-five radiation treatments and many doctor appointments, my husband continues to be my rock. The day I began chemotherapy, he quit smoking. His motto once again: "If you are going to feel bad, then I will feel bad with you." When I lost my hair and wasn't feeling great about myself, he joked, "Do you think I married you for your hair?" He continues to listen to all my fears, especially in the days leading up to my annual checkups. Although both of our scars have faded a bit, they continue to remind us daily how lucky we are. We battled cancer together. I couldn't ask for a better partner in this journey.

"…I am able to navigate patients through the maze of a breast cancer experience. I can address concerns by telling them about the programs and services at the Cancer Center."

— Cheryl Kott

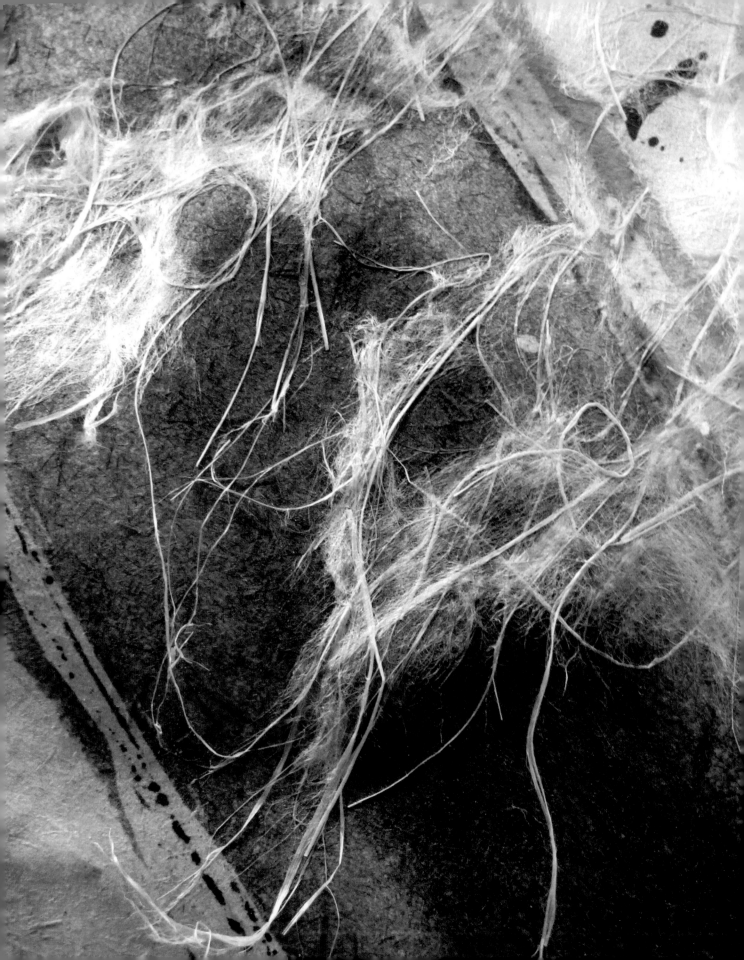

Another Yearly Mammogram

Sondra Schoenfeld

I answered the phone expecting a friend's voice but instead it was the radiology department secretary. "Mrs. Schoenfeld, we'd like to retake the mammogram you took a few days ago." I thought to myself, the technician must have made a mistake in procedure or perhaps I had moved, resulting in a blurred image.

It was November 1994. At age fifty-four, almost fifty-five, the furthest thing from my mind was breast cancer. My mother had lived to the age of eighty-nine with no major health problems and there was no history of cancer in my family; so naturally I assumed I would have the same good fortune. Nevertheless, I had routinely scheduled mammograms each year as recommended by my physician. I thought, just like the belief that carrying an umbrella sometimes prevents a downpour, getting a yearly mammogram would provide protection from having cancer.

Of course I retook the exam and it confirmed there was something on the X-ray that needed further investigation. What was it? Calmly, the doctor explained that there were various possibilities—benign cyst, calcification, malignancy—the only way to determine what was going on was to do further procedures: ultrasound and biopsy. What was it?

I was working five days a week and had no time to be sick. Initially I thought, this can't be happening to me! As kind and gentle as the doctors were, I somehow detached myself from facing the fear of a diagnosis of breast cancer. Thankfully, my husband came along with me for each procedure and, as we went forward, we discussed options and possible solutions. He was a source of great support as he faces life with optimism and, I must admit, I was in a doubtful frame of mind.

Why me? What was it?

Well, it was breast cancer! My doctor, Dr. Angela Lanfranchi, laid out my options in a caring, rational manner. I won't go into the medical details but it was agreed that for me a mastectomy with reconstruction was the road I would follow. Frankly, decisions were moving quickly and even though I was second-guessing myself constantly, I felt that I had to make a decision myself because ultimately it is the patient's responsibility, not the doctor's nor the spouse's. Thankfully, with the support of my husband and the guidance of Dr. Lanfranchi, I slid into a psychological comfort zone, ready to face any challenges. Knowing what I had was in many ways easier to deal with than not knowing. That was 1994. Now, years later, it seems like ancient history. Time has flown by so quickly!

My surgeries went well. I returned to my normal schedule. Six years later, I retired from my school position, still feeling vital and with energy to spare. This seemed an ideal time to try my hand in a different endeavor. I worked

CYST

Cysts are very common and rarely turn into cancers. It is extremely important to find out whether what you have is just a cyst or something else.

part-time as a jewelry sales associate for an upscale store. Then my husband and I reminded ourselves that there were many trips we had planned to take at this point in our lives, so we took the opportunity to travel the globe and fulfill our dreams.

As the years fly by, and I do mean fly, my life is full of continued activity. I find myself doing substitute teaching, which gives me some flexibility for travel. I play bridge with old and newfound friends; I enjoy grandchildren; I socialize with friends; I participate in a book club; I visit museums and attend concerts. Basically the spectrum of daily life is full. Rarely do I think or dwell on my encounter with cancer. It was a special experience in life, like others, that presented an obstacle one has to overcome. Then you go on! Each new moment is a gift I treasure.

Mammography, Ultrasound and MRI

Jane Tuvia, M.D.

"I wish to encourage women to rush to go see breast specialist (doctor) for timely examination… if/when you feel a hard piece inside your breast(s)."

— Naov Davin,
   Cambodian villager

Many women come to my office for routine mammograms or for a specific problem that either they found or their primary care doctor discovered. They often have many questions, especially about the diagnostic procedures that may be required.

The first step is screening mammography, the only proven method to detect early breast cancer and reduce deaths. Yearly mammograms can lead to early detection of breast cancers when they are most curable and breast conservation therapies are available. The most recent recommendations from the American College of Radiology, the American College of Obstetricians and Gynecology, the American Cancer Society and the Society of Breast Imaging, as well as from many other major medical associations, recommend women begin getting annual mammograms at age forty. Women with a strong family history of breast cancer, as well as women who have had radiation treatment to their chest for other medical conditions, should begin screening mammography earlier and should consult with their physician about when to begin.

Screening Mammography

Mammography is a specific type of low-dose X-ray imaging that is used to help detect abnormalities in the breast: these abnormalities may represent early breast cancer or may represent a benign (not cancerous) finding. Full-field digital mammography is a newer variation of this system where the X-rays are converted into digital signals and produce images of the breast on a computer screen instead of film.

The mammogram exam is performed by a radiology technician who has expertise in this field. The images are then reviewed by a radiologist with

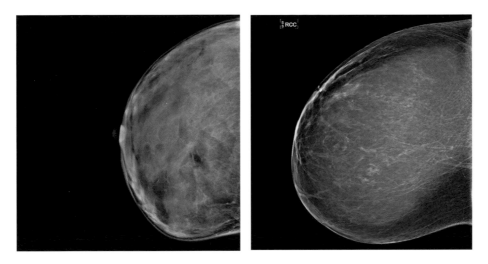

Left: Dense breast tissue may obscure an abnormality on mammography as there is no clear distinction between normal breast tissue and abnormal breast tissue. Right: Fatty breast tissue is less likely to obscure an abnormality.

experience in breast imaging and interpretation of mammograms. The facility where you had the mammogram will notify you, as well as your physician, of the results. All mammography facilities are regulated by a branch of the Federal Drug Administration (FDA) to ensure high-quality examinations and interpretations. The lowest possible radiation dose is used during mammography. Although exposure to high doses of radiation may infrequently cause cancers, the benefit of mammography far outweighs the risk of the low radiation. A false positive mammogram refers to what the radiologist suspects may be an abnormal finding, which may lead to biopsy. Most of the biopsies are normal and do not reveal cancer.

Diagnostic Mammography
Diagnostic mammography, unlike the routine yearly exam, is a procedure performed to evaluate a specific clinical problem, such as a breast lump or nipple discharge. It is usually performed with additional views if the radiologist has found an area on the initial images which may need additional evaluation. This occurs in about ten to fifteen percent of women undergoing mammography, and most of the time the results are normal.

Mammography, like all diagnostic procedures, has its limitations. It does not always reveal all breast cancers. This may be due to prior breast surgery, implants or, most often, dense breast tissue. Dense breast tissue is not abnormal; it just means that there is more breast tissue than fatty tissue. All cancers may not be detected on mammography, as they may be the same density as the normal tissue. Other findings, such as microcalcifications or architectural distortion, may be seen in spite of dense breast tissue. These findings do not necessarily indicate breast cancer but do require additional

"Reasons to obtain mammography in the male population include: a palpable mass, recent onset of breast enlargement or tenderness, changes in the skin related to the nipple-areola complex, nipple discharge or a history of previous breast cancer."

— Dawn Behr-Ventura, M.D.

workup. Since mammograms cannot detect all breast cancers, additional imaging techniques may be necessary.

If you have very dense breast tissue, or if the radiologist detects a possible abnormality, you may be referred for a further test, such as breast ultrasound to determine if there are any underlying abnormalities not clearly seen on the mammogram.

The treating radiologist will send the findings of these procedures to the referring physician, if there is one. If there is no referring physician, the radiologist may suggest further consultation with an oncologist and/or a surgeon for any further steps that may be required.

Breast Ultrasound

Breast ultrasound (sonogram) is an additional imaging technique that uses high-frequency sound waves to produce images showing the internal structure of the breast. There is no radiation involved. A sonogram may be performed to determine the nature of a breast lump, a nipple discharge, or an abnormality seen on mammography; it will help to determine if the lump is a cyst (fluid) or solid. Not all solid masses are cancerous. Ultrasound exams do not replace mammography and clinical breast exams; rather, they are used in conjunction with them when necessary.

The ultrasound exam is usually performed either by an ultrasound technologist or by a radiologist (who does the interpretation). It is important that this is done in a facility where the radiologist interpreting the ultrasound has experience in breast imaging.

Breast MRI

Magnetic resonance imaging (MRI) is a technique that uses a magnetic field and radio frequency pulses in conjunction with a computer to produce a series of images of the breast. It offers detailed information that may not be seen on mammography or ultrasound. It is not a replacement for mammography or ultrasound but is used as a supplemental study. The interpretation of the breast MRI is done by a radiologist with experience in breast imaging.

The MRI is a costly exam and not all insurance companies will cover it readily. Women who have an internal defibrillator or pacemaker, cochlear ear implant or some types of aneurysm clip cannot have MRI studies. Additionally, a breast MRI is very sensitive but not specific, meaning many areas will show up on MRI studies that are not at all cancerous. This may necessitate biopsy or follow-up MRI studies.

Breast MRI imaging is commonly used in the following situations:

- Screening for breast cancer in women at high risk for breast cancer, usually with a strong family history.
- To determine the extent of cancer after a recent diagnosis of breast cancer, as well as to determine if there are other cancers in the same breast or the other breast.

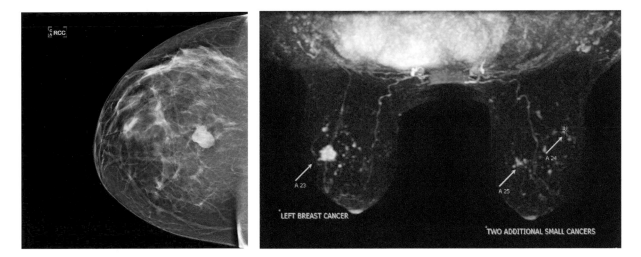

Left: Fatty tissue with suspicious mass. Abnormal mass is readily seen when background tissue is fatty. Right: Breast MRI shows a small cancer in the left breast and two small cancers in the right breast.

- To determine if there are enlarged lymph nodes in the axilla (armpit), which may indicate spread of the cancer.
- For further evaluation of abnormalities seen on mammogram and/or sonogram.
- To assess the results of chemotherapy for breast cancer treatment.
- To evaluate possible rupture of silicone implants.

The above breast MRI shows a small cancer in the left breast, as well as two small cancers in the right breast, none of which were seen on mammogram or sonogram. The largest mass in the left breast was detected only on ultrasound, not mammogram, and MRI was performed to determine if there were additional cancerous lesions.

Needle Breast Biopsies

Suspicious abnormalities identified in the breast are usually tested with a needle biopsy. This is usually done by the radiologist with guidance either from the ultrasound, mammogram or MRI unit, depending on which system showed it the most clearly. Local anesthesia is used and a small amount of tissue is removed from the questionable area and sent to pathology. This is generally an in-office procedure and takes fifteen minutes to one hour on the average. The radiologist and referring physician will receive the results within a few days.

The treating radiologist will send the findings of these procedures to the referring physician, if there is one. If there is no referring physician, the radiologist may suggest further consultation with an oncologist and/or a surgeon for any further steps that may be required.

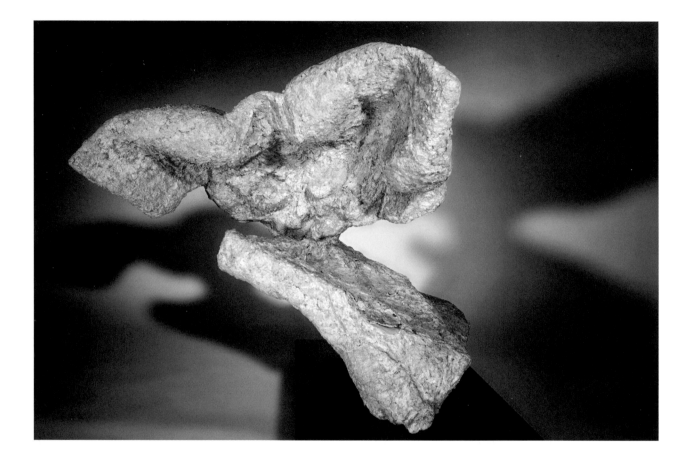

MAMMOGRAM MOMENT

A Radiology Technologist's Advice

Sandra Scott, R.T.(R.)(M.)

When I was a young girl l wanted to be a nurse or a nun. Even then, I had to be involved in taking care of people. Ultimately I started out in nursing, then switched to X-ray and from there specialized in mammography. What I do is more than pressing a button, more than positioning a breast; it is comforting others. I know one individual can make a difference in another person's life. I love it. I would not be in this field if I didn't.

Every mammography technologist needs to interact with the patient to keep her calm while doing the technical aspects of a mammogram. We do positioning and have to make sure the breast is placed perfectly in order to obtain the maximum amount of breast tissue on the image—knowing that a radiologist can only read what is actually on the film. The patient may complain about the compression, but compression is very, very important because it presses and separates the breast tissue, allowing for a clearer image. It also lessens the radiation that goes into the breast by minimizing tissue exposure.

When I started doing mammography I wanted to know what it felt like, so I had my co-worker position my breast as though she was actually doing a mammogram. That way, I got the sense of what the patient would go through. As a result, if a patient expresses discomfort, I really understand. The fact that I can focus on what she feels comes across. The optimal time to get a mammogram is probably a week after a period, but people vary. It's always important for a patient to relax, so I explain what's happening to calm down the patient. "I'm going to do your mammogram and I'm going to start with four views and this is how I go through it step by step, I start with the right breast then alternate." Everyone has their own way of doing a mammogram. The end result should be the same; the doctor should have a film that can be read easily.

We always advise the patient not to wear any lotions, creams or deodorants. Some lotions might have a little glitter or sparkle or something in it that shows up on a mammogram. Also, lotions tend to cause the breast to slip at times when you're positioning the breast and using the compression paddle. If the breast moves after compression during exposure, the mammogram must be repeated. This doubles the dose of radiation. Mammography is like taking a regular picture with a camera; if there's movement it will be blurry on the film. Deodorant will also show on the mammogram and looks like microcalcification, which can mimic an abnormality. Radiologists know the difference between deodorant and calcification, but deodorant near the real calcification can confuse the reading. Not every calcium deposit in the breast is bad. It depends on how the calcium looks. The radiologist determines if a biopsy is needed, so we don't want anything to mimic those conditions, which could lead to unnecessary biopsies. A biopsy is a sampling of the breast tissue in the area of clinical concern.

Q — Why is compression necessary when having a mammogram?

BIOPSY

A biopsy is a medical test that involves removal of tissue in order to examine it for disease.

In a private practice such as ours, the technologist also assists the radiologist with the needle-guided biopsies. Biopsies are usually performed under the imaging modality in which the area of clinical concern is seen. There is a mammogram-guided biopsy, which is called a stereotactic biopsy. Also, there is an MRI-guided breast biopsy and an ultrasound-guided biopsy. In some hospital settings a nurse may assist in this part. At our practice, I have the trays ready with everything that the doctor will need to do the biopsy, from biopsy probes to syringes with Lidocaine, which is a local anesthetic. It's my responsibility to prepare the jar for the specimen and to have the pathology requisition slip ready with the proper patient's name and identification numbers so that the radiologist can fill out his or her portion before sending the specimen off to the lab.

I also bandage the patient and give the instructions for aftercare. Our assistance is very important to the doctors. Without us, they cannot do their job as well. We all need each other. It starts with the front desk, then the technologist who assists the doctor by supplying the best images possible and by getting all the information so the doctor can read and render a report for mammogram results.

In this Internet Age, technology is readily at our fingertips. It's good that patients have access to information. However, over-researching can lead not to too much knowledge, but incomplete knowledge, which can result in patients coming in with incorrect ideas of how things should be done. This can create an incomplete understanding of the radiologist's and technologist's perspective.

I had a couple of patients recently who came in and said, "Do you have a shield to put around my neck?" Some of them didn't know that it's called a thyroid shield but they each told me, "My friend sent me an e-mail and said make sure to ask for the neck covering." I explained that in the first two views the shield will often show on the picture and block areas on the breast image. Leaving off the shield avoids having to repeat the mammogram in order to provide adequate images. If the patient wants the shield, she can have it for the other two views.

In my opinion, nothing has yet taken the place of mammography. The premise of mammography is to catch and detect cancers early. I don't want a doctor to find something when it's already broken out of the stables and galloped away. The government says mammography is still the best. Now, however, we also have the breast MRI and the sonogram. Each procedure has its place and works in conjunction with the mammogram. Each shows certain specific things in the breast. A sonogram would never show a calcification unless it's big. When you see this, it's benign. Some patients will say, "I want the sonogram, I don't want the mammogram." Then you have to explain to them each process has different capabilities. A sonogram ("sono") shows some things that a mammogram ("mammo") doesn't show and vice versa. After reading the mammogram, the radiologist renders the report with recommendations for the patient's next step.

No patient should go without the care they need unless it's the patient's choice. The patient should always be informed of what is needed next in the proper time, in order to be effective. Sometimes patients don't do things because they are scared. Sometimes a patient has had a mammogram and now needs a sonogram, but says to herself, "I'm not going to do it because they might find something worse, so I'm just going to forget about it." It is the job of the technologist, or the mammography coordinator assigned, to follow up with the patient and to make reasonable attempts to contact that patient in accordance with the policy and procedure of their facility.

We also have to make certain a system is in place to track a patient, to ensure that she follows all the recommendations for each step. We have to call a patient who doesn't show up for whatever might be needed as recommended by the radiologist. This also includes getting the surgical pathology report to be sure she understands her exact status.

In mammography, we are regulated by the FDA (Food and Drug Administration), MQSA (Mammography Quality Standard Act) and the DOH (Department of Health). Every year, each facility is inspected by the DOH. A technologist is assigned to perform daily, weekly and semi-annual tests on the mammography equipment to ensure the equipment is operating the way it should. From the mammography technologist to the radiation physicist and field service engineer, all of us work together to make sure our equipment is operating perfectly.

If the patient can't afford to follow up with the health professionals' recommendations, I help her find a place where she can get low-cost or free assistance. One way in New York City is to call 311. If the patient needs to go to a low-cost or free facility, there should be ways to facilitate her getting to the next step. Besides my work as a mammography technologist, I do health fairs at my church and invite other local churches and people in the area. The expenses all come out of my pocket but it's so important. I get people who have varied areas of expertise to give talks. I discuss breast cancer, the importance of having a mammogram, how essential it is to do a self-examination and actually show how to do it. The more you do self-breast exams the more you become familiar with your breasts and know when subtle changes occur.

There are three methods to perform a self-breast examination. You can do it in the shower, standing in front of a mirror or lying down. In all three, use the pads of your three middle fingers in a circular motion covering the entire breast moving from the chest wall and going towards the nipple or going up and down in a vertical pattern or in a wedge pattern. Also, when standing in front of the mirror, look for changes such as skin dimpling, pulling, discoloration and the like. For patients with difficult breasts, such as lumpy to the touch, my advice is to document where each contour is felt so that you are more apt to notice changes. Self-breast examinations should be done regularly. Remember always to use the right hand to examine the left breast and the left hand to examine the right breast.

"I wondered why I had not previously felt the mass since I had faithfully performed self-breast exams; yet I had missed it. A digital mammogram and biopsy confirmed my worst fears."

— Cindy Newsome

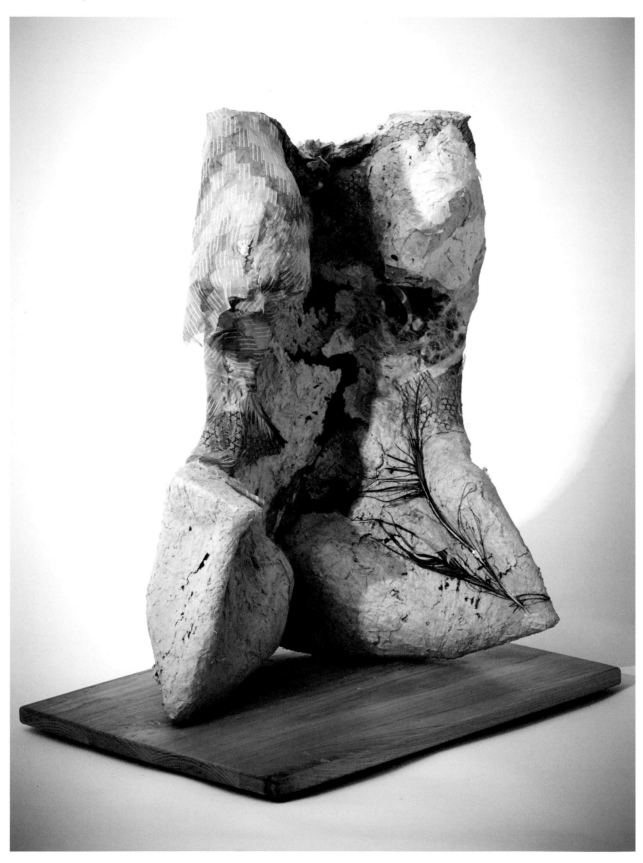

PULLING ONESELF TOGETHER

The Self-Exam

Keshia D. Hammond-Merriman

For some reason, I always performed breast self-exams when showering. The first time I felt a lump in my right breast I was thirty-one and I knew it meant trouble. Here I was—a single woman, living alone and scared out of my mind—wondering what to do. Finally, three months later, my close girlfriends convinced me to find out what the lump was. I called my primary care physician and made what seemed to be the beginning of endless appointments. Lesson number one in this journey: Whenever possible, have someone go with you to your appointments. It was a mistake thinking I could handle them by myself.

It became clear with my first mammogram and ultrasound that the journey was going to be an uphill battle. The radiologist, unaware of the mass I'd found, told me the mammogram was clear. At that moment I wanted to say "fine" and walk out of the office but didn't. I told the doctor, "The film may be clear, but I definitely felt a lump"—the same lump that appeared on the ultrasound. Now some of my fears were confirmed. There was a mass that had to be removed. My primary care physician thought it was a cyst, so she referred me to a general surgeon.

Lesson number two, learned after the fact: If there's a language barrier or if you feel uncomfortable with any doctor you see, find another doctor. The mass was removed. When I was in the general surgeon's office having the stitches removed, the doctor said, "I have the pathology report." What report was he talking about? For a short period I tried to believe the mass was just a cyst, thinking if anything was wrong he would have advised me to bring someone with me to the appointment. So I was calm. The stitches were removed and the doctor said, "Your report is not so good." When asked what that meant, he said, "You have cancer." At that point I fell apart and could not stop crying. The doctor went on to say he was going to schedule me for a mastectomy. I told him I couldn't talk about it then and would call the office the following week. Right then my concern was how to manage driving myself home and how to tell my family and friends. Somehow I did both.

My brothers (all three) went with me to the same doctor who had given me the diagnosis. Was it because they asked him so many questions that he no longer wanted to perform the mastectomy? In any event, he referred me to the Cancer Institute of New Jersey.

There, I met the oncologist I have to this day and the surgeon I see once a year. Both were very thorough, answered all my questions and were very patient. Both had that bedside manner that doctors should have. After all my research—reading books, articles on the Internet, whatever I could get my hands on—and after speaking with my doctors at the Cancer Institute, my decision was to have a lumpectomy instead of a mastectomy. Later, with the guidance of my

"Some cancers just don't show up on a mammogram but may be felt by you or your doctor."

— Susan McCoy, M.D.

oncologist, I decided to go through a rigorous course of chemotherapy followed by radiation.

After being cancer free for a little over three years, in 2007 I felt a lump in my left breast. My life was very different then because I was dating a wonderful man whom I later married. How was he going to handle all of this? He convinced me to move in with him so he could take care of me. I had to go through a similar course of treatment. Again my decision was to have a lumpectomy followed by chemotherapy and radiation. When my hair started to fall out (my second time being bald), my boyfriend shaved my head, cooked and cleaned. The only thing he couldn't do, because of his schedule, was go with me to my chemotherapy treatments. The following year we got engaged and in 2009 we were married. Now at ages forty and forty-one, we are trying to decide whether we are going to have children.

During this journey my oncologist referred me to the Sisters Network of Central New Jersey, who played a very supportive role in helping me deal with my breast cancer. Here, women share their personal experiences about anything and everything in dealing with cancer, from the initial diagnosis to the different treatments and post-treatment. The organization definitely plays a major role in the survival of many of its members and women in the surrounding communities. When you see all of the strong women and remember the ones who are no longer here, in spite of the obstacle (cancer), it makes you want to fight for life.

At the end of the day, you still have dreams. Your dreams may have changed, but that is a part of life. You still have fear of the unknown. My concern is whether to have children, and if so, will I be around to see them grow up? The biggest question of all is, will my cancer return? Let life be the driving force behind performing those breast self-exams and getting yearly mammograms. The key to fighting this deadly disease is early detection.

> *"... use the pads of your three middle fingers in a circular motion covering the entire breast moving from the chest wall and going towards the nipple or going up and down in a vertical pattern or in a wedge pattern."*
>
> — Sandra Scott

Watchful Waiting
Anne M. Johnston, Ph.D.

When I was diagnosed with breast cancer in 2002, my first reaction was, oh, I guess it's my turn, since one in eight women receive this devastating diagnosis. I was also one of the many who had taken HRT (hormone replacement therapy) for fourteen years, which studies show has a strong association with breast cancer.

My radiologist had been doing some "watchful waiting" for a year or two based on the myriad of calcifications that were revealed in my yearly mammograms. When the pattern changed, showing that some of the calcifications had aggregated, I knew it was time for a biopsy. The biopsy showed that I had invasive ductal carcinoma of approximately 3 mm—about the size of a sesame seed.

I wasn't happy about my diagnosis but I didn't go into panic mode either. I felt pretty savvy about breast cancer in general because I have two graduate degrees, an M.S. and Ph.D. in the medical science area, and worked the better part of my career as a director of immunology at a major medical reference laboratory. I was well aware of the BRCA1/BRCA2 gene mutations as well as the HER2 and estrogen receptor markers and felt comfortable reading the latest peer-reviewed literature on breast cancer. Most importantly, I knew my cancer was diagnosed early. This was reassuring.

I shared the news with my husband and two married daughters, who were very supportive. Our younger daughter is a physician specializing in pediatric infectious disease, so she immediately deluged me with the latest in literature on breast cancer, which I read and found helpful. I only shared my diagnosis with friends who had been through breast cancer, deciding that I would wait to tell other friends after I had made major decisions and knew more.

The biggest problem I faced was sorting through the many choices that needed to be made, including choosing the hospital for my surgery, the right physicians, breast surgeon and plastic surgeon and deciding whether a lumpectomy or mastectomy was right for me. If I chose the latter, what kind of breast reconstruction would be best? Armed with my husband as scribe, we began consultations with various doctors as to how to proceed. I found this to be a very anxious time. It helped a lot to talk with my "breast friends" as to how and why they had made their choices.

For a number of reasons, I chose to have a mastectomy and reconstruction with a silicone–saline combination implant. The surgery was no fun at all. I suffered for 24 hours with severe vomiting from the anesthesia and morphine drip. However, the good news was that results from the frozen sections of the sentinel node performed during surgery were negative. Okay, I thought, I'm on the right track—no need for chemotherapy, just anti-estrogen medication for five years.

I recovered quickly, only to receive a call from my surgeon who reported that the result from cytochemical testing performed on the remainder of the sentinel node was positive and that I needed to return to the hospital for a lymph dissection of the axillary nodes. I remember saying to my husband that what at first appeared to be a very early and simple breast cancer was now escalating into a more serious problem. I was disturbed because the thought of additional surgery, more positive nodes and a potential for lymphedema loomed large in my mind.

Waiting for the results of the lymphectomy, which took five days, was emotional agony. Happily the rest of the nodes were negative but unfortunately I developed lymphedema in my chest wall and arm. Now what? My cancer was stage 2, so even with only one positive node I might be a candidate for chemotherapy.

My husband and I began visiting local oncologists for their opinions. There are costs and benefits to chemotherapy and no one could give me a definitive

BRCA GENE TEST

The BRCA gene test is a blood test that uses DNA analysis to identify harmful changes (mutations) in either one of the two breast cancer susceptibility genes—BRCA1 and BRCA2 and should be checked. A BRCA gene mutation is uncommon.

"My primary care physician, who confirmed that there was a lump, made an appointment for me with the same breast surgeon who had performed a mastectomy on my wife several years earlier."

— Wilbur Dexter Johnston, Ph.D.

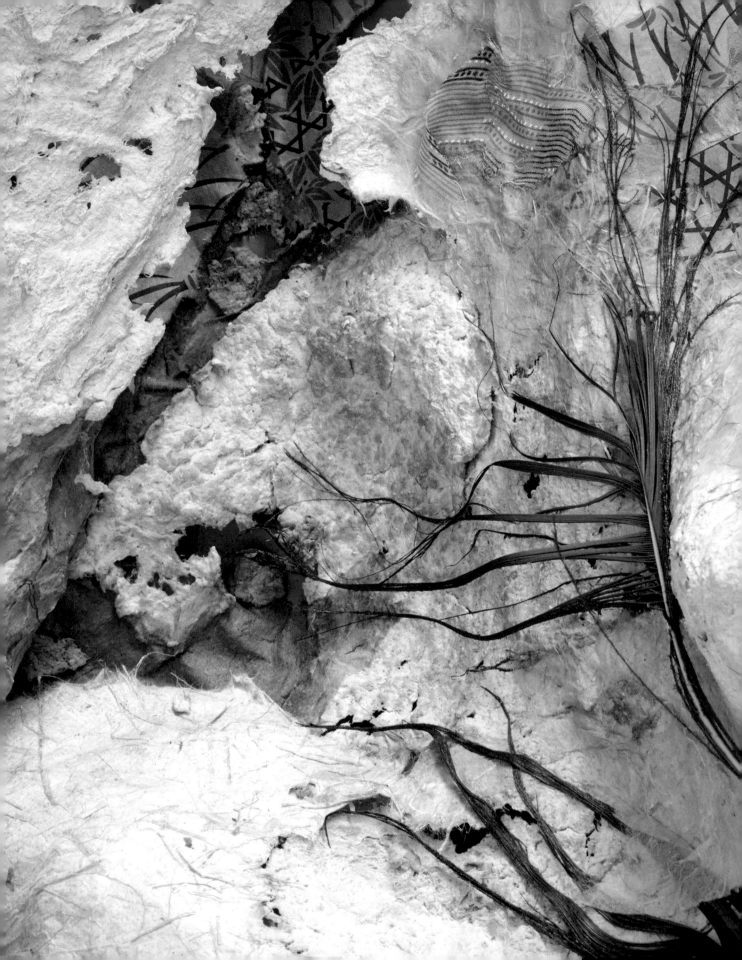

answer as to what to do. After discussing this with my "breast friends," I decided that I didn't want to be in the position of looking back one day, should the cancer recur, and regret that I had not gone through the chemotherapy. To be sure, there was pressure from my family to do everything I could to beat the cancer. I ultimately chose to have four cycles of Adriamycin/Cytoxin at Carol Simon Cancer Center, which offers many support programs for cancer patients. I participated in their Mind–Body program and found it invaluable.

Of course I lost my hair and noted, as I looked at my bald head in the mirror, that I have really nice ears! Chemotherapy treatment was not a big deal other than feeling fatigued on some days. When it was completed, my oncologist informed me that it was now time to begin taking Tamoxifen. I told her no, that I preferred to take Arimidex, an aromatase inhibitor. She insisted that Tamoxifen was the standard of care and I insisted that several clinical trials showed Arimidex to be superior to Tamoxifen. I won this argument and it's important because now the standard of care in post-menopausal women is the use of aromatase inhibitors, not Tamoxifen.

Lymphedema therapy and reconstruction followed my chemotherapy. The expansion part of reconstruction was not pleasant but the end result was a relatively normal-looking breast so it was worth it. Lymphedema massage eliminated the problem in my arm but I will forever have chest wall lymphedema.

LYMPHEDEMA

Lymphedema is a buildup of excess fluid in the body tissues, usually the arm, because of obstruction of lymphatic drainage back into the bloodstream.

A diagnosis of cancer forever changes one's life, in some respects, for the better. I have a whole different view of what is important to me and how to better prioritize my life. It's actually a very good feeling with which many cancer patients agree.

As a breast cancer survivor, I felt a strong desire to give back by helping other breast cancer patients. So I joined a New Jersey-based national organization, Cancer Hope Network (CHN), which uses volunteers to provide one-on-one anonymous counseling by phone. It's a user-friendly system. A patient calls a toll-free number and, following an initial interview, support is customized by one of the CHN patient services teams. A patient's profile is matched against an extensive database of cancer survivors. A volunteer is called with a patient's information, including his or her concerns, and in turn the volunteer calls the patient within forty-eight hours.

I have been a CHN support volunteer for over seven years. It's impossible for me to express how meaningful and rewarding this has been. I think I've heard every concern, fear, emotion, uncertainty and piece of misinformation that goes along with the diagnosis and treatment of breast cancer. I have learned that just listening may be one of the biggest benefits to patients, followed by a discussion of their specific questions. After completing a phone call, I reflect on what I've accomplished and how grateful patients seem to be to talk with someone who's been there. I'm thankful that I am healthy and able to help others—there's just no better feeling than that.

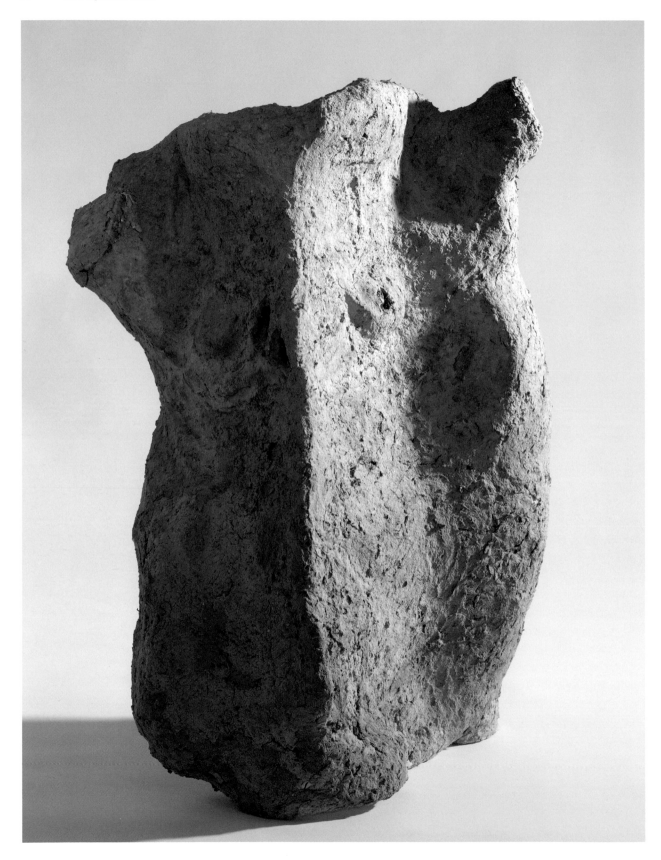

KERNEL OF CONCERN

Of Underlying Concern

Wilbur Dexter Johnston, Ph.D.

My situation: At age sixty-eight, while taking a shower, I noticed my left nipple seemed to be sticking out. I was not doing a chest wall self-examination, just washing. I followed it for a week or two, and noticed an underlying hemispherical lump, growing right under the nipple, had become about the size of a golf ball cut in half. At that point I was concerned because it was on the left side only, and I thought if it was a "male menopause" thing it would be symmetrical. (Not true, I learned: gynecomastia, which is what it turned out to be, is typically asymmetrical and related to hormonal imbalance, either at puberty or around age sixty.)

I made an appointment with my primary care physician, who confirmed that there was a lump, and made an appointment for me with the same breast surgeon who had performed my wife's mastectomy several years earlier. His comment was that we could watch and wait, but his recommendation was to remove the lump, since waiting would only result in a bigger problem later, both figuratively and literally, and regardless of the pathology, we wanted to get rid of the lump. The possibilities were, as he put it, gynecomastia, or a benign tumor, or a precancerous growth, or something more serious, in descending order of probability. He recommended a mastectomy, as that would give the most definitive diagnosis as well as the best solution to the problem. It turned out it was not cancerous, and he did not remove the nipple (just all the rest of the breast tissue) so there was no need for reconstruction.

I had been with my wife through her mastectomy, the uncertainties, the waiting for results of various tests and the travails of chemotherapy, so I knew what I could expect if that path had to be taken. In my case the period of uncertainty was brief, less than two weeks from the appointment with my primary care physician to the pathology results confirming the absence of cancer. My wife was much more anxious about the situation than I was. Nevertheless, I was glad and relieved that I would not have to undergo chemotherapy. My wife and I may now be one of the very few married couples in the world, I imagine, who have matching left breast mastectomies.

IV

A Different Kind of Challenge—
*Lack of diagnostic support in
a developing country*

A Hard Place in My Breast

Men Salath

Editor's note: The following was translated in Cambodia, directly from the original interview that took place in a Cambodian village. This account offers a unique insight into the challenges faced by breast cancer patients in developing countries.

My name is Men Salath. I am a woman of fifty-one years old. I have four children. I am resident of Soken village, So Kong commune, Kang Meas district, Kompong Cham province, Cambodia. I am a farmer.

In 2008, I got to know that I had a hard piece in my breast. First, a piece of about the size of the smallest finger emerged, and I went to Krou Khmer, a Khmer traditional healer who gave me Khmer traditional medicine. I took this medicine for two years. First, I felt better. Later on, the problem came back. I felt pain again.

My neighbors had suggested that I go for an operation. I went for an operation because the medicine that I had taken did not work for the piece. The doctor did not tell me what it was. The doctor at [the] hospital did not say anything but felt (touched) my breast and operated on me. Initially, I was asked to pay $120.00. But, it cost me (I paid) $100.00.

I requested the doctor to examine the piece that they had taken out from me. But, they did not let me know what had happened even 10 days after. The doctor told me that he would have to see it first, and then they would use laser or radiation but I never went back.

I understand that our medical person is not like that of other countries. I wished they look at me with machine. There are women with such pain like me. But, they are simple; they live far away from my place. They are not sure if they would go for an operation as they are afraid it might come (keep coming) back. I did not feel so painful with it, but after the operation I still feel something hurt in me.

"The Nobel Prize made it possible for me to meet with top medical leaders in various countries and become acquainted with international health problems, among them cancer."

— Andrew V. Schally, Ph.D.

What Happened To and In Me?

Naov Davin

Editor's note: The Cambodian-language text, which appears on the adjacent page, was written in a Cambodian village; the text below was then translated in Cambodia from the original. This account offers a unique insight into the challenges faced by breast cancer patients in developing countries.

My name is Naov Davin. I am forty-nine years old. I am resident of Ampe Phnom village, Svay Kroavann commune, Chbar Morn town, Kompong Speu province, Cambodia. I have had breast cancer since 2009.

It was probably a year before I discovered I have breast cancer, I had felt there was a small hard piece (approximately the size of our human smallest finger) in my breast. Gradually, I could feel the hard piece becoming larger and larger, while at the same time, I also felt fatigue, and my body was then with constantly high temperature (mild fever). Then, I did not know for sure what had happened to and in me?

The hard piece did not constantly make me feel very painful but only mild from time to time. Later, when I could feel the hard piece becoming larger, my nipple sank. I was very frightened, and I rushed to go to a hospital for examination. Then, I was told I have breast cancer. My panic prompted me to go see cancer specialist (doctor) who put me in a scanner to find out if the cancer cells have spread to other parts (organs) of my body. The examination indicated that there was no spreading. I felt so relieved with the result. The doctor told me that it is 85% good that I could have hope.

Many friends of mine encouraged me to make myself happy (no desperateness) for maintaining my good health. I had undergone two-week treatment through intravenous injections of medicines. Later on, after six intravenous injections have been done, gradually, my hairs lost till no more hairs in the head, meanwhile, I feel so stressful and nauseated, but it does not come out, and I felt fatigue and depressed. I underwent an operation with one of my breasts removed. I have become disabled. I cannot do anything, as I had done before, as I wished. I, later on, have undergone laser treatment that made me very tired (my knees weakened) as I could not even walk forward. My neighbors have often said to me that I would not survive. But, I encourage myself by listening to Dharma. Since the treatment has been started until this month of August 2011, I have undergone two-year treatment already. I do not know what will happen to me in the next three years. The question is that whether my cancer would be cured?

I wish to encourage women to rush to go see breast specialist (doctor) for timely examination and treatment if/when you feel a hard piece inside your breast(s).

"When women (in Cambodia) are diagnosed with breast cancer, certainly less than 50% of them are able to discuss the diagnosis with their husbands...who often then leave their wives."

— Sedkai Meta, M.D.,
as told to Charulata Prasada

Naov Davin's original text in Khmer script

នាងខ្ញុំឈ្មោះ នៅ ដាវិន អាយុ ៤៩ឆ្នាំ មានទីលំនៅក្នុងភូមិអំពែភ្នំ ឃុំស្វាយក្រវ៉ាន់ ក្រុងប្ប៉ាវមន ខេត្តកំពង់ស្ពឺ។ នាងខ្ញុំ មានជម្ងឺមហារីកសុដន់ នៅឆ្នាំ ២០០៩។ មុនពេលដែលខ្ញុំដឹងថាមានជម្ងឺមហារីក នោះ ប្រហែលជាមួយឆ្នាំមុន ពេលនោះសុដន់របស់ខ្ញុំមានដុំរឹង ប្រហែលប៉ុនកូនដៃ ក្រោយមកដុំនោះ រឹកធំទៅៗ ពេលនោះខ្ញុំមានអារម្មណ៍ថា អស់កម្លាំង ស្លុតឈ្លើ សាច់របស់ខ្ញុំភ្លៅស្ទៀង ។ ក្នុងពេលនោះ ដែរ ខ្ញុំក៏មិនទាន់ដឹងថាយ៉ាងម៉េចដែរ។ ព៌ីព្រោះដុំនោះមិនធ្វើឲ្យខ្ញុំឈឺចាប់អ្វីទេ ប៉ុន្តែដុំនោះធ្វើឲ្យខ្ញុំដឹងថា ចាប់ឈ្លៀបៗ ម្តងម្កាលដែរ។ បន្ទាប់មកទៀតដុំនោះរឹកធំទៅៗ វាក៏បានទាញក្បាលដោះលិបចូលទៅ ក្នុង។ ខ្ញុំក៏ចាប់ផ្តើមក័យយ៉ាងខ្លាំងហើយក៏បានទៅមន្ទីរពេទ្យធ្វើការពិនិត្យ ទើបដឹងថាខ្ញុំមានជម្ងឺមហារីក សុដន់។ ខ្ញុំមានអារម្មណ៍ក័យតក់ស្លុតយ៉ាងខ្លាំងពេលនោះខ្ញុំក៏បានទៅជួបគ្រូពេទ្យផ្នែកជម្ងឺមហារីក គាត់ ក៏បានឲ្យខ្ញុំធ្វើ   ដើម្បីឲ្យដឹងថាកោសិកាមហារីកបានសាយកាយទៅសរីរង្គទៃទៀតឬអត់។ ក្រោយពេលធ្វើការពិនិត្យរួចហើយ   ឃើញថាមិនមានការសាយកាយទៅសរីរង្គផ្សេងទៀតទេ ខ្ញុំក៏មានកម្លាំងចិត្តបន្តិចមកវិញត្រូវពេទ្យបានប្រាប់ថាខ្ញុំសង្ឃឹមជាបាន៨៥% ពេលនោះមិត្តកត្តិជាច្រើន បានឲ្យកម្លាំងចិត្តថា កុំអស់សង្ឃឹមពេក ត្រូវធ្វើចិត្តឲ្យស្បាយដើម្បីកុំឲ្យសុខភាពយេីងចុះទ្រុងទ្រោម។ ខ្ញុំក៏បានព្យាបាលដោយការបញ្ចូលថ្នាំតាមសរសៃបានព៌ីរសប្តាហ៍។ ក្រោយមកសក់របស់ខ្ញុំក៏ចាប់ផ្តើម ជ្រុះបន្តិចម្តងៗ។រហូតទាល់តែអស់។ខ្ញុំមានអារម្មណ៍តានតឹងក្នុងខ្លួនចង់ក្តួតតែក្តួតមិនចេញ អស់កម្លាំង ទន់ដៃទន់ជើងពិបាកក្នុងខ្លួនពេលធ្វើការបញ្ចូលថ្នាំតាមសរសៃចំនួន៦ដងមក។ ខ្ញុំបានធ្វើការវះកាត់ ដោយការកាត់សុដន់មួយចំហៀងខ្ញុំក៏បានក្លាយជាជនពិការ មិនអាចធ្វើអ្វីកើតតាមតែចិត្តខ្ញុំចង់ធ្វើបាន ដូចកាលពេលមុនទៀតទៅ។បន្ទាប់មកទៀតខ្ញុំបានធ្វើការព្យាបាលដោយបាញ់កាំរស្មី ពេលនោះទន់ ជន្ធង់ដេីរមិនចង់ទៅមុខទៅ។ អ្នកជិតខាងតែងនិយាយថា ខ្ញុំមិនសង្ឃឹមរស់ទេ ប៉ុន្តែខ្ញុំបានស្តាប់ធម៌ដេីម្បី ជួយជាកម្លាំងចិត្ត។ ចាប់តាំងព៌ីពេលដែលធ្វើការព្យាបាលរួច រហូតមកដល់ខែ សិហា ឆ្នាំ២០១១ ខ្ញុំបានព្យាបាលអស់រយៈពេលព៌ីរឆ្នាំមកហើយខ្ញុំមិនទាន់ដឹងថា   ៣ឆ្នាំទៀតយ៉ាងណានោះខ្ញុំក៏មិន ដឹងដែរ។ តេីជម្ងឺមហារីករបស់ខ្ញុំអាចជាសះស្បើយបានដែរ ឬទេ?

នាងខ្ញុំក៏សូមធ្វើការផ្តែផ្តាំទៅស្ត្រីគ្រប់រូបដៃទៀត   ប្រសិនបេីមានដុះដុំរឹងនៅក្នុងសុដន់ សូមប្រញាប់រួសរាន់ទៅជួបគ្រូពេទ្យផ្នែកពិនិត្យសុដន់ ដើម្បីធ្វើការព្យាបាលឲ្យបានទាន់ពេលវេលា ។

Cancer in Cambodia: A Doctor's View

Sedkai Meta, M.D., *told by Charulata Prasada*

Cambodia is a country of 14.5 million people, of which 30.7% live below the poverty line.[1] Almost 20% of the population is urbanized.[2] Malnutrition amongst children is prevalent, as 40% of children under age five are stunted, and 14% are severely stunted.[3] Rates of maternal mortality and under-five mortality for children are improving but remain high. The focus of the health care system is directed at primary health care and communicable diseases. There has never been a national study on breast cancer. The Ministry of Health is in the process of developing a strategy on breast and cervical cancer. Plans are underway to develop a national cancer institute but presently there is only one fully functional oncology ward in the country.

Over the past twenty years, Dr. Sedkai Meta[4] has treated women with highly progressed stages of breast cancer. Dr. Meta reflected on the Cambodian health system and Khmer society's response to breast cancer for over an hour with the goal of improving early detection, diagnosis, treatment and care for women as follows:

The health system's capacity to prevent and respond to breast cancer and cervical cancer has been limited due to lack of adequate financial resources. Much donor assistance thus far has been targeted at the HIV/AIDS epidemic with good results in that area.

Every year, I would treat between ten to fifteen woman with highly progressed (stage 3 and 4) breast cancer. I believe that the number of women seeking treatment is small because many women deny or limit their contact with the health system. This is primarily due to the relatively high costs of health care. Most women are simply too poor to seek diagnosis and follow through on treatment and care.

Knowledge and understanding about breast cancer also remain limited. To date, breast cancer has never been introduced as a public health concern. Khmer society is still quite traditional. This influences norms around women's decency. Many women, particularly older women, are too shy to reveal their undergarments, let alone have breast examinations with a man or woman doctor. This hesitation is a key barrier to early detection. When women are diagnosed with breast cancer, certainly less than 50% of them are able to discuss the diagnosis with their husbands. There are numerous experiences where husbands leave their wives when they are found to have breast cancer. This is known to happen across socioeconomic classes.

Poor families often lack the resources to take care of women with breast cancer. There is some discrimination against women when they are unable to work and fulfill their traditional roles and responsibilities.

We have very competent doctors with international degrees and training. However, many of our doctors divide their time between government hospitals

"I got to know that I had a hard piece in my breast. First, I went to Krou Khmer, a Khmer traditional healer who gave me Khmer traditional medicine… First, I felt better. Later on, the problem came back."

— Men Salath

and private practice. The bedside manner of doctors is a deterrent to patients. Communication is limited and patients are frequently too intimidated to ask questions about their diagnosis or discuss treatment options with their doctors.

We have equipment, albeit dated, about ten years old. We also lack resources for maintenance within our hospitals. There are times that I use my own money to make small repairs that I require.

Those who can afford it travel to Vietnam or Thailand for health care. There is a disinterest in the national health care system because the facilities in these other countries are updated and plentiful.

We need raised awareness and a behavior change here in Cambodia. Women and men need to be informed about breast cancer and early detection. It is important that men are also targeted to support making women's health a priority within the family and to increase the utilization of health services. Television and radio would serve as excellent channels for such a campaign.

There also needs to be behavior change amongst doctors themselves: away from a strictly disease-driven approach to a patient-centered, more communicative and compassionate bedside manner. This will encourage greater use of health care amongst women and the poor especially.

1. Unicef Cambodia:2011:10 Cambodia Country Profile.
2. IBID.
3. CDHS:2010:147.
4. This is a fictional name to preserve the anonymity of the person interviewed. Sedkai Meta means compassion in Khmer. The doctor's reflections were motivated by deep concern and a constructive commitment to improving health care for women in Cambodia.

V

Major Treatments—
*Explained by specialists and
described by survivors*

Medical Options
Richard Margolese, M.D., C.M., F.R.C.S.(C.)

Patients are so overwhelmed by the diagnosis of cancer that the complicated array of choices and decisions they face is all the more difficult. The first thing a patient needs in an oncologist is someone who realizes this and meets the patient's need for communication and understanding. Careful and detailed explanations and patience in answering questions are key in reaching the best decision. Treatment choices are often a synthesis of medical options and patient conditions and preferences. For a condition such as appendicitis, there are no confusing choices to make. Everyone knows the patient needs a simple operation and will get better. For cancer, where outcomes differ and no single treatment stands out as guaranteeing a cure, there are choices to be made.

Strategies
There are two strategies for control of breast cancer: Local control (choice of surgery) and systemic control (consideration of adjuvant treatments).

1. Local control
What extent of surgery is necessary to control the tumor in the breast? It is now very clear that cure rates with mastectomy are not better than with breast conserving surgery (lumpectomy), which should be the treatment of choice whenever feasible. Some patients will have tumors that are too extensive or are multicentric so that a lumpectomy is not possible. While radiation therapy is always given after lumpectomy, it is sometimes necessary after full mastectomy.

2. Systemic control
What other treatments should be given (hormonal or chemotherapy) to control any cancer cells that might have metastasized (spread) to other organs? These cells would not be influenced by the surgery or radiation. To answer this question, some estimate of the risk of metastasis is necessary. The classical step in this evaluation has been to examine the lymph nodes under the arm. If cancer cells are present in these nodes it means those cells have traveled from their primary site in the breast, and having done that, they could have traveled to other sites as well. Today, this operation has been significantly reduced in scope so that instead of removing all of the nodes in the region, surgeons can identify the sentinel node and base the decision for chemotherapy on that. The point is that a small number of metastatic tumor cells growing in other places, like lungs or bone, would, in time, become fatal, but can often be eliminated if treated with appropriate adjuvant therapy before they grow too large. This is similar to putting out a small fire with only one bucket of water, but if the

"The initial trauma of a malignant diagnosis is undoubtedly one of life's worst experiences and will remain so until a cure for cancer is found."

— Joe Wojtowicz

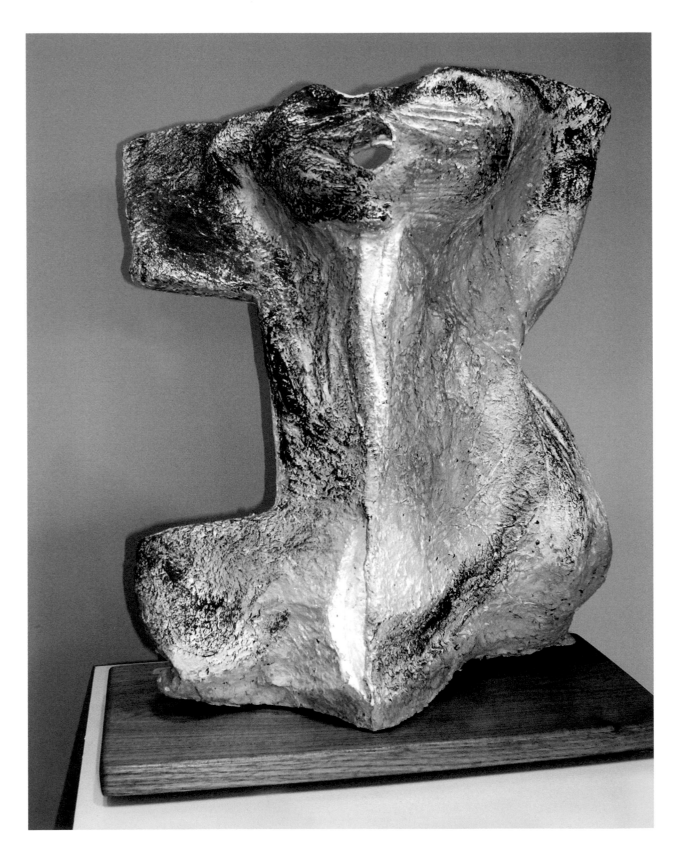

MOMENT OF ANXIETY

fire spreads and is too large, this will not work. The two main types of adjuvant treatments are hormones and chemotherapy.

Many tumors show a sensitivity to estrogen (positive estrogen receptors) and cure rates can be improved by administering anti-estrogens. One of these agents is Tamoxifen. Tamoxifen has been in use for thirty years and works by blocking the growth-stimulating effect of estrogen on any existing cancer cells. Newer drugs like anastrozole (Arimidex) or letrozole (Femara) work by blocking the manufacture of estrogen at its source. These drugs are all effective and have very few serious side effects.

For many patients, especially those who have low estrogen receptors, post-operative chemotherapy will also improve long-term survival results. Even some patients with estrogen sensitivity will benefit from adjuvant chemotherapy. This is often a difficult decision where the benefits must be weighed against the downside of discomfort and risks from side effects.

Today, more sophisticated approaches are being developed where tumor cells can be analyzed for the activity of specific genes known to be active in proliferation and metastases. This analysis produces a risk score that can be used in deciding whether or not to recommend chemotherapy.

Prevention

The old cliché about prevention being better than the cure is apt here. In the 1980s, we treated 3,000 women with Tamoxifen in a clinical trial evaluating Tamoxifen after breast surgery. This trial was successful. Tamoxifen reduced the treatment failure rate by 25%. Most interesting was the unexpected finding that these women were much less likely to develop a new cancer in the opposite breast over the next several years. Working on the suspicion that Tamoxifen was suppressing the evolution of precancerous cells into cancerous cells, the Breast Cancer Prevention Trial was developed to confirm this hypothesis. A group of 13,000 women at high risk for cancer were divided into two groups, to receive Tamoxifen or a placebo. The breast cancer incidence was reduced by 50% in the group taking Tamoxifen. There is a low risk of possibly serious side effects so it is important to assess the cancer risk against the risk for adverse events, but in general, this is a safe and effective intervention for most women at an elevated risk for breast cancer. High risk may be signified by significant family history or findings of precancerous changes on biopsy. A second trial confirmed the benefit and showed that another drug, Raloxifene, was nearly as effective and had somewhat less risk of adverse effects.

Clinical Trials

Much of the above information comes from a scientific tool called a clinical trial. This is a method of comparing two treatment choices in a population of patients. Medical science has come to rely so much on clinical trials that no new medication or intervention is likely to be adopted unless it is validated by a clinical trial. Generally speaking, it is usually better for patients to participate in trials than to receive standard treatment, partly because one of the choices, known as arms, in the trial is likely to be a new treatment that might prove to be more effective. In order to prevent bias in conclusions, it is most important that patients be randomly assigned to one or the other of the treatments. For example, if we were to compare surgery versus medical treatment for heart disease and allow participants to choose their therapy, we might find that younger and healthier patients were more likely to choose surgery. We could find a difference in outcome without ever doing any treatments, just the selection of patients would make the difference. Randomizing the assignments assures that the two groups are the same except for the different treatments.

In addition, clinical trials are supervised by monitoring committees that ensure that the protocol is followed carefully, all required testing is carried out and evaluated in a timely fashion and any adverse reactions are quickly spotted and handled appropriately. A further advantage is that in trials of newer agents, some of which are very expensive, there is usually no cost to the participant.

Q — What is HER2?

An outstanding example of all these advantages was a clinical trial aimed at improving survival for breast cancer patients whose tumors carried an increased level of a protein called HER2. When present in excess amounts, HER2 indicates a more worrisome prognosis, but the development of an antibody, Herceptin, aimed at neutralizing HER2, led to a clinical trial where patients received standard chemotherapy with and without Herceptin. The result was a dramatic improvement in survival for patients receiving Herceptin, so that this is now standard treatment for women whose tumors are HER2 positive. It is true that only half of the women in the trial received Herceptin, but no one outside the trial received Herceptin until the trial was completed and analyzed, so many of the participants did gain from being in the trial.

Most clinical trials in cancer are carried out under the supervision of agencies like the Clinical Trials Group of the Canadian Cancer Society Research Institute or the National Cancer Institute in the United States. Sites participating in clinical trials can easily be found at the websites of these organizations or of university hospitals in your area.

Where to go? As with any health problem, highly specialized centers are more likely to have access to sophisticated diagnostic and treatment tools and to have personnel who are active in research and in a position to evaluate newer approaches. But the most important ingredient is empathetic communication between doctor and patient, which allows the full benefit of the expertise and resources to help the breast cancer patient achieve the best possible outcome.

Uphill Imperative

Monica Becker

My life before breast cancer: avid gardener, insane hours doing yard work, ceramic artist, mother and stepmother, OCD housewife, Bible-study leader, exercise fanatic.

My life after: reading all I could about cancer, trying to do all I did before my diagnosis and feeling like crap most of the time; couldn't lift a gallon of milk; switched to using left hand for a lot of things; couldn't pick up full garbage cans or carry grocery bags—that bothered me a lot. Tried to go back to weight-lifting with bad results. No gardens for years. Disbelief and fear. Letting my already long hair grow even longer. Getting overly involved in Relay for Life, with very mixed emotions. That's a whole other tale.

Reactions after surgery: surgeon in recovery room after excisional biopsy, "I'm 95% sure it's not cancer." The surgeon then leaving for a black-tie event. My husband reading model railroad magazines, me trying to tell the nurse what to do before I go into shock and there's no oxygen. The surgeon returning because I'm hemorrhaging, throwing his tie over his shoulder, complaining that I'm giving him trouble. Later, I read my hospital record and it said, "Patient tolerated procedure well." Two weeks later a phone call from the surgeon, "Do you want the good news or the bad news first?"

My church's reaction: casseroles, a few visits, phone calls, cards. My friends: the ones who disappear and the ones who don't when they hear the word cancer. My mother-in-law's first words to me: "Don't you dare die; my son and the boys need you." My eight-year-old son's question when I told him I had cancer, "People die from cancer, don't they?" I said, "Yes, but I'm not going to." His older brother, age ten, asked, "Are you worried about it?" I said, "No." He said, "Then I won't either." But then he wrote about it in school and the teacher put a big red slash through the whole page because he didn't double space the story.

I had complications. My daughter and her husband, who was stationed in the Navy in Ballston Spa, New York, brought their six-month-old son and helped run the house. The after-surgery bra, swelling and icepacks made me look as endowed as Dolly Parton. I required a second surgery to remove blood clots and clean up the margins. Total fiasco. My husband went to work. Two female friends from church brought me for same-day surgery and we prayed aloud in the waiting room. I was given only local anesthesia. No barrier, as requested. Instead, the surgeon actually tossed a piece of gauze on my face. I listened to Elvis singing gospel on a portable CD player so I couldn't hear him talking about his vacation.

My younger sister's initial response was, "Great, now my daughter has double the chance of getting breast cancer." But she got a mammogram the very next day. Her friend and colleague in Virginia, a surgeon, offered to do a double

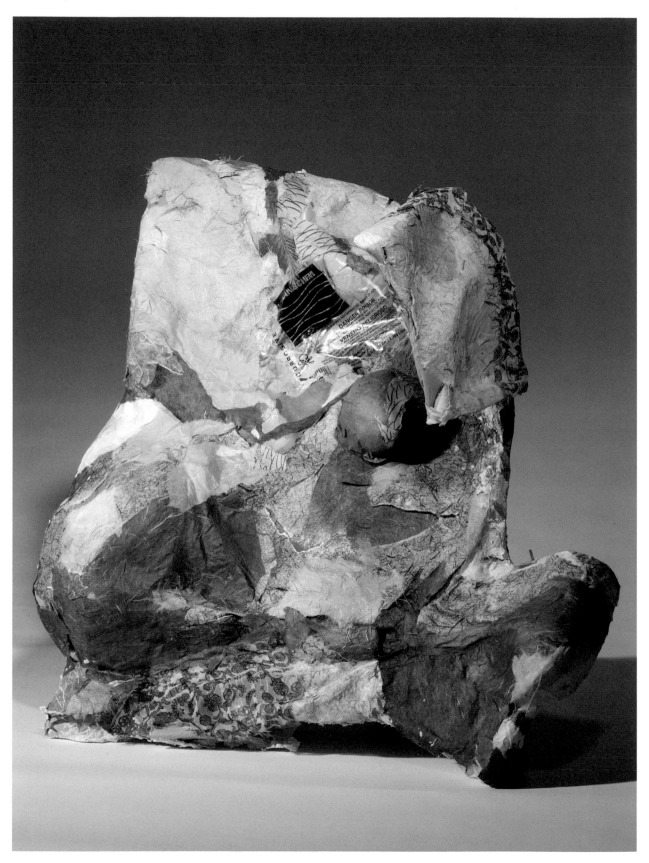

TOXIC

mastectomy and reconstruction for free. My other younger sister, in Rochester, sent me fancy pajamas and asked if there was anything else I really wanted. I said, "Clean windows," and she paid a local company to clean all thirty-six windows in our house. I read everything I could in medical journals and agreed to participate in a ten-year study for DCIS: excision only, no radiation, no chemo.

Ways I coped: in retrospect, I should have allowed myself some pampering and definitely more time for recuperation, but my absurd determination/independence, or as my mother calls it, my "uphill imperative," kept me from feeling sorry for myself and probably set an example to others, I hope. I would handle it differently now though. Found a fabulous shop in New York City—Ripplu on Madison Avenue—where the staff help you purchase bras that fit well and make you look and feel better (even making adjustments with a sewing machine on the spot). This became a mecca (and family joke, as I now had cleavage due to the bras' construction). Went from a 32A to 36C with no padding—go figure, and I had been upset because after the second surgery they removed just a few more centimeters to clean up the margins.

All in all, I was lucky. My cancer was caught early. It was confined in an otherwise benign growth and considered DCIS, barely stage 1. I found an excellent oncologist who continues to monitor me. I did end up taking Tamoxifen for five years, which at first made me miserably nauseated. Tried splitting the dose to morning and night, then was doubly nauseated. Figured out if I timed the split dose until after eating breakfast and before a mid-morning snack, then later between a mid-afternoon snack and dinner, I barely had any nausea.

My advice: learn as much as you can regarding your particular situation. Talk about it. Find a good doctor—good bedside manner is a plus. Throw out the ugly after-surgery bras as soon as possible and splurge on sexy, well-made bras in colors you've never worn before. (I went from traditional black, nude and white to navy blue, maroon, hot pink and orange, with lace.)

If you're pre-menopausal, watch out for menopause. My oncologist did not recommend HRT, bio-identical hormones or even herbal estrogen-based products. For me that's been hell. Get a monthly massage, read about or talk with other women about their stories (this was not commonly talked about, even twenty years ago); keep up the aftercare of blood-work and mammograms, and make use of, or at least try, alternative things like acupuncture and meditation. Don't be afraid to go to a support group, a private psychologist or psychiatrist, or now the Internet. (I haven't done the last because by the time I was computer-literate enough, I had mostly dealt with the grief, fear and anger.)

Don't expect your spouse, family or even close friends to understand or be the support you need. They most likely will be trying to deal with their own feelings. There are exceptions; I'm just saying... Also be prepared for old feelings to resurface when you least expect it. Twelve years later, I read in the initial office visit notes of a retiring doctor that I had no right breast. I was furious! My right breast may have a scar but it's still there.

DCIS

Ductal carcinoma *in situ* (DCIS) means that the cancer starts inside the milk ducts, carcinoma refers to any cancer that begins in the skin or other tissues (including breast tissue) that cover or line the internal organs, and *in situ* means "in its original place."

Last but not least, when asked if I wanted to tell my story for this book, I said yes enthusiastically, but inside my head and heart I heard these questions: do I really want to revisit that time in my life? How can I write it in an encouraging, positive way, but also include the bad parts? Should I risk telling the truth, even if it offends family, friends or the medical profession?

Be forewarned: people will say incredibly insensitive things. "You shouldn't be feeling so much pain. You don't have large enough breasts" (by a doctor). "You'll probably get heart disease too" (by a long-time female friend who was into Eastern stuff at the time and believed my overly caring nature caused my breast cancer, related to some chakra or something). "Be thankful it wasn't in both breasts" (by a man). I thought, uh, one is more than enough. I wish I had said to that man, "That's like telling a guy with testicular cancer they only have to remove one of his balls." "Be grateful it wasn't worse" (by several people). Any day a doctor says you have cancer is not a good day. "Cancer is caused by stress. You need to handle stress better." Yeah, and you need to stick your head up your rear end.

My own personal theory on why I got cancer: I was born and lived the first eight years of my life in Levittown, Long Island (a known hot-spot). In my early twenties I was subjected to radiation on my right heel for an obstinate case of plantar warts. In my thirties and early forties I was put on various birth control pills to regulate and control dysmenorrhea (didn't help, and the weight gain and nausea eventually made me give up that route). As far as dietary factors, I was a vegetarian/health-nut from age sixteen. I breast-fed all three of my children. Prior to me, there was no family history of any kind of cancer. Does it ultimately matter why? I don't think so, although a lot of magazine articles, time, research and money are spent on this. I have come to believe that what matters is how you live through the diagnosis, what you learn about yourself and, finally, how you choose to use the experience to help others.

A Breast Surgeon's View
Christine Rizk, M.D., F.A.C.S.

Breast cancer is the most common and most curable cancer women can contract. In the U.S., one in eight women will have breast cancer over the course of her life. It is perhaps one of the most stressful experiences a woman and her family can go through. Often the worst part of it is the diagnosis because of the amount of fear, apprehension, anxiety and uncertainty it creates.

Surgeons are frequently at the front line and the first health care team member a patient meets. Most women facing breast cancer will initially have a team of two or three members that may include a surgeon or surgical oncologist, a medical oncologist and a radiation oncologist. The key is the word in front of oncologist; so for example, the surgical oncologist treats cancers surgically, the medical oncologist treats cancers with medications sometimes including chemotherapy or other medications and the radiation oncologist treats them with radiation. Surgeons need to obtain and confirm the diagnosis of breast cancer so that they can accurately stage the cancer and then initiate treatment.

Diagnosis

Diagnosis starts with a suspicion either on examination or on a mammogram. Women have an extraordinary ability to be in tune with their bodies and know when something is off or just not right. The most important advice I can give to women is to have an awareness of your body and know if anything has changed. While a lot of women have anxiety about doing a breast self-exam, they should be encouraged so they can discuss this with their physician, including the family doctor, a gynecologist or a breast surgeon.

Sometimes we can detect cancers before they are even felt on examination by either the woman or any of her physicians. This can be particularly difficult for women because some may come in and say, "but I don't feel a lump. How can I have breast cancer?" That is because not all breast cancers are the same. In fact, there are many different varieties. A good analogy is that of something as simple as an apple. You can imagine the many different types of apples that we have; Granny Smith, Red Delicious and yellow apples as well, and yet we call them all apples even though they look and taste different.

Breast cancers are an extremely diverse group of diseases that are treated very differently depending on their type. Therefore, proper diagnosis is essential. When there is an area of suspicion on the mammogram or on examination— when something is new or different or is of concern—it calls for another mammogram and an ultrasound as well.

"Often the primary care physician is the doctor who begins the investigation of a problem, orders a test and then refers the patient to a specialist for an appropriate procedure."

— Barrie Raik, M.D.

Biopsy

Once an abnormality is detected, a tissue segment is taken involving a special type of needle called a biopsy needle. The surgeon or radiologist will first numb the skin with something similar to Novocaine, then sample the area. This process is usually painless, especially when adequate and appropriate numbing medicine is given. Tylenol can be taken ahead of time to manage pain if the patient is feeling apprehensive. However, no kind of Advil, ibuprofen, Motrin or aspirin should be taken before a biopsy because it can promote bleeding.

Taking multiple samples enables adequate coverage of the suspicious area. It does not give all the answers but it allows us to have some pieces of information analogous to connecting some pieces of a jigsaw puzzle. While a biopsy obtains a few pieces of the puzzle, we don't get the big picture or see the entire puzzle until the time of surgery. At that time all of the tissue of interest is removed and analyzed in the lab by a doctor called a pathologist who is specially trained in analyzing tissue and giving us the results, which are critical to determining the treatment.

Unfortunately, sometimes the biopsy needle can just graze the area of interest as opposed to hitting it head-on and sometimes we will have a result that is discordant, which means the results did not come back the way we anticipated based on the imaging. In a discordant result, the surgeon and the radiologist must carefully discuss the case to ensure that the surgeon removes the entire area of interest because otherwise the area of concern would be under-diagnosed and the appropriate diagnosis would be missed.

Lymph Nodes and Staging
Lymph nodes are located throughout our bodies. If you have ever had a bad cold, you may have noted swelling in your neck. This swelling was due to the expanded lymph nodes located in your neck, which were filtering and trapping the bacteria that made you sick.

On the issue of staging, many factors must be considered, particularly the size of the tumor and the status of the lymph nodes. Lymph nodes tend to cause a lot of anxiety among women because there is often the impression that if the cancer is in the lymph nodes it is essentially an incurable situation. This is completely false. If there is cancer in the lymph nodes, it certainly is harder to cure, and will often require some additional form of chemotherapy as part of the treatment, but it is quite likely curable.

In a breast cancer situation, lymph nodes can swell. If cancer cells are trying to escape the breast, the first place they will stop is the lymph nodes. The cancer cells travel on highways in the breasts called lymphatics that empty into the lymph nodes. The job of the lymph nodes is to filter the drainage of the breast and prevent any breast cancer cells that have left the breast from traveling beyond the lymph nodes.

A lot of women will ask, "What stage am I?" In general, there are stages 0, 1, 2, 3 and 4. Staging is a classification of how advanced the disease is and helps to determine the prognosis, treatment and treatment options. Women with stage 0 breast cancer are treated very differently from those with stage 3 breast cancer.

Q — What are the various cancer stages?

We are particularly interested in lymph nodes when we are trying to obtain a stage. If lymph nodes are involved it is usually a stage 2 or, based on the number of lymph nodes involved, it could potentially be a stage 3. This becomes very important for treatment and treatment strategy planning. Therefore, part of any cancer operation should include some type of evaluation of the lymph nodes. Most commonly, we will perform what's called a sentinel node evaluation, which involves checking the first few lymph nodes underneath the armpit to look for cancer spread from the breast.

We think of nodes as being arranged like beads on a string or like dominos. If cancer spreads, it spreads in a very orderly progression, going to the first lymph node in the chain. While it may just rest there, it may go to the second node, then on to the third just as dominos fall in a chain, one behind the other. If we can identify the sentinel nodes, which are the first few lymph nodes in the chain, and can actually check them during surgery, we can determine if the cancer has spread to the other lymph nodes. If it has not spread, this is very good news for the patient. It is excellent as far as her prognosis and we do not need to remove all of the lymph nodes as was traditionally done up until the mid-1990s.

Sentinel node biopsy usually involves injection of one or possibly two dyes. One dye is a nuclear dye and is injected just behind the nipple. Some surgeons will also use a second dye—a blue dye that can turn your urine blue-green the morning of surgery—either one called Lymphazurin or another called methylene blue. All of the dyes travel on the lymphatics and enable a surgeon to identify and check the sentinel nodes at the time of surgery.

If we do find cancer in the sentinel nodes, we do not know how far down the chain it has gone. So we remove all of the lymph nodes under the arm near the affected breast and test all of them to find out how many are involved. Clearly, the fewer involved the better. One or two is better than three or four, which is better than five or six, and so on. If any of the lymph nodes are involved, some type of chemotherapy will often be suggested or even required. Thus in staging, we look at the nature of lymph node involvement and whether cancer has spread to any of the organs, such as the liver, the lungs, the bones or the brain.

The breast is predominantly made of three things: fat, milk glands and milk ducts. The milk glands make milk when a woman is pregnant and the ducts are sort of like straws for the milk to get from the gland to the nipple. While most of the ducts end at the nipple, they crisscross a woman's breasts completely and breast cancers can occur anywhere throughout a woman's breast.

Where we find calcifications, which look like little specks of salt on a mammogram, there will often be what's called *in situ* disease. Ductal carcinoma *in situ* or DCIS, for short, is stage 0: where the cancer cells are completely contained within the duct and have not escaped the milk duct. Another term for this is the non-invasive variety of breast cancer. It is extremely curable and has an excellent prognosis.

Most commonly, women will fall into the stage 1 category where they will see the word "invasive" on their pathology results. That word is particularly frightening for many women because it suggests that cancer has spread throughout the breast or the lymph nodes or even their bodies; *but that is not the case*.

Invasive ductal carcinoma simply means that the breast cancer cells started in the milk duct, blew a hole through the milk ducts and landed in the surrounding fat.

Invasive lobular cancer means that it started in the milk gland and went into the fat as well. It does not mean that cancer has spread to the lymph nodes.

Treatment

Treatment is dependent on the type of breast cancer, as well as its size and the size of the woman's breasts. Sometimes the disease is confined only to one part

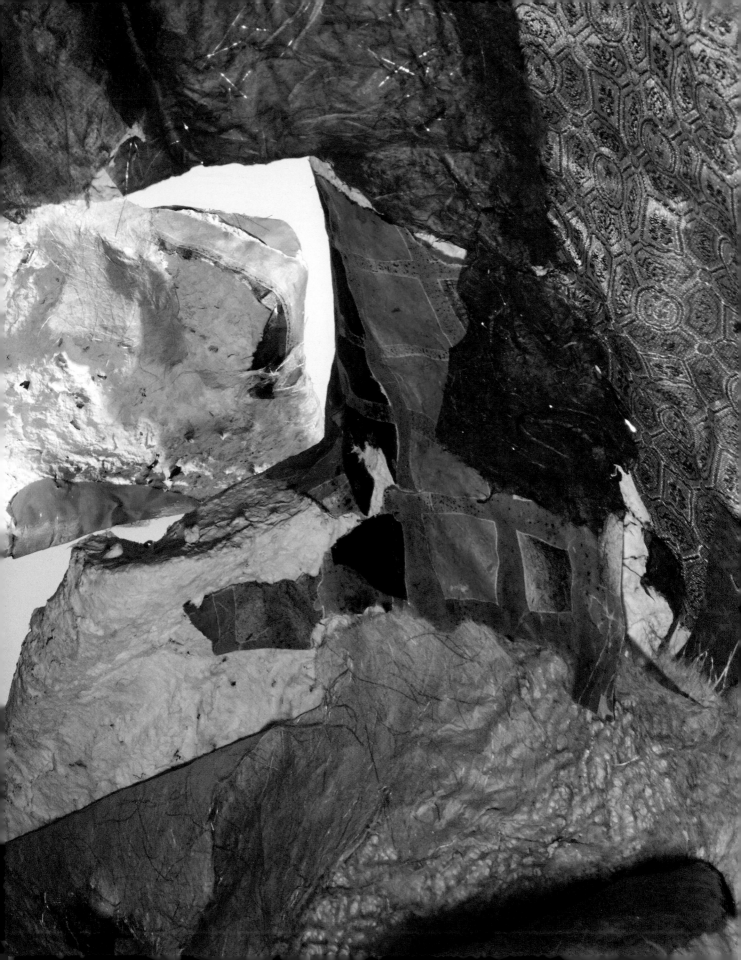

of the breast or one quadrant of the breast. If disease is contained within one quadrant, particularly if a woman is large breasted, a good choice of treatment is breast conservation or lumpectomy, which means removing only a part of the breast, as opposed to the entire breast.

Removal of an entire breast is called mastectomy. An important factor here is not only the woman's choice but whether she is agreeable to radiation after lumpectomy. This procedure is needed in order to sterilize the remainder of her breast. Since lumpectomy removes only the area of disease, the remaining breast needs to be protected or sterilized. On the other hand, if a woman is small breasted or if the tumor is quite large compared to the size of her breast, a better result may occur if the woman has a mastectomy to remove the breast and then reconstruct it.

There are different types of mastectomies. If possible, we will perform a skin-sparing mastectomy. Most often skin, the outer shell of the breast, is not the problem. Imagine a hard-boiled egg. You have the shell and then you have the actual egg inside it. When performing a mastectomy, we try to preserve that outer shell (the skin with a very thin layer of fat just below the skin called the subcutaneous tissue), but remove all of the breast tissue from within.

There are other options. A simple mastectomy is where the nipple and the areola (or the dark skin around it) are removed, as well as a fair amount of skin. If the tumor is close to the skin or involving the skin, this is the preferred approach. There is also a nipple-sparing mastectomy, which is somewhat controversial. It is not for all women with breast cancer, but is a reasonable option for women who have preventive surgery, such as those who have been informed that they have a genetic predisposition to breast cancer.

In discussing lumpectomy with radiation versus mastectomy, one must realize that they are equivalent as far as survival is concerned. Some women think if the breast is removed they will not need chemotherapy. This is not necessarily the case.

Chemotherapy decisions are based on a variety of factors including the stage, the size of the tumor, the lymph node involvement and most recently the results of a new test called Oncotype DX. This is a test that looks at the genetics or DNA of the tumor and allows us to stratify women as far as their risk of recurrence of the disease. It also allows us to estimate the benefit of chemotherapy in these women. Radiation is important to prevent the disease from returning in the breast or the lymph nodes if the woman has had a lumpectomy. Of course, in some groups of women who have had a mastectomy, we may recommend radiation based on the tumor size and lymph node involvement, as well as patient age and other health problems.

One last thing to consider about lumpectomy is that it will sometimes cause a divot in a woman's breast, a little dimple or a depression. This is why the result of a lumpectomy tends to look better and work better in women who are larger breasted. Keep in mind that your surgeon is not just removing disease but also providing a clear margin surrounding the area of disease. Consider a sunny-side-up egg, with the yolk and the surrounding egg white.

"I had been with my wife through her mastectomy, the uncertainties, waiting for the results of various tests, and the travails of chemotherapy, so I knew what I could expect if that path had to be taken."

— Wilbur Dexter Johnston, Ph.D.

The tumor is like the yolk, but we need not only to remove the yolk but also the white around it, which is similar to a clear margin where a line of healthy normal tissue is obtained around the tumor. This means removal of not only the tumor but also a rind of healthy tissue without cancer that surrounds the area of interest.

Three to four weeks of resting and recovering and recuperation after surgery is a good idea. During that time, there should be consultation with either the medical oncologist or the radiation oncologist or both. The medical oncologist needs to make decisions regarding chemotherapy. Today, many of the side effects of chemotherapy can be prevented. Therefore, the most common side effect we see in women now is fatigue.

Radiation planning involves consultation with a radiation oncologist. Radiation is essentially an X-ray beam that is pointed at the breast to prevent cancer from coming back. It does not cause hair thinning or loss but can cause temporary skin changes such as a sunburn-like appearance to the breast.

There are two situations where chemotherapy and/or radiation will precede surgery: if the tumor is particularly large, compared to a woman's breast size, and in cases where there is inflammatory breast cancer where the breast in fact looks red and swollen and inflamed. In both cases chemotherapy may be used first. This will serve to shrink the tumor down and help obtain a clear margin to help take less of the breast out and improve the cosmetics of the breast after lumpectomy.

Reconstruction

Reconstruction can take two forms. One is with an implant, otherwise known as a tissue expander, which is gradually built up over time to expand the breast to whatever size a woman would like. The second major option is called a flap reconstruction in which fat is taken from a woman's belly, for example, and moved to reconstruct the breast. While this is a lot of surgery, it allows a woman to have a tummy tuck and a breast reconstruction in one setting. These options should be discussed pre-op with your breast surgeon as well as with the plastic surgeon, particularly where partial or complete reconstruction is to occur in the same setting immediately after mastectomy.

Delayed reconstruction is also a possibility. That is where, after surgery, chemotherapy, and potentially even radiation, the patient comes back in a year or so, after the tissues have recovered, to have reconstruction. It is important that women know that reconstruction is almost always an option. The question is the timing. If a patient chooses not to have reconstruction, she can be fitted with a special bra that will allow her to look essentially symmetrical. If she has her clothes on, it would be difficult to tell she has had any surgery.

Genetic Testing

Those who are forty or under, or have a very strong family history of breast or ovarian cancer on either side of the family, should consider genetic or BRCA testing. This testing may determine the presence of a gene that increases risk for both these types of cancer. It would have particular impact because both breasts are at very high risk when that gene is present. This is something certainly to discuss with your breast surgeon or ask to see a geneticist in your community.

In Conclusion

The information contained in this article is basic and general. It is not a substitute for individualized treatment that can only be provided by the team of doctors who will look after you. Many women who go through the journey of breast cancer have incredible strength and courage. Nonetheless, they need not only the support of their families and friends and co-workers, but they should also know that there is support available through the American Cancer Society and through many local support groups. Sometimes women prefer a buddy, which offers more one-on-one interaction. This can be arranged, for example, through the American Cancer Society or the Hope Network, where women are matched for disease and age and can talk one-on-one on the phone rather than in a support group setting.

Breast Reconstruction

William L. Scarlett, D.O., F.A.C.S., F.A.C.O.S., F.A.A.C.S.

When I discuss breast reconstruction with patients, I review all of the options available to them and then help them make a choice. We discuss what surgeries can be done for their specific situations and circumstances. Then they choose which option is right for them. The breast reconstruction can be started the same day as the mastectomy (immediate reconstruction) or weeks, months or even years after the mastectomy (delayed reconstruction). We know that, psychologically speaking, women feel better if we are able to begin the reconstruction the same day as the mastectomy. To waken from surgery and see the beginning formation of a breast mound makes women feel more whole; however, there are circumstances when we have to delay reconstruction. The most notable instance is for people who have inflammatory breast cancer. This means that the cancer involves the breast skin. In this instance it is not recommended that we do immediate reconstruction, but wait at least 24 months—after the conclusion of chemotherapy and radiation treatments.

When we talk about reconstruction options, we break them down into two groups: autologous reconstruction (using your own tissue) and reconstruction with implants. According to the American Society of Plastic Surgeons, 80% of reconstruction in the U.S. is done with implants. There are also certain circumstances where we combine using a person's own tissue and an implant to achieve the desired result.

"Now I'm concerned with the present and the future. I'm going to a plastic surgeon next; at least I want my nipple back! In our society, women usually wear tops at the beach, men often don't."

— Rich Loreti

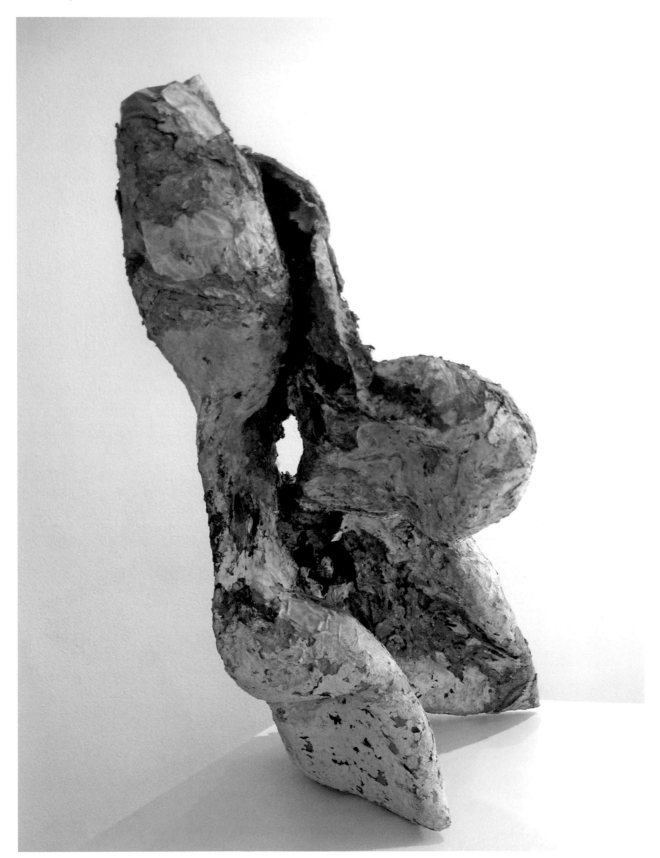

PRERECONSTRUCTION

Tissue from the abdomen, back or thigh can be used for reconstruction with various techniques and recovery times. When using implants, we will sometimes start by stretching the skin with a tissue expander—this process can take several weeks. When the breast reaches the desired size, the surgeon replaces the tissue expander with a permanent implant. While some women choose to enlarge their breast size with this surgical opportunity, others elect to be reduced in size and lifted. Plastic and reconstructive surgeons should be instrumental in taking the negative cancer situation and turning it into an opportunity to improve a woman's self-esteem.

Some women elect to stop after this first stage of reconstruction. They are pleased with the look of the breast mound in clothing and bathing suits and they do not want to pursue further surgery. Others want their new breast to look as natural as possible. The next step can be the reconstruction of a nipple and subsequent tattooing. There are many techniques to create a new nipple by using an individual's own skin. We can take skin from another place (armpit or groin); we can use skin from the opposite nipple; or we can use the skin from around the scar of the mastectomy. Tattooing adds coloration to the newly created nipple. If nipple projection is not a concern, the woman can skip the nipple reconstruction surgery and proceed directly to tattooing. Three dimensional tattooing gives the illusion of having a projected nipple.

For women having a one-sided mastectomy, we can perform a number of different procedures to make the other breast match. This can include breast augmentation, breast reduction or simply a lift to match the height of the reconstructed breast. For women undergoing a lumpectomy with radiation, the size and shape of the breast may change. They may need a symmetry procedure after treatment to make the breasts match in shape and size.

It is important to remember that breast reconstruction has no effect on the treatment of cancer—positively or negatively. The reconstructive surgeon should always take a back seat to the treatment plan of the oncologist. If someone is undergoing chemotherapy or radiation, we do not proceed with any further reconstruction until they have finished their treatment and the oncologist has given us clearance to do so. It is critical that the entire care team communicate and coordinate the treatment plan effectively. Weekly team meetings can help to facilitate this open communication and planning.

The breast surgeon and the plastic surgeon must be able to work collaboratively in order to schedule the reconstruction at the same time as the mastectomy. Also, both surgeons must understand the woman's goals for the surgery and work together to achieve those results. There are techniques that each surgeon uses that are complementary to each other in order to achieve outstanding results. Unfortunately, almost half of the women undergoing mastectomies in the U.S. are not offered reconstruction. This could be due to the lack of a solid medical team. The patient may need to be her own advocate when choosing her surgeons.

The most important thing to remember about breast reconstruction is that all decisions are individual. Find a plastic surgeon who will review all of the

"A year later, despite my initial hesitancy, I had reconstructive surgery… At thirty-five, it boosted my self-esteem and morale."

— Peggy S.

options with you and help tailor the surgery to your needs and wants. If you do not feel that the surgeon or their staff has given you the information or the time needed to help make your decision, then seek out a second opinion. Other breast cancer survivors and support groups are also a great source of information. Breast reconstruction is all about the individual being pleased with her new appearance and feeling whole again—in mind and body.

Breast Cancer and Lymphedema
Marcy McCaw, B.Sc.P.T., C.L.T.

The earlier cancer is caught, the lower the chance that it has moved to the lymph nodes and therefore the lower the chance of lymphedema. Women who have had any removal of lymph nodes, either sentinel or axillary node dissection from breast cancer surgery, are at risk for lymphedema.

What is lymphedema?
Lymphedema is swelling that occurs as a result of a compromised lymphatic system. There are two kinds of lymphedema—primary and secondary. Primary lymphedema is caused by a genetic disorder where one is born with an abnormal or underdeveloped lymphatic system. Secondary lymphedema is the result of damage to the lymphatic system seen primarily in patients who have had removal of lymph nodes as a consequence of cancer surgery. This swelling is much different from that which is seen in an injury (such as an ankle sprain) where the swelling is due to inflammation. Lymphedema is a protein-rich swelling. Due to the compromised lymphatic system, fluid can build up in the interstitial space, where the stagnant lymph fluid containing proteins and debris causes the swelling of affected tissues. The overall risk of lymphedema for all cancers is reported to be 15–30%.[1] There is no cure for lymphedema and it is a progressive condition.

How does the lymphatic system work?
The lymphatic system is made up of lymph vessels and over six hundred lymph nodes. There are lymph nodes throughout the body. The main location of nodes is in the abdomen, groin, neck and armpits. This system transports fluid throughout our bodies and back into the circulatory system, or it is eliminated by the body. There are deep lymph vessels and some that are very close to the skin. When the lymphatic system is healthy it pumps two to four liters of lymph each day. The heart regulates 90% of the fluid and the lymphatic system regulates 10% of fluid exchange. The lymphatic system has three primary functions. First is its immune response, which is our primary defense against bacteria, viruses and fungi. For this reason the lymphatic system could also be

"Waiting for the results of the chemotherapy, which took five days, was emotional agony. Happily the rest of the nodes were negative, but unfortunately I developed lymphedema in my chest wall and arm."

— Anne Johnston, Ph.D.

referred to as our immune system. Second, it returns protein-rich fluid that has escaped from the circulatory system. If the system is compromised, the protein can remain in the interstitial space in the affected area. This protein attracts water into the affected area, resulting in swelling. Third, the lymphatic system is involved in the transport of select nutrients from the digestive system to the circulatory system.[2]

What are the signs and symptoms of lymphedema?

1. Slow onset
2. Pitting in the early stages
3. Heaviness, achiness
4. Skin changes
5. Cellulitis, which commonly starts around the elbow area and is progressive

Management and control of lymphedema

If detected early, lymphedema can be treated, managed and controlled. The average time it takes for lymphedema to develop is six to eighteen months after cancer surgery. However, due to the damaged lymphatic system, a person is at risk for lymphedema for the rest of his or her life.

The following are risk reduction practices that one should follow:

1. Wear garden gloves in the garden.
2. Be careful when shaving with a razor.
3. Wear sunscreen and insect repellant.
4. Avoid tight, constricting clothing.
5. Do not allow needles or blood pressure measurement on affected arm.
6. Watch for infection, cellulitis, acute rapid onset of redness, map-shaped pattern, an area feeling warm to touch, swelling, flu-like symptoms and fever.
7. Learn self-massage.
8. Practice dry self-brushing.
9. Use deodorant that does not contain aluminum compounds.
10. Get early treatment for sub-clinical lymphedema.
11. Monitor measurements from three months post-treatment up to a year.
12. Have physical therapy, manual lymphatic drainage (MLD) and wear compression garments.
13. Wear compression garments for air travel.

The standard of treatment for someone who develops lymphedema is called Complete Decongestive Therapy (CDT).

This treatment is a two-phase treatment protocol.

Initial Phase (for two to four weeks depending on the severity)
1. Manual lymph drainage (lymphatic massage)
2. Compression bandaging
3. Remedial exercises
4. Skin and nail care

Maintenance Phase
1. Garments (day time)
2. Bandaging (night)
3. Exercise (daily)
4. Skin and nail care
5. Manual lymph drainage, as needed
6. Follow-up visits

Patients need to follow up with their therapists every six months once they are in the maintenance phase. They will also need to be re-measured for new garments every six months. This continual monitoring and compliance can help patients manage their lymphedema without complications.

There are other lymphedema treatments, which include a pneumatic pump to mechanically stimulate manual lymphatic drainage, debulking surgery, liposuction, node replacement surgery and pharmaceutical therapy. These approaches can be used in conjunction with the standard CDT treatment but are not a cure for lymphedema.

CDT is a very effective treatment for a patient who has lymphedema, but there has been more focus on prevention of lymphedema and early intervention before a patient develops clinical lymphedema. Clinicians are trying to establish the practice of doing pre-operative measuring of patients and then following up with patients and monitoring their measurements over time. If we can detect any change in measurements early, we can prevent and reduce the progression of lymphedema.

The NIH (National Institutes of Health) and the National Naval Medical Center Breast Care Center conducted a five-year study on the prevention of progression of lymphedema for patients at risk. This study showed that if subclinical lymphedema was detected and intervention treatment promptly initiated, the affected arm's volume was reduced to nearly that of the unaffected arm. This subclinical lymphedema is not visibly noticed and there are no symptoms. If the measurements showed an increase of 83 ml or a 3% volume difference of the arm, compared to the pre-operative measurements, this indicates that the patient has subclinical lymphedema. These patients were treated with off-the-shelf compression garments for four weeks. After this time their volumes had decreased.

Conclusion

In conclusion, pre-operative assessment in the context of a prospective surveillance model enables the early detection and management of subclinical lymphedema. An early intervention protocol with a 20- to 30-mm Hg compression garment significantly reduces the affected limb's volume to near baseline measures and prevents progression to a more advanced stage of lymphedema for at least the first year post-operatively. Further research is warranted to confirm the long-term clinical and cost effectiveness of this surveillance model compared with a traditional impairment-based model in treating breast cancer lymphedema.[2] Exercise has been a concern regarding its effect on lymphedema. However, more studies have shown that exercise helps reduce the risk of lymphedema as well as helps those who have lymphedema. Inactivity can cause a sluggish lymphatic system; obesity can also increase the risk of lymphedema. This is why exercise has now become an important factor for breast cancer patients.

Breast cancer survivors with lymphedema who started with a slow, progressive weight lifting program had no significant effect on limb swelling and showed a decreased incidence of exacerbations of lymphedema, reduced symptoms and increased strength.[3] Therefore women who get involved in a progressive weight training program reduce the chances of increased arm swelling by as much as 70%. Exercise needs to be an integral part of any lymphedema patient's lifestyle.[4]

Lymphedema is a chronic condition that has to be monitored. Patients can be proactive by practicing risk reduction strategies to prevent lymphedema. Exercise and early detection are important. It is hoped that one day a cure for lymphedema will be found. More studies need to be done on the lymphatic system to truly understand its role in effecting a cure.

1. Incidence of Breast Cancer Related Lymphedema, Petrek, J.A. Heelan, M.C.: Cancer, 83 (12 Suppl American) 2776–2781(1998)
2. Lymphatic Enhancement Technology, Aetiology, USA manual, Desiree De Spong, 4, 2011
3. Weight Lifting in Women with Breast-Cancer-Related Lymphedema, Kathryn H. Schmitz, Ph.D., M.P.H, et. al, *N.Eng.J.Med*; 361:664–73 (2009)
4. Preoperative Assessment Enables the Early Diagnosis and Successful Treatment of Lymphedema, Nicole L. Stout Gergich, P.T., M.P.T., Cancer 112, 2809 (2008)

Chemotherapy:
What Is It and How Should You Prepare for It?
Myra F. Barginear, M.D.

Chemotherapy is the use of medicines or drugs to treat breast cancer. Many times this treatment is just called "chemo." It is used to treat early-stage breast cancer after surgery to reduce the risk of the cancer coming back. Chemotherapy is also used to treat advanced-stage breast cancer to destroy or damage the cancer cells as much as possible.

Depending on the stage of breast cancer, the goal of chemotherapy is one of the following:

- **Cure cancer**: meaning to kill cancer cells to the point that your doctor can no longer detect them
- **Control cancer:** to keep cancer from spreading or to slow its growth
- **Ease cancer symptoms:** to shrink tumors that are causing pain or pressure.

What are the stages of breast cancer?

Stage 0: Stage zero (0) describes disease, such as ductal carcinoma *in situ* (DCIS) or lobular carcinoma *in situ* (LCIS), that is only in the ducts and lobules of the breast tissue and not in the surrounding tissue of the breast. It is also called non-invasive cancer.

Stage 1: The cancer is no larger than two centimeters (approximately an inch) and has not spread to surrounding lymph nodes or outside the breast.

Stage 2: Breast cancer is divided into two categories according to the size of the tumor and whether or not it has spread to the lymph nodes:

Stage 2A: The tumor is less than two centimeters (approximately an inch) and has spread up to three axillary or underarm lymph nodes. Or, the tumor has grown bigger than two centimeters, but no larger than five centimeters (approximately two inches) and has not spread to surrounding lymph nodes.

Stage 2B: The tumor has grown to between two and five centimeters (approximately one to two inches) and has spread to up to three axillary (underarm) lymph nodes. Or, the tumor is larger than five centimeters, but has not spread to the surrounding lymph nodes.

Stage 3: Breast cancer is also divided into two categories:

> *Stage 3A:* The tumor is larger than two centimeters but smaller than five centimeters (approximately one to two inches) and has spread to up to nine axillary lymph nodes.

> *Stage 3B:* The cancer has spread to tissues near the breast including the skin, chest wall, ribs, muscles or lymph nodes in the chest wall or above the collarbone.

Stage 4: The cancer has spread to other organs or tissues, such as the liver, lungs, brain or bone.

How does my doctor decide to recommend chemotherapy?
Breast cancer is a heterogeneous disease. It differs by individuals, age groups and even the kinds of cells within the tumors themselves. Other factors taken into consideration include menopausal status, general health, the size and location of the tumor and the stage of the cancer. Certain features of the tumor cells (such as whether they depend on hormones to grow) are considered as well.

Q — Are there different types of cancer?

There are also molecular tests to help you and your doctors decide if chemotherapy is beneficial. The molecular tests currently commercially available are Oncotype DX® and Mammaprint®. These tests are most helpful in women with negative lymph nodes and estrogen receptor-positive breast cancer. These tests are used in addition to the standard clinical variables mentioned above and are still under investigation in clinical trials to see who benefits the most from these tests.

How is chemotherapy given?
Chemotherapy medicines come in many forms and can be given in many ways: Intravenously (IV) as a slow drip (also called an infusion) through a thin needle in a vein in your hand or arm or through a port (sometimes called by brand names such as Port-a-Cath or Medi-Port) inserted in your chest during a short outpatient surgery. A port is a small disc made of plastic or metal about the size of a quarter that sits just under the skin. A soft thin tube called a catheter connects the port to a large vein. Your chemotherapy medications are given through a special needle that fits right into the port. You also can have blood drawn through the port. When all your cycles of chemotherapy are done, the port is removed during another short outpatient procedure. Chemotherapy can also be given by mouth (orally) as a tablet or capsule.

Q — What is a port?

Chemotherapy medicines can be given one at a time, which is usually the case in metastatic or stage 4 breast cancer, or are given in combination, which means you get two or three different medicines at the same time. Standard chemotherapy treatments may include one or more of the following medications:

- Abraxane (paclitaxel)
- Adriamycin (doxorubicin)
- Carboplatin (Paraplatin)
- Cytoxan (cyclophosphamide)
- Doxil (doxorubicin)
- Efudex (fluorouracil or 5-fluorouracil)
- Ellence (epirubicin)
- Gemzar (gemcitabine)
- Halaven (eribulin)
- Ixempra (ixabepilone)
- Lapatinib (Tykerb)
- Methotrexate
- Navelbine (vinorelbine)
- Taxol (paclitaxel)
- Taxotere (docetaxel)

It is also important to note that chemotherapy works best when you get the recommended dose of medication, on time, with no major delays, for the number of times or cycles.

What are the side effects?

Chemotherapy is effective against cancer cells because the medicines target rapidly dividing cells. However, normal cells in your mouth, intestinal tract, blood and hair also divide rapidly—so chemotherapy may affect them too, causing mouth sores, diarrhea and/or gastrointestinal upset, decreased blood counts and hair loss. Decreased blood counts refer to anemia (decreased red blood cells) and neutropenia (decreased white blood cells).

Other side effects you may have from chemotherapy depend on the medicine itself. The side effects you have may be different from someone else who is on the same treatment. Most side effects are anticipated by your doctor and will be discussed in great detail prior to your treatment. Medications can be given to either prevent the side effect (nausea) or treat the side effect (anti-diarrhea medication). Most chemotherapy side effects resolve shortly after chemotherapy has been completed, but some side effects may take several months or longer to go away completely. When you and your doctor are deciding on a chemotherapy regimen, weighing the benefits versus the risks of side effects is part of the process.

Can I work during chemotherapy?

Most people can work during chemotherapy treatments. It is a personal decision. It also depends on the chemotherapy treatment plan. It is not common for the chemotherapy itself to produce side effects that would make it impossible to keep working, but sometimes it does. In general, however, the side effects from chemotherapy can make it hard to keep up your daily routine, so you might

"When chemotherapy treatment was completed, my oncologist informed me that it was now time to begin taking Tamoxifen and I told her, 'No, I prefer to take Arimidex,' an aromatase inhibitor."

— Anne Johnston, Ph.D.

want to take care of a few things before treatment such as getting your teeth cleaned and having a complete dental checkup. Also, ask for help around the house and consider joining a support group.

Fatigue is a common side effect with chemotherapy treatments; unfortunately it has not been well-studied and is not well-documented in all cases, but it is reasonable to expect some degree of fatigue with chemotherapy treatment.

Conclusion

I often tell my patients that breast cancer will frequently be on your mind, yet it need not diminish the quality of your long and healthy life. Everything that is done in the world is done by hope. Breast cancer treatments have become significantly more effective and less toxic over the past few decades. Improved therapies are due in large part to the many brave women who have participated in clinical research trials. Research and clinical trials are fundamental in our efforts to better understand the biology of breast cancer as well as to improve current treatments.

Q — What side effects may come from chemotherapy?

The Port Is a Great Invention

Annelise DeCoursin

After a routine mammogram, in February 2000, microcalcifications were discovered and I was sent to the hospital for a biopsy. This was a very painful procedure in which, unfortunately, they discovered a small, quarter-inch malignant tumor. I was happy that the tumor had been found early and eager to take care of the problem before the cancer spread. After all, it doesn't magically disappear, and one must face up to the necessity of action.

Within no time at all, many good things happened. The tumor was removed, along with fourteen lymph nodes. Since I would be having chemotherapy, I had a port put in. The port is a great invention because the patient is spared the unpleasant mess of needles in their veins. For me, the only downside of having a port was that I couldn't ski.

Q — Is some cancer treatment being given as outpatient treatment?

After thirty days I had three more chemo treatments. All food except Mountain Dew and pizza tasted awful. Being an independent person, I never brought my family with me to treatments. I felt more in charge of my care if I went by myself.

It's not necessary to do fancy exercises to get your arm working again. I placed things in the kitchen on the upper shelf so I'd have to search for them. Luckily, I'm a violinist and play many concerts. This was good exercise and gave me other things than my illness to think about.

My hair fell out but there were wigs that looked much better than my own hair. It was fun buying wigs.

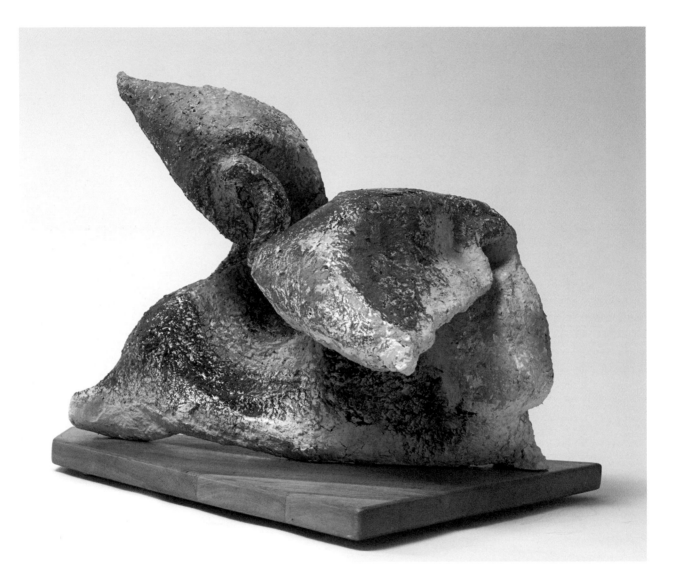

A year later, thirteen tumors were discovered on my bones, one on my liver and one on my lung. That was disappointing. I was then given chemo six times a month and several bone and CAT scans were taken every year.

During the nine years I had this treatment a few things went wrong. Herceptin, a perfect chemo drug for me, damaged my heart, closed my tear canals and filled my lungs with water. My lungs were tapped and the Herceptin discontinued. Another problem was that my wonderful port was placed in the same spot where I put my violin. I didn't want to play the violin in pain and had the port moved to another spot. It was right in the middle of my chest and was great for a few years.

Then disaster struck. The port got infected. I checked into the hospital in the middle of the night, with blood pressure of 60/40 and a temperature of 103°. I had septic shock and MRSA. Nasty!

The doctors were great and I survived. I was in isolation for a few weeks. It was boring. The most exciting thing was to fill out the menu. A technician, a young man, found out that I liked music. He'd sing to me while snapping his fingers. A one-man band! He liked that I played "gigs."

All this is now behind me. I don't have cancer any longer. No more chemo, but I see my oncologist every third month. My port is not being removed since I never know if there will be a recurrence. I have been well for twenty-eight months.

I've never felt sorry for myself because negative thoughts only make things worse. If you're tired or unhappy, don't just sit there. Go for a walk and be happy you're alive!

"Your chemotherapy medications are given into the port. When all your cycles of chemotherapy are done, the port is removed during another short outpatient procedure."

— Myra F. Barginear, M.D.

When Pink Was Just a Color

Paula Flory, *as written in her diary*

Saturday, October 15, 2011, 5:54 P.M., EDT

I own a few pairs of pink boxing gloves. Almost a decade ago, when my life as a "gym rat" began, I fell in love with boxing. After my first boxing class or two I'd decided it was time for me to purchase my own gloves. At the sporting goods store I obviously went straight to the pink ones. God they're cute. In addition to being the right weight, they were most certainly the perfect color. Those gloves presented me with so many opportunities for putting together coordinated workout ensembles. In addition, just like a fresh pair of kicks makes you feel like you could run a marathon, those gloves made me feel like Cassius Clay in boxing class. (Yeah, I'm old school!) Of course they garnered attention. Everyone loved them and most women wanted a pair for themselves. Jab, cross, hook, uppercut, bobbing and weaving. Damn, that was fun. Over time, when the first pair of pink gloves had seen better days, I went out and purchased a second pair, punched the crap out of those and went on to purchase another. Always pink, always cute, and always made me feel strong and powerful.

You'd think I'd have known that the gloves were constructed of pink leather for a reason other than because it was a color that appealed to women. You'd think I'd been hanging around this earth long enough to recognize that the pink gloves were created as a breast cancer awareness fundraising product. Apparently, I'd been living in my own little protective bubble. Yes, of course I was aware of breast cancer. You can't live in the U.S. and not be aware. I got my mammograms, did my "selfies," donated money, participated in the Race and supported my sister Kathy, who, for years, has donated her valuable time and amazing talents to the Susan G. Komen Foundation. And despite the fact that I had known people with breast cancer and did what I was told I should do to keep this disease at bay, pink, to me, was just a pretty color and a singer. Then in April 2011, I found my unusual and unwanted armpit dweller.

October is Breast Cancer Awareness Month but I was made well-AWARE on May 12, 2011. I feel guilty that I'd been swimming through the beautiful sea of life without an appropriate level of sensitivity to the many, many women and men who have suffered and to the many, many women and men who have died, and to the family members who have suffered and grieved along with them. Every Saturday morning at 7 A.M., for years and years, I would wrap my hands and pull on those pink gloves and punch away. I had no clue whatsoever that those gloves would become a symbol for what the rest of my life would be like. A fight in Pink.

I've been through a lot since May of 2011. On both a physical and psychological level I've gotten pretty beaten up. One big surgery down and seven "Bad Titty Bombs" completed. In a little over a week I'll receive my last Taxol treatment. I know it's only one more but that doesn't mean I don't dread it. And I mean DREAD. The first hour of infusion is all pre-meds: Oral steroids, a steroid drip and an anti-acid drip. This first long hour puts me in something of a coma. My husband, Chuck, and sister, Rosalie, can attest to the fact that I'm a bit of a melancholy drunk by the time the last drip is pumped into my port. I'm dizzy and can't think straight. Sleep doesn't come. I feel as though I'm being submerged in a pool of thick pink sludge. I've tried watching TV and leafing through magazines and I just can't focus. Rosalie tries so hard to make it okay. She shops online and shows me the stuff, trying to get me excited about a purchase, but it brings no relief. She offers me ice pops, blankets, breadsticks, encouraging words. She gives of herself completely and tearfully tells me that she would trade places with me if she could and I know she means it. She covers me with love and concern and compassion and still, I feel like crap. And this is all before the actual Bad Titty Bomb is hooked up and pumped in over a three-plus-hour period. Those hours are tedious, painful and mind-numbing. And the actual infusion is only the beginning of the difficult days that follow. How in the hell could I have lived my whole life with so much insensitivity? Perhaps that's the wrong word. Obviously I had compassion for people with cancer.

"Side effects can come together in a perfect storm, to create lack of appetite and compromised nutritional status. During this time the most important piece of advice is to eat."

— Karen Connelly, R.D., C.S.O.

Obviously I knew that it was a horrible disease. But how dare I wear those gloves thinking they were produced because they were a pretty color! Ignorance is bliss, I suppose.

I know that with the completion of chemotherapy I will have reached a significant milestone in my treatment plan; however, I'm not feeling the relief that I thought I would feel as I head towards this finish line. Is it because I know there is so much more to come? Another surgery is scheduled, a tedious and rigorous radiation schedule and a couple more surgeries after that. And then hormone therapy in the form of a pill. A drug like Tamoxifen taken daily for five to ten years. Okay, I think I know where my lack of relief stems from. It's the five to ten years of hormonal therapy. Yes, I am grateful that I have an estrogen-receptor positive cancer and that there are pharmaceuticals that act as an insurance policy of sorts. The Tamoxifen will prevent the flow of estrogen, which will hopefully prevent more cancer. Key word, "hopefully." I still have a right breast, bones, a liver, lungs and, oh yeah, I almost forgot, a brain. All are there as patient and willing hosts for cancer cells. So I will endure the wrath of hormone therapy, which I hear can be pretty damn awful, and I will pray every single day that it is working. The only diagnostic testing I will receive once the hormone treatment begins is a yearly mammogram of my right breast and basic blood work. No bone scans, no PET or CT scans. I will live my life assuming the cancer is suppressed unless my body tells me otherwise. A survivor friend told me that I will without a doubt wake up one day and NOT have cancer be the first thing that enters my mind. I want to believe her but when I take that pill each and every day when I wake, how will I not hope, pray and wonder what, if anything, is brewing in my body?

TAMOXIFEN

Tamoxifen is a drug that blocks the actions of estrogen and is used to treat and prevent some types of breast cancer.

It's October and you can't turn on the TV, cruise the web, open a newspaper or magazine without reading stories about breast cancer. Right now, the stories that stick with me and re-run over and over in my mind are the stories about the women who were through their treatment and feeling well until the cancer returned, either in the once healthy breast or in a more remote part of the body. Did you know that my chemotherapy drugs do not prevent cancer cells from crossing the blood–brain barrier? I do. How will I ever let that thought go? "FDF" (Fantastic Doctor Fox, the nickname I gave to my medical oncologist Dr. Kevin Fox, Head of the Rena Rowan Breast Cancer Center at Abramson Cancer Center at the Hospital of the University of Pennsylvania) tells me this will be my biggest challenge. Keeping my head free and clear of these negative thoughts will be how my personal fight will continue well beyond the debilitating side effects of the BT Bomb.

My pink boxing gloves are resting on a shelf in my bedroom closet. I see them every day and think about the strength and power I possessed when I wore them in class. I can't help but wonder, as I sit here today with saggy muscles and a back that is severely weakened by the Taxol, if I will ever don those pink gloves again and pack a mighty punch. All those years in the gym, training my body—I never knew that I was actually training for the fight of my life. The fight FOR my life.

Early on in my treatment I said I would never become one of those "pink ribbon people." That I would never define myself by my disease; and this remains true. But I will forever be a fighter. I now understand WHY my gloves were pink, but man how I wish I could go back to a time when to me, pink was just a color.

Tuesday, October 25, 2011, 12:18 P.M., EDT

I dream of a grandmother in a warm kitchen baking chocolate chip cookies with her small grandchildren. Just as she is about to take the last batch out of the oven, she says, "Stand back kids, the oven is hot." Before she opens the oven door she gathers her hair back into a ponytail and fastens it with the hair tie she has around her wrist.

Her brown-eyed granddaughter says, "Granny, you have pretty hair, and it's kinda long. Do you like your hair long, Granny? Why do you like your hair long?"

She tells the little one that when she was younger she got very sick and in order to get better the doctors had to give her medicine that made all of her hair fall out. And as she gestures in a circular motion around her entire head, she tells her granddaughter that she was totally bald. She then explains that when her hair finally grew back, she was so thrilled to have it that she decided to grow it on the long side. And she liked it so much that she's kept it pretty long for all these years.

With that being enough of an explanation for her young brain, they then decide to go outside to play while the cookies cool down. Her grandson asks, "Granny, can you teach us to jump rope all fast and fancy like you do it?"

"Of course I can teach you to jump rope all fast and fancy!"

The Grace of Caregiving

Tobias D. Robison

My wife, "B," was in the kitchen, yelling, angry with me, upset. This had to be an emergency. I ran downstairs—I'm sixty-nine, but yes, I ran—to see.

"B" had just prepared her breakfast. She had cut a ripe pear into neat little pieces. She added some banana and a nice helping of Cheerios. And then she took my buttermilk out of the fridge, mistaking it for her skim milk. She poured my buttermilk all over her cereal.

"B" hates buttermilk. She will have to throw her entire breakfast out and start over, and there was only one ripe pear. She's in tears, and it's all my fault. What made me decide to buy buttermilk anyway?

"And I feel terrible!" she says.

"I know," I say. "I'm sorry."

"You have no idea how I feel!" she says, and of course, she's right.

She's in chemo. It robs her of all energy at unpredictable times. And while the chemotherapy is digging out and destroying her cancer, it is ripping into her guts.

"I don't have cancer," she says. "I have chemo!"

Sometimes she's her old self, accomplishing everything she wants to do in a day. But when she's overwhelmed, how can I help? Well, here's what I've learned: it takes a while to understand what that means, *to help.*

My wife had breast cancer many years before, and that first time, she only needed radiation. The new breast cancer fell on my wife nine months ago, and the treatment had to be more aggressive. We dreaded chemotherapy. I knew that I must be prepared for anything. I started to shed commitments and responsibilities, to set aside time for my wife's needs. It was not hard to lighten my own load. I'm nearly retired, and my busy life is full of self-appointed commitments, plans and deadlines. I regretfully shucked many of these, and I thought, I'm ready.

I did not yet understand.

I saw a friend at the local hospital. He and my wife were both having tests. I told him about my wife's cancer. He looked right at me and said, "your job is to be The Rock."

I liked the sound of that. I told "B" about my desire to be The Rock. She understood what I meant. As we prepared to face chemo, we joked about it. Sometimes I reviewed my least helpful behavior and wondered if I am really The Rock?

My friends misunderstood. "You're going to be unemotional like a rock? You're going to withdraw? Nothing will affect you?"

No, of course I didn't mean those things; I meant that I would always be there, never frazzled. Arguments might *almost* erupt. But I would be the serene pillar of strength.

I had the right idea, but I still did not understand.

I was there for my wife again and again. The night before the first treatment, she had to sign a release form. I was hoping she wouldn't read it, but she did. The form detailed the many ways her chemo drugs could poison her and worse. "They're going to kill me," she said. I opted for common sense, arguing that if the drugs were worse than the cancer, no one would administer them. But wow, that release form scared me, too.

Sometimes, I was there so that my wife didn't have to argue with herself about whether to take Compazine. Sure, it would control her nausea, but she would get sleepy and be able to accomplish nothing. *Nothing*, did I understand?

The cancer center gave us four pages of symptoms to watch for. If any of these struck, I was to call the Nurse's Hotline, or dial 9-1-1 or, in the worst cases, call a hearse. I taped those pages to a wall. As "B" grumbled about her miserable symptoms, I checked those pages again and again to make sure we weren't having an emergency. I picked up dropped forks, refilled drinks and did little tasks that she has always done for herself, to help her conserve her energy.

"Cancer impacts... every aspect of life; for example home life, parenting, social life, work and interpersonal relationships."

— Vilmarie Rodriguez, M.S.W.

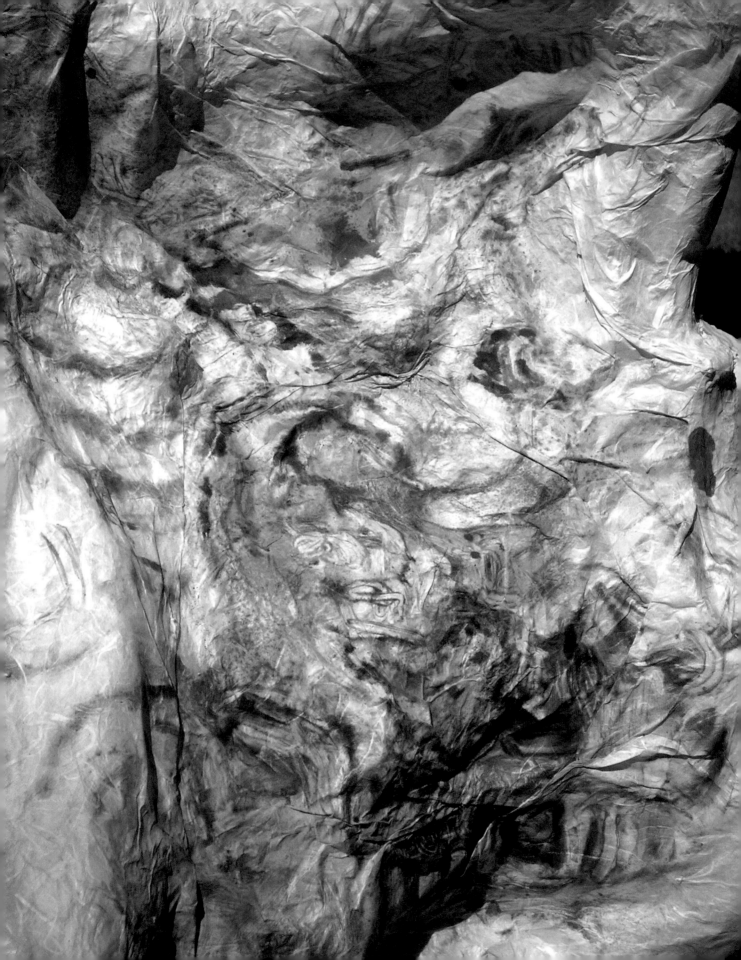

Only once did I make the mistake of eating fish at home. "B" hates the smell of fish, and the chemo chemicals had enhanced her fine sense of smell.

I couldn't help thinking about what I was *not* accomplishing. I know: I said that I had shed my commitments, to have time to do what I was actually doing. Still, I was depressed that my own goals for the year lay in tatters. A novel lurked on my computer, unedited. I was afraid to make appointments that might conflict with my wife's needs. I had expected a few accomplishments for this year, and none of them happened.

Time is precious, especially if you measure it against what's not getting done. I got annoyed, bitter and angry. But I kept it to myself because I was The Rock. To make matters more painful, I understood that I was one of the lucky ones. My wife never dominated all my time. She always gave me great chunks of respite to do as I pleased. But she was at the mercy of the demands that the chemo medicines made on her body, at unanticipated moments, arriving in irregular rhythms, wrecking my attempts to create my own continuity, distracting me from what I had planned.

Eventually I understood. My wife's priorities, great and small, trumped every one of mine. *Of course* it was going to be impossible to live my life as I had planned. My opportunities to help and care for her should always come first.

Why had I taken so long to understand? Like many people, I felt that I could always take on something else *in addition*. If, like me, you're an optimist, it's hard to see the limits that twenty-four hours a day, minus the time to eat and sleep, engrave on your life.

Sigh. I'm human, and I shall remember one blunder during "B"'s treatments. Three evenings after the penultimate chemo, she was miserable, and quite vocal about it. "See you in a few hours," I said as I rushed off to a class that I really wanted to take. When I returned, she was still miserable, and still vocal about it. How could I have deserted her? There were ways I could have helped her before I left, and I hadn't even offered. I knew my priorities, but it's so human to be selfish. I had fallen off The Rock, and I hastened to remind myself who came first.

It made an enormous difference to me to accept that I must surrender my own priorities, *all of them*. It's wonderful to ease another's burden with joy and grace. The moments of ease that I've brought to my wife during her treatment are a reward I shall treasure. "B" will recover, and there'll be more time for my goals.

Radiation Therapy
Mitchell K. Karten, M.D.

The treatment of cancer utilizes three modalities: Surgery removes the tumor, surrounding normal tissue and nodes. Chemotherapy preferentially destroys cancer cells and is used systemically to treat metastatic cancer or as adjuvant

Q — What is conservative
radiation therapy?

*"I was lying on the
table, anchored in a
blue plastic cradle,
looking around ....
Halfway up the right
wall, stacks of blue
cradles filled layers
of shelves. There were
so many cradles!"*

— Marion Behr

therapy. Radiation therapy is similar to surgery, in that it only treats a limited region of the body. It is used for definitive treatment in breast cancer or palliation of symptoms from metastatic disease, such as bone pain. Any or all of these modalities may be used in the treatment of a particular patient.

Radiation therapy may be used in conjunction with two treatment options: mastectomy or local excision (lumpectomy) with preservation of the breast (conservative therapy). These treatments have equivalent overall survival (OS) and disease-free survival (DFS) rates. Following mastectomy the tumor cannot recur in the breast; however, the tumor may recur in the chest wall, skin or lymph nodes. Many mastectomy patients will receive radiation therapy to the chest wall and lymph nodes. In conservative therapy, radiation therapy is used to treat the remainder of the breast after lumpectomy. Most surgeons recommend conservative therapy.

Radiation therapy to the breast begins four to six weeks after surgery or the last dose of chemotherapy. Before treatment starts, a planning process called simulation is necessary to set the machine properly for each patient. Photographs of the area of treatment may be taken to record the treatment. Skin marks and small permanent tattoos (the size of a period in a sentence) may be used to mark the skin for setup purposes. Immobilization devices, such as slant boards or cradles, are used to ensure consistent positioning throughout the treatment. A non-contrast CT scan (no dye injection or drink) is often performed to aid in planning. The CT scan does not provide diagnostic information; it is used to determine the shape of the breast or chest wall, lung and cardiac volumes, so that the treatment computer can customize the plan for each patient.

Radiation therapy to the intact breast has to mimic a mastectomy; therefore the entire breast (including the skin and nipple) and sometimes the lymph nodes are treated with X-rays. This is usually followed by a boost using an electron beam to the area of excision. The radiation oncologist will prescribe a dose of treatment, which is delivered over thirty to forty treatment days. Treatments are given five days a week, Monday through Friday, with holidays and missed days being made up at the end. A course, including planning and treatment, may take eight to nine weeks. Daily visits last twenty to thirty minutes, but the actual treatment is about two to three minutes long. The experience is similar to a chest or dental X-ray. Shielding gowns are not needed, as the head of the machine contains a blocking mechanism that shields normal areas from radiation. No burning sensation or pain occurs during treatment. The machine is open and no parts touch the patient, but some patients may note a faint odor of ozone.

Radiation therapy treatment to the breast will not cause nausea, vomiting, diarrhea or hair loss. Because bone marrow cells are not in the treatment field, there is no significant effect on the immune system. Nevertheless, all cancer patients should avoid obviously sick visitors and should practice good hand washing and respiratory hygiene. Contact with pets is permitted but contact with litter should be avoided if possible. Patients receiving radiation therapy to the breast are not radioactive and are not any danger to visitors or children. Sexual intimacy is allowed but non-hormonal barrier birth control (e.g., condoms but not birth control pills) should be practiced. Your oncologist should be consulted. A balanced diet is recommended, and a stress multivitamin supplement may be used. You may feel generalized fatigue or tiredness, especially if chemotherapy was just completed.

Side effects of treatment may include skin darkening, slight changes in the shape or contour of the breast or peeling of the skin. These effects only occur in the treatment area. Although the effect is similar to sunburn, radiation skin reaction is caused by a different mechanism; therefore, sun-blocking ointments will not prevent a reaction. Fair-skinned women may not have a reaction and dark-skinned women may. No creams, lotions, perfumes, hair removal products or antiperspirants should be used in the treatment area as they may irritate the skin. Corn starch, baking soda or Tom's of Maine Sensitive Skin Deodorant (an aluminum-free product) may be used for personal hygiene. Should skin peeling occur, the physician will prescribe creams or a short break from treatment. I prescribe steroid creams and Aquaphor for mild reactions and antibiotic ointments for skin peeling. If axillary surgery for nodes was performed, straight razors are not recommended due to the risk of nicking. Wet electric razors, showers and mild soaps are permitted. After treatment is completed, the patient can resume using personal care products. Sun exposure to the treated fields should be avoided for one year.

An initial follow-up visit is scheduled one to three weeks after the treatment to monitor resolution of treatment effects and then every two to three months for the first two years. Patients occasionally feel anxiety and depression at the end of treatment because they are no longer coming daily for treatment and interacting with a supportive staff. "Did the treatment work?" and other questions cannot be answered by testing immediately after therapy. The answers require the passage of time and a continued dialogue with the oncologist. Mammograms are performed every six months or annually.

It should be remembered that the majority of patients have an excellent result and a prolonged disease-free survival and quality of life.

Q — What are side effects from radiation? Can they be controlled?

Surviving Cancer
Evie Hammerman, M.S.W.

I am a very lucky seventy-four-year-old woman who has had two cancers in the past five years. The first was breast cancer and then, two years later, colorectal cancer. Early detection was the key to discovering the equivalent of a cure in both cases. In both situations the cancer was self-contained and surgically removed.

The breast cancer was discovered during my annual routine mammogram in a rural community hospital in New Hampshire. I elected to go to Boston, MA, which is seventy miles away, for further diagnosis and treatment, feeling it would be wise to get the best care possible. Boston is a major medical center for cancer treatment within an integrated system of hospitals.

Fortunately, one of my sons lives in Boston. He or his wife accompanied me to all appointments and procedures. Having someone with you is very important. It's difficult to be a patient and process all the information alone. After my mammogram I was told that I had stage 1 invasive ductal carcinoma breast cancer and was referred to a surgeon.

My surgical appointment was several weeks later. It was psychologically and emotionally hard to wait. During this time I looked up information on the Internet, spoke with people who had breast cancer and consulted a psychotherapist. I knew I could have a lumpectomy or a mastectomy and found out that I could have contaminated lymph nodes in my armpit. Some lymph nodes would have to be removed and tested and would be an indicator of the extent and possible spread of the breast cancer.

At my surgical appointment we went over the options. My surgeon was impressed that I was informed about my cancer and the various choices. We all agreed that a simple lumpectomy was the right procedure, given the small size of the cancer and the fact that it had been found very early. The surgery was scheduled for two weeks later as an outpatient procedure. Again, my family came and stayed with me until it was time to go into surgery.

My recovery was easy. Fortunately, the cancer in my left breast had not spread to the nodes. I was able to eat and do all activities, making sure not to lift or strain my left side or arm. As a left-handed person it was important to avoid edema (swelling). However it turned out that the surgeon had not gotten sufficient margins for the cancer and I needed to go back and have another similar procedure two weeks later. After recovering from the second procedure I was referred to an oncologist. The doctor recommended radiation treatment followed by oral hormone therapy.

I live in New Hampshire, where the state motto is "live free or die." I was feeling resentful about further treatment. My cancer was small and had been surgically removed. I am a widow living alone. All my decisions about this cancer were made by me alone. My three sons and their wives were always there for me, supportive of whatever procedures I decided to take or not take.

In general, I did not tell people about my breast cancer, feeling I couldn't cope with their questions and concerns. I didn't want people asking, "How do you feel" and treating me as if I were ill. Psychologically, having radiation was a very difficult decision for me. The percentage of success by having radiation was only three to four percent better than not doing it. Was it worth it?

It was important to take care of myself, not for a spouse or family members, but for me. In the end I decided I did not want a recurrence of breast cancer and would dot every "i" and cross every "t." I had been lucky this time and was

"It is now very clear that cure rates with mastectomy are not better than with breast conserving surgery (lumpectomy), which should be the treatment of choice whenever feasible."

— Richard Margolese, M.D.

afraid about taking care of myself alone if there were a recurrence that was worse.

I decided to do radiation locally and drove thirty minutes for treatment four days a week for eight weeks. I found the radiation dehumanizing. People undressed and walked to and from the radiation room in hospital gowns. The therapists were patient and empathetic, but I felt like cattle going to slaughter. I did drive myself to all my treatments, despite the fact that I experienced great fatigue by the end. In retrospect, it would have been better to ask people to take me to the appointments.

Subsequently, I started the hormone therapy and was able to tolerate it well. I took Tamoxifen for two and a half years and then switched to an aromatase inhibitor, which I was told would be necessary for another five years. Because of adverse symptoms from taking the aromatase inhibitor, I have stopped all hormone therapy after a total of five years.

It is more than five years since the breast cancer diagnosis and I feel like a true cancer survivor. I am glad that I did the radiation and the oral chemotherapy. Breast cancer is serious even if it is the simplest form.

Two years ago I went for a routine colonoscopy. The doctor discovered a mass in my rectum and recommended an MRI to see if it had spread. The MRI showed the mass to be contained in the colon but indicated possible problems on my ovaries and an enlargement of the uterus lining. I was completely overwhelmed. Even though my breast cancer was under control, I felt filled with uterine and colon cancer and was really scared.

My son and I went to see a colorectal surgeon. He confirmed that there was a mass in my rectum just where it connected to the sigmoid colon. He felt it was self-contained but probably had an early cancer in the middle of it. He scheduled surgery and arranged for a gynecologist to do a hysterectomy at the same time. He also told me that there was a slight chance of my having an ileostomy, but that it would be reversible. I would be in the hospital for four to five days and then recuperate at home for a month or two.

The surgery went well but I did have an ileostomy. The doctor reported there was a self-contained mass and the biopsy showed a spot of cancer in the center. No further treatment was required since the surgeon had removed all of the mass.

For the first couple of weeks after surgery, my children stayed with me to help. After my children left, though I had never asked for help before, I asked some of my friends to each give me one day of care. Originally, I asked about a dozen friends to come in the morning to help me shower, cook, and feed me lunch and dinner (because of the ileostomy I needed to eat pureed food) and stay overnight. As it turned out, I could shower myself and no one needed to sleep overnight. I found someone being with me from lunch through the evening was too long. I needed to nap and have quiet time in the afternoon. So people came mid-afternoon and cooked and fed me dinner, then went home.

Friends were delighted to do this. Many people told me how pleased they were to be asked for their help. It made them feel good to know that they could do something and I learned how important it is to ask.

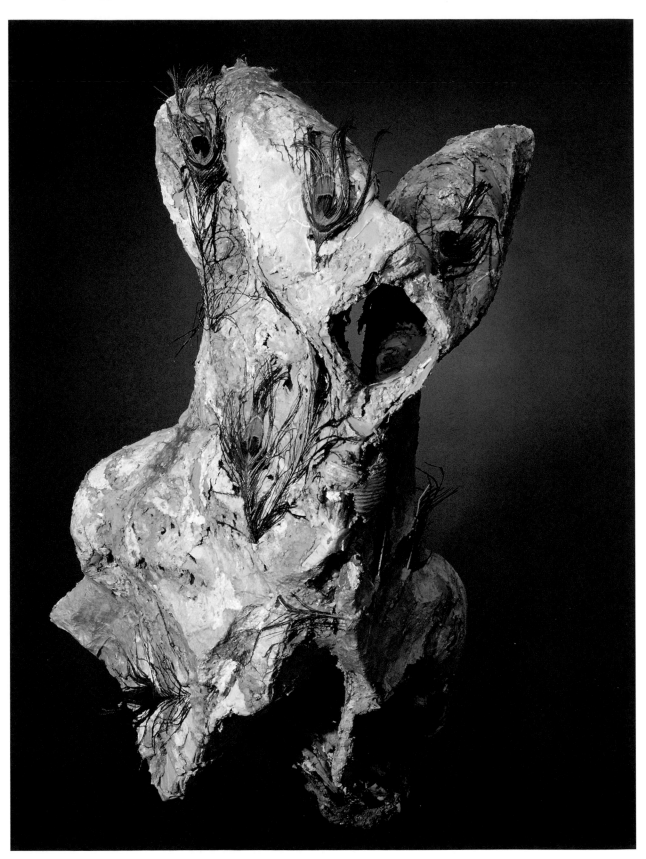

CANCER SCARES

The visiting nurse came for six to seven weeks and taught me how to change the ileostomy myself. I gained enormous respect for anyone who has a permanent ileostomy or colostomy. It is a difficult lifestyle to cope with. At eight weeks my ileostomy was reversed. This took another surgical procedure and recovery. Then it was necessary to learn how to eat regular food again and get back to a normal life.

The recovery from the colorectal surgery was long and complex, involving my whole digestive and excretory systems. Now I am back to normal and able to engage in all my activities. The difference is I know that I can have something life-threatening happen to me, so my aim is to live life as fully as possible. I feel totally cured and definitely a cancer survivor.

Here are some lessons I learned that I'd like to pass on:

1. Early detection is essential for the best treatment and cure. Because of early detection I was able to have surgery in both cases; the cancer had not metastasized and was able to be totally removed surgically, enabling me to be cured of cancer.

2. It is important not to panic when you hear the word "cancer." You need to investigate and find the right doctor and hospital to get the best care possible. Be sure to explore all available resources. As it happened, I was able to consult with a cousin who is an oncologist in another state. Referrals from your own doctor and recommendations from other people who had similar experiences are important resources.

3. It is normal to feel anxious and scared. You need to find a way to cope by seeing a psychotherapist, talking to others with similar experiences, joining a group, talking to friends and family and following your own self-care activities, i.e., reading, journaling, listening to music and physical activities.

4. Always take someone with you to doctor appointments. One day I went alone and had a misunderstanding with the doctor, so I learned to always take someone. You might even bring a tape recorder to the appointment if it is okay with the doctor.

5. Ask for help in dealing with your illness and in recovery. It is an important thing to do for yourself, and it is a gift to others to tell them what you need and how they can help you.

Being a cancer survivor has enabled me to enjoy my family and friends, to do volunteer activities, to travel, to be physically active including playing tennis and swimming regularly and to do all the things I want to do. I've learned to not put things off and to do everything I can while I am healthy and able. My life is very good and I am grateful for it.

"I'm allergic to latex. At one point a technician taking blood was wearing latex gloves; fortunately, my husband, who was with me, asked about this."

— Marion Behr

Heart
Michael Carr

You are concerned about my heart because
it's partly yours. After all, you are my mother.

You are concerned with my heart because
of the drugs that killed and cured.

You are concerned that my heart will break
one day, but don't worry because I'm tough.

You are concerned that I've given my heart
freely over the years, but this time it's for real.

You are concerned that my exercise routine
is far too strenuous so you bought me a monitor.

You are constantly and completely consumed
with the safety and protection of my heart.

I ask you, is it because you have so much
love in your heart that you needed a second?

Is it because you remembered the time
when we once shared the same heart?

I'd like to think so. Because that seems
like a forever kind of thing.

The Man in the Vinyl Chair

Michael Carr

I will see him there always, rustling, struggling to
steady the troubled, mortified soul constantly shouting
obscenities in his ear. Restless evenings become
endless, zombie mornings for the man in the vinyl
chair, unable to leave the side of a son, so cut up
and sick that for the man, the vinyl
chair doesn't seem so inconvenient.

The dialogue is simple most nights.
The man squeakily finds a restful position
as he folds out the chair and then he turns toward
the hospital cot, reassuring himself that the son
is indeed still breathing, equal chest rise
and all that. "I'm fine," is the son's stoic
mantra and the man usually agrees.

The good days will be relearned, the life lessons,
interrupted by cruel disease, will continue.
The son takes comfort, finds solace in knowing
that one truth is always constant:
There is a man in a vinyl chair ready to fight the night and stay beside him
until the morning.

VI

Further Guidance—
Essential advice for the road to recovery

Oncology Social Workers and How We Help

Vilmarie Rodriguez, M.S.W., L.C.S.W.

Oncology social workers generally have a master's degree in social work (M.S.W.) and are trained in and knowledgeable about assisting cancer patients and their caregivers. We are members of the health care team and, as such, can help navigate the health care system and intervene with day-to-day challenges that accompany a cancer diagnosis. We practice in many different settings such as hospitals, local community cancer centers, social service agencies and organizations like CancerCare, which are able to provide free professional support services to anyone affected by a cancer diagnosis

A cancer diagnosis changes everything. Cancer not only impacts the individual but the entire family and support network involved. It not only touches on health issues, but every aspect of life; for example home life, parenting, social life, work and interpersonal relationships. It is difficult for the cancer patient and the caregiver to enter the cancer journey not knowing what to expect, realizing that the world they once knew will change forever. It is here that oncology social workers become a valuable resource. When you speak to one of us, we will ask, *"How are you coping?"* This generally opens the door of communication and enables us to ask other questions to ascertain whether there is a good support system in place, what practical services need to be addressed, what psycho-educational matters we need to focus on and what individual coping styles may be. We look at the individual as a whole and work together to achieve a healthy balance.

Q — How does an oncology social worker provide help for a cancer patient?

When someone hears that they have cancer, it is as if time stops and everything occurs in slow motion. This is when speaking to an oncology social worker can make a huge difference in how patients cope and how prepared they are for the journey to come. We help patients understand the information and treatments for their specific cancer, options provided, resources available and how to communicate with the health care team. As part of the health care team, we know how to navigate the medical and social services systems and can identify local and national resources for services such as transportation, lodging while in treatment, financial resources, referrals and linkages to other organizations. We make the journey a little easier by providing emotional support, practical resources and guidance along the way.

Communication with the medical team and family members becomes incredibly important at a time when decisions need to be made and support is needed. Patients are not only faced with learning a new medical language, but also with learning to become more assertive, by asking questions within a system that may be intimidating and overwhelming. Most doctors will address questions and concerns, but patients may find it difficult to ask. We help patients shape and prepare their questions and give practical tips about

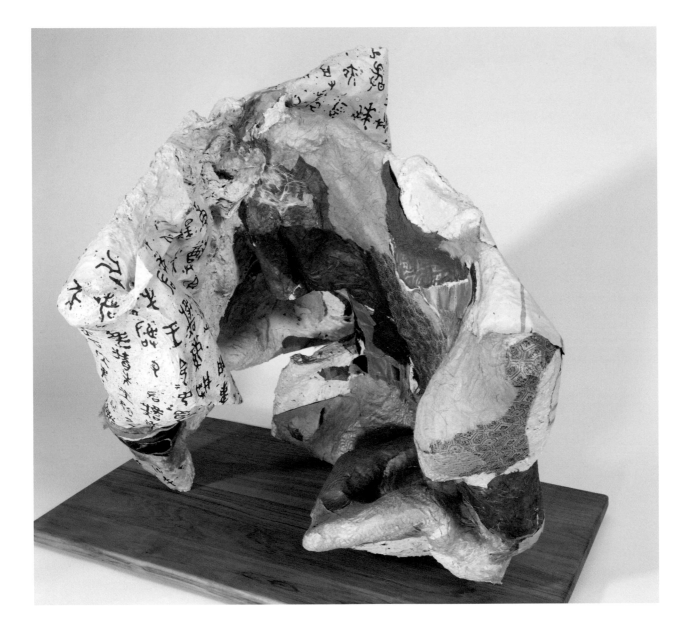

KIMONO DANCE

communicating so that they feel more informed and empowered. Similarly, speaking with your family members and friends can be another instance in which speaking to one of us can be helpful. Many people find it useful to process their feelings with us because they do not feel required to disguise their emotions. We allow patients to become more aware of their true feelings and engage in effective ways of coping. Sometimes talk therapy, role playing or discussing and practicing what will be said to family and friends with an oncology social worker can help alleviate anxiety and provide the clarity needed to determine what information will be disclosed to whom and when. Accepting that this is your journey and that you are in control is sometimes challenging in a new world, where one's control has been suspended for a limited time.

We can assist you at every phase of treatment from initial diagnosis, through active treatment, into the post-treatment survivorship phase. Cancer survivors often experience different sets of questions and concerns. When you are no longer going to your doctor on a scheduled basis and are being seen at a three-month, six-month and yearly interval, it can cause anxiety and some patients feel that their safety net has been removed, leaving them stranded. This is not so. We can provide you with the reassurance you need to reengage in your previous activities, address interpersonal relationships that were placed on hold and, most importantly, help you with your self-esteem and body image issues, if any are present. There are many organizations out there solely dedicated to cancer survivorship that provide a varied scope of services. Transitioning to the role of cancer survivorship is a process. We are here to help.

The financial costs of a cancer diagnosis are significant and continue well into survivorship. According to a Cancer Trends Progress Report, the U.S. estimated national cost for cancer care in 2006 was $104.1 billion. The economic burden that patients face can sometimes affect treatment decisions, or their ability to adhere to their medical regimen. Day-to-day living expenses are often impacted, retirement and pension funds may be drained. Patients are often faced with entering the social service system not really knowing what to ask, where to go or what's available. While there are programs that assist patients with the cost of screening, treatment and medications, the public often is unaware of these resources. Oncology social workers are instrumental in making these linkages.

"I am determined to advocate until African-American women no longer have the highest death and shortest survival rates."

— Dorothy Reed

Resource List

Financial Support

American Cancer Society — 1-800-ACS-2345

CancerCare, Inc. — 1-800-813-4673
www.cancercare.org

Medicare — 1-800-633-4227
www.medicare.gov

Medicaid — 1-800-492-5231 ext. 2
www.cms.gov

Social Security Administration — 1-800-772-1213

Veterans Benefits — 1-800-827-1000

Catholic Charities — 1-703-549-1390

United Way — 1-651-291-0211
www.unitedway.org

National Care Assistance

Cancer Financial Assistance Coalition — 1-800-813-4673
(CFAC)
www.cancerfac.org

National Coalition for — 1-888-650-9127
Cancer Survivorship
www.canceradvocacy.org

American Cancer Society — 1-800-227-2345
www.cancer.org

National Cancer Institute's — 1-800-4-CANCER
Cancer Information Service
www.cancer.gov

Medication Assistance

Needy Meds-Drug — 1-800-503-6897
Assistance Programs
www.needymeds.org

RX Hope — 1-877-267-0517
www.rxhope.com

General/Concrete Needs

American Cancer Society — 1-800-227-2345
www.cancer.org

St. Vincent de Paul — 1-314-576-3993
www.svdpusa.org

Helplines/Support

CancerCare (all types of cancers) — 1-800-813-4673
www.cancercare.org

Susan G. Komen Breast Care Helpline — 1-877-465-6636
ww5.komen.org

Cancer Support Community — 1-888-793-9355
(all types of cancers)
www.cancersupportcommunity.org

Livestrong (all types of cancers) — 1-855-220-7777
www.livestrong.org

Cleaning Assistance

Cleaning for a Reason — 1-877-337-3348
www.cleaningforareason.org

Co-Pay Assistance

CancerCare Co-Pay — 1-866-552-6729
Assistance Foundation
www.cancercarecopay.org

Patient Advocate Foundation — 1-800-532-5274
www.patientadvocate.org

Partnership for Prescription — 1-888-477-2669
Assistance
www.pparx.org

Chronic Disease Fund — 1-877-968-7233
www.gooddaysfromcdf.org

Help with Legal Issues

Cancer Legal Resource Center — 1-866-843-2572
www.disabilityrightslegalcenter.org/
cancer-legal-resource-center

The Importance of a Nurse Navigator

Sherry Melinyshyn, R.N(EC)., B.N.Sc., C.O.N.(C.), P.H.C.N.P.

Facing a cancer diagnosis and navigating the health care system can be an overwhelming and stressful experience for both patients and family members. A professional health care provider, such as a nurse navigator, can assist in this journey and reduce the complexity and anxiety of the process for everyone involved.

A nurse navigator's role is to serve as a patient liaison and help navigate the complexities of a health care system.[1] The concept of a nurse navigator was introduced in the early 1990s to help patients obtain the highest quality of care, through breaking the perceived barrier of medical-specific knowledge.[2] Nurse navigators work as members of multi-disciplinary teams that include, for example, other health care providers such as surgeons, radiologists, oncologists and family physicians. They are required to be experts and leaders in their field, using advanced practice nursing knowledge and evidence-based findings in the delivery of patient care.

The primary focus of the nurse navigator is assessing the patient's needs during a visit to a health care facility. Education is a key element with each visit and it is vital that patients are provided with the information they need to make informed decisions regarding the management of their care. In addition to education, nurse navigators provide supportive care to patients through the use of cancer-specific guides such as the Supportive Care Framework.[3] They offer necessary services that focus on meeting all the needs of patients, from the physical to the spiritual, throughout the entire process of treatment and beyond.[4] Receiving compassion from health professionals and obtaining a diagnosis as quickly as possible are the primary supportive care needs of patients during the time prior to diagnosis.[5]

Assessment of the patient at each visit allows the nurse navigator to evaluate the patient's supportive care network, level of understanding of the diagnosis and need for medical treatment. Clinic appointments are scheduled in order for the patient to have the necessary time to ask questions and review the information received. Having this additional time with a nurse navigator helps to reduce anxieties, as well as provide the patient and family members with the opportunity to review and reflect on the patient care plan.

Nurse navigators collaborate with other members of the health care team for many steps of the cancer journey. For example, nurse navigators help organize radiology investigations, surgical consultations and obtain pathology findings. Timely follow-up to investigations and prompt booking of appropriate appointments provide a seamless navigation for patients.

Nurse navigators understand the importance of providing a careful balance in the amount of information provided to patients. Too much information can be overwhelming, especially when patients are experiencing high levels of anxiety.[6] However, it is still important to discuss the diagnosis and proposed treatments. The nurse navigator helps the patient understand the educational materials provided to them and tailors the information to their individual learning needs. Women diagnosed with breast cancer rank "knowledge of how and where to get information" as their highest informational need.[7] If the supportive care needs of patients remain unmet, they may continue to experience emotional distress, which can escalate and affect compliance with their care plan.[8]

Telephone contact with patients is a significant component in the role of a nurse navigator. Patients should be encouraged to call with any concerns, including pre- or post-operative care questions, review of provided information or to receive reassurance. The benefits of telephone assessment and management include continuity of care and prevention of problems without the limitations inherent in a scheduled visit.[9]

My personal journey as a nurse navigator has been very rewarding. My expertise was founded on my prior clinical position as an oncology nurse in an outpatient cancer center, where my primary focus was breast cancer and pediatric oncology. Every day I learned a new life lesson, and every day I felt grateful for my health and the health of my family. I quickly learned that good health should never be taken for granted. If I was to name heroes, I would name all the patients whom I helped navigate and who faced their cancer diagnoses and treatments each day with optimism and courage.

When I transitioned to the role of nurse navigator, I had the expertise to educate patients about what they could expect regarding the multiplicity of cancer therapies. My knowledge base was enhanced through other health care providers as well, including the radiology team, secretaries and community health care providers. However, it was the patients who taught me how to be the nurse navigator they needed to meet their physical and emotional needs. No two patients had the same experience, and having the understanding, information and compassion to meet the many different needs of patients and their families was the greatest lesson I would learn. The position was truly very fulfilling. Nurse navigators are invaluable members of the health care team. They make a significant contribution by providing supportive care to patients and families navigating our complex health care system.

1. The Ontario Breast Assessment Collaborative Group. (2001). *Multidisciplinary roles and expectations for Breast Assessment in Ontario.* Toronto: Author.
2. Psooy, B.J., Schreuer, D., Borgaonkar, J., & Caines, J.S. (2004). Patient Navigation: Improving timeliness in the diagnosis of breast abnormalities. *Canadian Association of Radiologists,* 55(3), 145–50.
3. Ontario Cancer Treatment and Research Foundation. (1994). *Providing Supportive Care to Individuals Living with Cancer.* Toronto: Author.
4. Ibid.

5. DeGrasse, C.E., Hugo, K., & Plotnikoff, R.C. (1997). Supporting women during breast diagnostics. *Canadian Nurse, 93*(9), 24–30.
6. Denton, S. (1996). *Breast Cancer Nursing.* London: Chapman and Hall.
7. DeGrasse, *loc. cit.*
8. Cancer Quality Council of Ontario. (2003). *The Quality of Cancer Services in Ontario.* Toronto: Author.
9. Cooley, M.E., Muscari Lin, E., & Hunter, S.W. (1994). The Ambulatory Oncology Nurse's Role. *Seminars in Oncology Nursing, 10*(4), 245–53.

The Contributions of a Patient Navigator

Cheryl Kott

When I was diagnosed with breast cancer in May 2007, the American Cancer Society's Patient Navigation program had not yet been introduced in the area where I live, and I was unaware of the many programs and services available to breast cancer patients. My friend Cathy, an eight-year breast cancer survivor, listened, located a wig provider dedicated to cancer patients, listened, brought me eye makeup to replace my disappearing brows and lashes, listened and gave me hope. When I had an opportunity to become a volunteer patient navigator in the newly formed program at the Carol G. Simon Cancer Center at Morristown Medical Center, I knew that this was my chance to be "Cathy" to other women; by helping them go through breast cancer treatment the way my friend helped me—by listening, by identifying resources and by offering hope.

Through my work as a patient navigator…

…I am able to help patients navigate the maze of a breast cancer experience. I can address concerns by telling them about the programs and services at the Cancer Center, from support groups, to mind/body programs, to child life services, to nutritional counseling, to music, art and writing therapy. Each patient is more than just a patient and there is more to her experience than medical treatment.

…I am able to refer patients to Reach to Recovery (American Cancer Society) or the Cancer Hope Network, and they are able to connect with survivors who share similar diagnoses and treatments, giving them information and hope to better empower themselves.

…I am able to tell patients about the American Cancer Society's wig services, so that they are able to select a wig and have it professionally styled, all free of charge. No patient who wants a wig needs to go without because of financial constraints.

"2.5 million survivors of breast cancer in our country need to know there are a number of wonderful national survivorship programs with branches throughout the United States, programs that help women to overcome the challenges of survivorship."

— Angela Lanfranchi, M.D.

…I am able to refer patients to Look Good Feel Better. One patient, who always seemed so sad, broke into a huge smile when she told me about her Look Good Feel Better experience. She told me that after the program had armed her with a complimentary makeup kit, she felt beautiful for the first time since starting treatment and, more importantly, she recognized herself again when she looked in the mirror.

When I was going through breast cancer treatment, I felt so fortunate to be surrounded by family and friends who gave me infinite love and support. Now I have the opportunity to help others become aware of the support and programs available to help during this difficult and stressful time. My goals are twofold: first, to ensure that a woman going through breast cancer treatment does not feel that she is going through it alone, and second, as someone who has been through it, to offer hope.

Look Good—Feel Better

Michele Capossela

Cancer can rob a woman of her energy, appetite and strength, but it doesn't have to take away her self-confidence.

"Emily, is that you?" her husband asked as she emerged with ten other cancer survivors who had attended the Look Good Feel Better session. "I didn't recognize you! After sixty-two years of marriage, I thought they changed my wife in that room behind those doors."

Emily is an eighty-year-old lung cancer patient who felt a strong sense of urgency to look the way she did before her chemotherapy treatments. Her oncologist advised her that she would lose her hair and incur some skin changes as she began her six-month regimen of chemotherapy. "Having heard that my appearance would change so quickly, I knew I had to do something to be sure I didn't look old and like cancer has gotten me."

Thankfully, her medical team realized just how important her self-confidence was to her recovery. They shared their stories of others who had been through treatments and how much they appreciated the free two-hour makeover session that truly saved their lives! Emily heard about the survivors before her who were helped to manage the temporary appearance-related side effects of cancer treatment: how to put on eyebrows, how to moisturize dry, patchy skin, how to know the difference between a human hair and a synthetic wig and how to wrap a turban out of a T-shirt when you just don't feel like wearing a wig. All of those examples motivated Emily to call the American Cancer Society (800-ACS-2345) and register for the upcoming free session.

"I bought a wig that perfectly matched my hairstyle, and later bought a second, cheaper wig just to wear to the gym. I learned makeup techniques to mask my missing eyebrows and lashes, and continued in my job."

— Kathi Edelson Wolder

Walking into the room, she was surprised to see smiling faces, welcoming volunteers, beautiful makeup, mirrors, hats and turbans. All she needed to do was sit and enjoy the time and learn the techniques that would allow her to feel herself once again. The two hours flew by; there was laughter and emotion; there were smiles and tears; but most of all, there was hope.

As Emily left the room, with several phone numbers of newly formed friends who were now joining in her battle, she emerged from the room, smiling, and with a skip in her step. A volunteer in the session said to her as she exited the room, "Oh Emily, you may want to take your name tag off now," to which Emily replied, "If I take it off, how will the nurses know it's me, I look so beautiful!"

Look Good Feel Better is a non-medical, brand-neutral public service program that teaches beauty techniques to cancer patients to help them manage the appearance-related side effects of cancer treatment.

Look Good Feel Better group programs are open to all women with cancer who are undergoing chemotherapy, radiation or other forms of treatment. In the U.S. alone, more than 700,000 women have participated in the program, which now offers 14,500 group workshops nationwide, in more than 3,000 locations.

Thousands of volunteer beauty professionals support Look Good Feel Better. All are trained and certified by the Personal Care Products Council Foundation, the American Cancer Society and the Professional Beauty Association/National Cosmetology Association at local, statewide and national workshops. Other volunteer health care professionals and individuals also give their time to the program.

Nutrition and Cancer
Karen Connelly, R.D., C.S.O.

Everyone eats. This is a fundamental truth that runs through every culture, religion and race. Exactly how we view the food we eat and how we interpret the impact of the nourishment our bodies receive differs from person to person. The origin of the importance of food in one's life most likely was established in infancy. The importance of food and nutrition in one's cancer journey draws its strength from this core foundation. After a breast cancer diagnosis, women are often told by their medical team which treatment modalities are best suited for their type and stage of cancer. At the conclusion of these treatments, women are placed in yet another new position at a new frontier called survivorship. This segment in the cancer journey can be frightening as well as empowering. It is here that women can make critical lifestyle changes that can enhance the outcomes of their conventional treatments and provide a safeguard against future recurrence.

Breast cancer treatment can include surgery, radiation and chemotherapy, or some combination of these three modalities. Nutritional status before, during

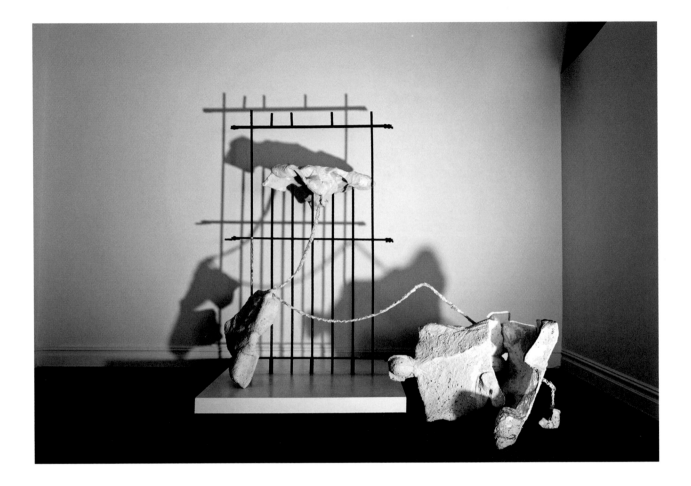

OVER THE BARRIER

and after treatment is one factor that impacts all aspects of treatment tolerance and recovery. Surgery is demanding on the body and adequate nutritional status can help expedite recovery. Chemotherapy is a systemic treatment and therefore affects every part of the body, in addition to the breast. Taste changes, nausea, vomiting, diarrhea, constipation, fatigue and cytopenias can come together in a perfect storm of side effects to create a lack of appetite and compromised nutritional status. During this time the most important piece of advice is: eat! The foods chosen at this time might not be ideal food choices; however, the goal now is to nourish your body with an adequate amount of calories and protein.

All preconceived notions you have about the foods you love or the foods you think may be helpful to your cancer diagnosis are null and void. The word normal no longer exists and should not exist as its disappearance from your vocabulary removes the potential bias that otherwise might prevent your embrace of new foods and dietary habits that will help keep you nourished through your treatment. For example, taste changes are a common side effect. In order to manage them you may need to look to foods that you would not or did not eat, but may now find tolerable and possibly enjoyable. This newfound favorite food may change to the most disliked, unappealing food overnight. Be ready to accept these constant changes as part of your evolving dietary plan.

Nausea, vomiting, diarrhea and constipation are the most common forms of gastrointestinal distress during chemotherapy. Adjustments to the fiber content of the diet can help alleviate diarrhea and constipation. Nausea is best managed by avoiding foods with strong aromas and those that are spicy, fried or overly sweet. If your appetite is very poor, try to put yourself on a schedule to eat or drink every hour. This helps to keep the habit of eating a regular part of your day and not something you allow yourself to skip. Most importantly, do not underestimate the need for hydration. If you are unable to maintain sufficient fluid intake due to the side effects of treatment, talk to your oncologist, as you can be put on a schedule to receive intravenous hydration supplementation during this difficult time.

Dehydration can cause a host of problems such as electrolyte abnormalities, fatigue, alterations in blood pressure and heart rate, dry mouth and decreased urine output. Arranging set times to receive intravenous hydration takes the pressure off you to consume the increased amount of fluid needed to counter vomiting and diarrhea, or just the lack of desire to eat or drink that results in dehydration. For many women, radiation treatment is a common part of the breast cancer treatment plan. Radiation treatment does not produce the same level or variety of side effects as chemotherapy since radiation is targeted therapy. Only the treatment area is affected by radiation, therefore side effects are localized to that area. The other major complaint from radiation treatment is fatigue. Maintaining a healthy diet at this time can be helpful in combating the fatigue and helping the body stay strong.

Once all treatment is completed, women may ask, "What's next?" Survivorship is a new chapter in their cancer journey. One in which they now govern. If a

"Only once did I make the mistake of eating fish at home. 'B' hates the smell of fish, and the chemo chemicals had enhanced her fine sense of smell."

— Tobias D. Robison

woman has not already been in touch with a registered dietitian during active treatment, it is imperative that she seek their guidance in survivorship. A registered dietitian, with the certified specialist in oncology nutrition credential, is the optimal professional to provide women with breast cancer the most reliable and most recent recommendations on nutrition and cancer. The goals of dietary intervention by the dietitian include: assisting women in identifying the foods/food groups that are abundant in cancer-fighting compounds, interpreting the latest research and extrapolating the relevant information on the relationship between nutrition and cancer and formulating a plan based on these findings for each individual person.

For example, dietitians can help women understand the ongoing controversy between soy and breast cancer or explain the effect of cruciferous vegetables on estrogen regulation. If you have been recently diagnosed or are currently under treatment, ask your cancer center or medical oncologist if they have a registered dietitian on staff. Every cancer center is different, some have dedicated oncology dietitians on staff and some may refer you to a dietitian located in the community or at your local hospital or clinic. Coverage for services provided by a dietitian varies among insurance companies. Call your provider to determine how much is covered and how many visits you are entitled to. Some cancer centers that have a dietitian on staff charge for their services and some do not; the only way to find out is to call. The Oncology Nutrition Practice Group, a sub-unit of the Academy of Nutrition and Dietetics, has a website (www.oncologynutrition.org) that includes a search engine to find a registered dietitian who is a certified specialist in oncology nutrition in your area. If financial constraints prevent a woman from obtaining the assistance of a registered dietitian, there are other resources to explore. The Cancer Support Community is an international non-profit organization dedicated to providing support, education and hope to people affected by cancer. This organization provides support groups, counseling, education and healthy lifestyle programs. The programs offered at the Cancer Support Community are an invaluable resource for women at every stage of their cancer journey, and all of their services and programs are free of charge. Each state is listed individually on their website for easy identification of a local chapter in your area. The American Cancer Society, CancerCare and the National Cancer Institute are also great resources that can connect women with reliable nutrition information.

Q — Are there special foods one should eat while getting chemotherapy?

The current recommendation by the American Cancer Society is that it is safe for women with a history of breast cancer to consume up to three servings of whole soy foods per day. Fat and alcohol have also been studied at great length. Recommendations vary depending on the type of breast cancer. Research changes but public opinion and outdated advice is slow to change, which is why guidance from a nutrition professional is essential. The ideal diet for cancer survivors is the same as for cancer prevention. The diet should be based on whole foods, including at least nine servings of fruits and vegetables a day, with a focus on cruciferous vegetables (broccoli, cauliflower, cabbage and dark leafy greens), high in fiber and whole grains, legumes, teas, lean protein and low-fat dairy products. Vitamin D and calcium supplements are also a necessary part of this diet. Exercise is the other vital component in a breast cancer survivorship plan. Research has shown that regular exercise can help reduce the risk of recurrence. Women need not get discouraged if they are exercising and not losing weight as current research suggests there are protective benefits to exercise regardless of initial weight status or evidence of weight loss.

It is important to seek a nutrition professional who will meet each woman mentally, physically and spiritually, wherever she may be on her journey. This is a fundamental characteristic to find in health care practitioners because they are the ones who can identify the prominent place nutrition holds and use that information to strengthen the importance of making necessary dietary and lifestyle changes that safeguard against a future recurrence. Women are survivors from the day of diagnosis, and power over their future health status may be just a spoonful away.

Understanding Cancer-Related Fatigue
Meryl Marger Picard, Ph.D., M.S.W., O.T.R.

If you feel exhausted as you traverse this cancer journey, you are not alone! The majority of people diagnosed with cancer experience a specific form of fatigue during their cancer experience called Cancer-Related Fatigue (CRF). Fatigue is the great disrupter of life roles, habits and routines. It is debilitating and is often the most stressful symptom cancer patients identify. Many women are unaware that addressing any of the medical causes of CRF, along with simple lifestyle changes, can increase their overall energy.

What is Cancer-Related Fatigue?
Cancer-related fatigue is different from feeling tired because you worked too many hours, painted the kitchen or did not have a good night's sleep. The National Comprehensive Cancer Network (NCCN) defines CRF as a "distressing, persistent, subjective sense of tiredness or exhaustion related to cancer or cancer treatment that is not proportional to recent activity and interferes with usual functioning."[1]

Addressing CRF by resting or decreasing your daily activities may not leave you feeling any more refreshed. The most typical experience of CRF is feeling as though you are about to come down with the flu or, as one friend described it, falling off a cliff in the middle of the day. Typically, CRF will not impact your ability to care for yourself, but you may see changes, due to fatigue, in your ability to work, manage the household, socialize with friends, or take part in leisure activities. CRF is differentiated as a clinical diagnosis from Chronic Fatigue Syndrome, which cannot be related to a cancer diagnosis or treatment, although they both share the symptom of significant feelings of fatigue.

Causes

CRF is complex and occurs for a multitude of reasons; therefore it is critical to inform your oncology team about changes in your usual energy level. Your oncologist will review your lab tests to ensure that you are not suffering from treatable medical conditions that result in fatigue. There are specific medications that address anemia secondary to cancer or cancer treatment. Chemotherapy may leave you feeling more tired within the first few days after infusion, but you will probably note improvement in your energy toward the end of each week as your next treatment session approaches. Fatigue from radiation therapy tends to build slowly over time and you may not notice any effects until several weeks into treatment.

For the majority of women, CRF resolves within the first year after completing treatment and you will find that you are able to resume your prior activities. There is a smaller group of women, approximately one-quarter to one-third, who continue experiencing mild to significant fatigue after treatment concludes. This prolonged fatigue can impact the quality of your life and future plans. It does not matter if you are five weeks into treatment or five years after treatment concludes. It is important to verbalize what you are feeling and to understand your management options.

If you undergo surgery, expect to have fatigue following the surgery and while you are recovering. There is also a strong connection between having pain and feeling fatigued. Tell your team if pain at your surgical site or in your arm is interfering with daily activities or sleep, since there are medications and rehabilitation treatments that can reduce these symptoms. Rapid onset of menopause, accelerated by some chemotherapy drugs, can reduce your quality of sleep, resulting in daytime fatigue, as can an undiagnosed sleep disorder. Feelings of sadness, depression and anxiety are common reactions during diagnosis and treatment. Depression can make you feel exhausted, making it difficult to engage in activities you want or need to do. There are support groups available in most cancer centers, through private organizations and online communities. Your cancer center may also provide access to a social worker to discuss problems you are having adjusting to the cancer diagnosis and treatment.

Managing Fatigue

Slowing down during the roller coaster of diagnosis, surgery or treatment may be a matter of necessity or choice. Recognize that CRF is a variable, not static, state. Become attuned to subtle or overt shifts in your energy level during any given day or week. Be proactive! Managing fatigue after you are depleted will not balance your reserves.

"I did four rounds of chemotherapy. The first two days weren't bad. The third day felt like I had hit a wall. The exhaustion was like nothing I had ever experienced."

— Rich Loreti

How you typically spend your day changes from the point of diagnosis and is initially dominated by physician visits, tests and treatment appointments. Aside from managing these scheduled events, create a working calendar of the tasks that you want to do, have to do (absolutely no one else can complete them) and need to do each week. Friends and family are probably asking how they can help. Accept their assistance with gratitude and become the team manager, rather than requiring yourself to be the worker responsible for every task. Or better yet, assign someone close to you to manage the team.

Keep track of a simple daily one-to-ten fatigue scale with a score of one as the equivalent of having your usual level of energy prior to your cancer, versus a ten, defined as the worst, most debilitating fatigue you have ever had. Note the scores in a datebook or electronically and share this information with your providers. Fatigue is gauged by your perceptions. If you are tired, no matter what the score, reprioritize your activities.

Conserving Energy

Energy conservation is about learning to thoughtfully use available energy and balancing periods of less demanding tasks with more physically demanding activities. Visualize your energy level as a pot of gold. You can quickly deplete the entire pot in a few hours or pace removing the coins throughout the day. Some days, such as the day after chemotherapy, there are few coins in the pot, while other days will yield more. For women adept at handling challenges at home and work, this deliberate decision-making process about how you use your energy, instead of doing it all, is initially unsettling. Give yourself permission to decide how you spend your time. If attending a friend's birthday dinner or watching your child's softball game is more important than doing the laundry, then adjust your task expectations accordingly.

Pace yourself. You may not be able to do it all. If you want to or can continue to work through treatment, you may need to adjust your household chores. Do not start a heavy physical task that you cannot easily end. It is possible to vacuum one room, but not the entire house. Dishes dry themselves. Frozen vegetables come pre-chopped. Crock pots can cook dinner, as can friends and family. The bed police do not knock at your door if you do not make the bed. Groceries can be delivered, along with prescribed medications. There are volunteer agencies throughout the country that provide free house cleaning while you are in treatment. Type "free house cleaning for cancer patients," along with your home state, into a web browser or ask your oncology social worker for information. Instead of updating everyone each day, start a personal web page or send group e-mails or texts.

Exercise and Stress Management

Research supports the use of exercise to help lower levels of CRF and stress. The key is finding a form of exercise you enjoy. If you exercised regularly prior to diagnosis, there is a high likelihood that you can continue, although initially

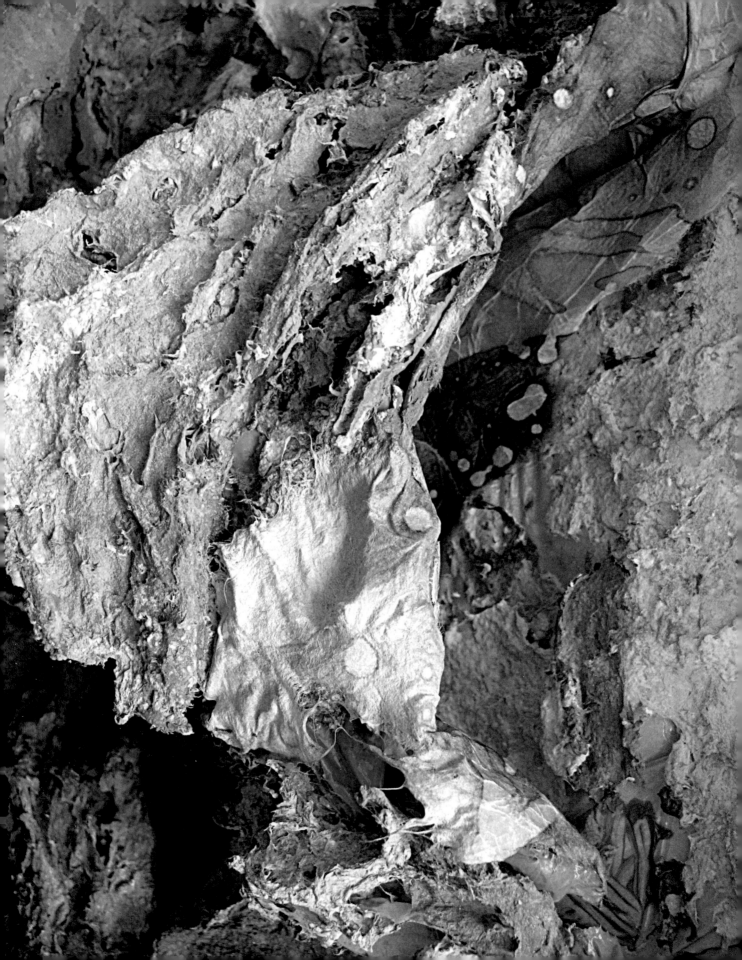

at a less intense level. If you exercise infrequently but feel well enough to do so, consider walking, Tai Chi or yoga. It is critical that you speak with your physician, occupational or physical therapist before starting a new exercise regimen. It can feel counterintuitive to exercise when you are fatigued, but the evidence points to better CRF management with an appropriate level of activity. If you are very active, you may wish to wear a compression sleeve on your arm to help prevent lymphedema. If your CRF increases for more than one to two hours following exercise, decrease the amount or intensity. Many cancer centers offer mind/body therapies that address both gentle exercise and stress management. Consider other forms of stress management including meditation, support groups, patient education groups, art therapy or journaling.

You Are in Charge!
Empower yourself by creating a written plan for how to address your CRF symptoms that incorporates your support system. Review any fatigue symptoms as part of every clinical conversation. The increased focus on survivorship research, including long-term quality of life, means that oncology teams are more attentive than ever to helping you address your ongoing fatigue needs. Finally, treat yourself gently and compassionately and use your energy for the life tasks and events you truly want to enjoy!

1. www.jnccn.org/content/8/8.toc and www.jnccn.org.content/8/12.toc

VII

The Whole Person—
Addressing the mind, body and spirit

Breast Cancer and Spiritual Care
Nomi Roth Elbert, M.Ed., Spiritual Care Provider

What is spiritual care, and how can one weave it into his or her work with women who have been diagnosed with breast cancer? Spiritual/pastoral care is providing spiritual support to the individual (and/or family members) in need. It is important to listen effectively while providing a care plan that can utilize religious and spiritual resources while considering cultural and socioeconomic factors. It is my intention to try to create a "holy space" between the pastoral care provider and the individual in need. Using the individual as a "human text," I attempt to establish a spiritual/holy interaction using my toolbox of religious and spiritual resources such as text, song, prayer and storytelling, thus creating a bond that will assist those in need. I ask the women how they are, "Where are you at this moment?" I allow them to be with whatever feelings they are having at the time, be it anger, fear, denial, hope.

Working with women who have been diagnosed with breast cancer requires specific and special understanding. The breast is what nurtures the child. The breast is nurturing physically, emotionally and spiritually. For women, the breast is a part of their body that often identifies them as women in relationship to their sexuality and as mothers. The breast is often associated with the ability to offer safety, nurturing and fulfillment. The breast is associated with a woman feeling attractive, wanted and needed. It can be traumatic for a woman to be told she needs to have surgery, treatment and possibly removal of her breast, threatening the essence of her being, traumatizing her world of feeling safe and loved.

As girls we realized we were different from boys, and one of those differences is that we have breasts. From our breasts comes the milk we can feed our newborns, from our breasts women define their attractiveness and femininity. From our breasts comes partial definition and spiritual connection to our womanhood.

Our society, our world, makes us fear cancer. We are afraid of illness, dependency, change and perhaps even death. Breast cancer for a woman (and we acknowledge that men can also have breast cancer) compounds these fears and changes. Any time a woman goes for a mammogram, there is this fear, and one out of eight women may be diagnosed with breast cancer. At the moment she is told that she has cancer the fear becomes even stronger. With that fear, her spirit and soul is touched at a different level. It is that depth, that level, I wish to share with you, the reader.

When providing spiritual care and/or counseling with a woman who has been diagnosed with breast cancer, I have found that using guided imagery has a profound effect. Movement, art, the study of Jewish, Christian and Muslim texts and poetry have all provided tools to connect the individual woman with what she is experiencing spiritually, during the time we are working together.

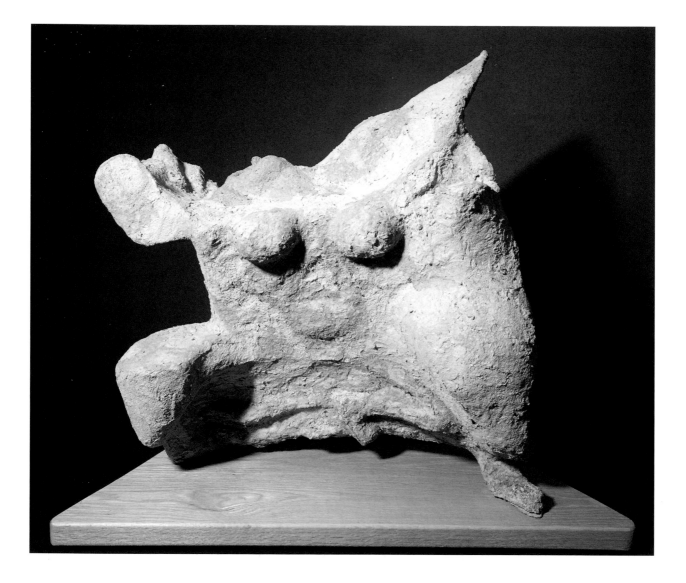

PRAYING

Often women blame themselves for having breast cancer. One woman, "M," felt that she was being punished after the death of her son. For her, the ocean and water were sources of healing. We used guided imagery to help cleanse and heal her and her spirit, and to allow her to accept the treatments she was receiving and acknowledge that they may indeed help her.

"J" was able to alter her self-image and sense of herself. She was able to accept the changes that had occurred and see greater beauty and strength inside of her and towards the world at large.

"A," upon early detection, decided to have a total mastectomy before beginning any form of treatment. She had experienced other acute trauma and death in her family and wanted to attempt whatever was possible to save herself. For her, prayer, reading Jewish texts and song gave her strength, hope and the ability to cope through these times.

Once diagnosed, the fear of the cancer returning often sits at the back of the mind. I found that by providing the opportunity to work with breathing exercises, before and immediately after a return examination, the patient was able to relax and eliminate some of the mounting anxiety.

The combination of acceptance, strength of hope and fighting the cancer; the acceptance of assistance from family, community and, if available, a spiritual support system, offers enormous help during the time of treatment and afterwards.

What does it mean to have spiritual support? It means to *be* with the person, not to advise, judge or counsel. Whatever their belief system is, my attempt is to open up a window to their heart and spirit, to allow them to listen and be with what it is they are experiencing and to know that I am there with them during this part of their journey.

The lesson of courage, fear, strength and celebration of life that occurs with women and their families over the course of diagnosis, treatment, remission, reoccurrence and death is part of life's journey. How one travels this journey, the team support from the medical, family and spiritual members involved, contribute to the purpose and meaning of one's life on deeper and new levels, which can contribute greater awareness and appreciation of one's existence, even during difficult times. There is no greater gift than having the opportunity to work with, and touch, the human spirit of another.

"The love and support of my family, friends and church got me through this emotional roller coaster."

— Peggy S.

The Role of the Oncology Social Worker
Elisabeth (Elsje) Reiss, M.S.W., L.C.S.W.

I was born and raised in Amsterdam, in the Netherlands, where I was trained as a midwife. In 1978 at the age of twenty-eight, I developed cancer and needed chemotherapy. It was scary and made me feel very much alone and different from my peer group, many of whom were having babies at the time. There were no support groups or organizations to help me get through this difficult period. I promised myself that, if ever there came a time when it was not possible to practice midwifery, I would devote myself to working with cancer patients. When I came to the U.S. in 1982, my midwifery degree was not accepted. I then decided to go to graduate school to obtain an M.S.W. (Master in Social Work) to specifically work with cancer patients. I chose to specialize in oncology social work and spent several years working in the cancer unit of the Yale-New Haven Hospital as a member of the oncology team.

My role on the oncology unit was to listen to each cancer patient, and to understand them and their concerns. These included fears and uncertainties regarding pain, how long they would live with the disease, what treatments would still help them, how they would die and how family members would cope, to name a few. In addition, these patients were confronted directly with their own mortality as well as with existential issues. They would ask themselves, "Who am I? Why am I here? What has been the purpose of my life? How can I create more purpose in the time left?" Helping patients process these issues was one of my tasks. For one patient, the greatest concern was that he wouldn't continue to be in the life of his seven-year-old grandson. We talked about the fact that his grandson wouldn't know him well. The patient then started a journal for his grandson. This provided a great sense of relief for him.

After working in hospitals, I am now in private practice and counsel adult patients. We discuss every phase of their experience with cancer. I see patients who have just been diagnosed, those in the middle of treatment, and those who are in the terminal stages of their disease. Sometimes, patients come to me after completing treatment to process unresolved feelings and issues. My sessions sometimes include spouses and adult family members and even sometimes children. I advise parents on what to tell their children about their cancer and give them suggestions on how to have these conversations. For example, it is important not to avoid the word cancer and to explain what it is. Children overhear the use of the word, and what they imagine is often far worse than the reality. It is also important to provide opportunities for the children to ask any questions they might have. Parents must be honest with their kids and use language that is age appropriate. Honesty fosters trust between parents and children for the rest of their cancer journey together. It is also helpful for parents to inform their children's teachers and guidance counselor.

A good deal of my work consists of educating patients and their families in the process of the disease and medical decision-making. I am able to do this because of my strong medical background. Very often, newly diagnosed cancer patients are overwhelmed and fear that a cancer diagnosis equals death. In reality, many patients who are diagnosed with cancer do not die of the disease. I am often able to clarify what the physicians have told them and help them decide what treatment to choose.

After the initial shock of the diagnosis, it is my hope that my patients can learn to focus on living with the disease instead of dying from the disease. Since grieving is a natural response to loss, patients need the time to mourn their losses. This can be loss of health, loss of energy or loss of a job, to name a few. Family members go through their own stages of grieving and sometimes have different time frames than the patient. This needs to be acknowledged and respected.

People who are ill with cancer often feel very much out of control. The social worker can help the person regain as much control as possible, which is very important. Well-meaning family members sometimes take away the little control the patient still has. This can include, for example, what and how much to eat, continuing treatment or not, who to visit and how to spend one's time. A good example of a patient taking control is that of a dying woman who wrote her own obituary and, as a gourmet cook, supervised the making of appetizers for her memorial service. This meant a great deal to her. Patients who are close to death are usually aware of the fact that they are going to die. Very few are in denial. Although some patients may not want to talk about dying, most feel a need to do so. The social worker's role is to give patients the opportunity and respect they need to process what is happening to them in their own time and way.

I might ask patients, "Are there things you need to finish, things not said to people?" If they say they are afraid, the next question might be, "What are you afraid of?" They can be afraid of many different things—of being in the ground, of experiencing pain, of not seeing family members any more. Sometimes it is sufficient to just sit and hold their hands. It all depends on what the person's needs are.

The issue of hospice care comes up with terminal patients. A lot of people go into hospice care far too late. Physicians tend to push for treatment. The social worker can intervene and let the physician know if the patient doesn't want treatment any more. In the hospital setting, social workers can play a valuable role as a member of the treatment team—physicians talk to patients; social workers let patients talk. In some instances, team members asked me to talk to a patient if the patient wasn't able to deal with the situation. In others, the patient had decided he or she wanted to go into hospice and I spoke to the physician who would then agree with this decision.

In most cases the patient should make decisions about hospice based on what the physician says. Patients have a number of choices on how to use hospice services. Besides free-standing in-patient hospices, some hospitals have dedicated hospice in-patient units or hospice beds and some nursing homes offer in-patient hospice services. Alternatively, the patient and their family may opt to have the patient at home with home hospice services.

There are rules governing hospice and it is important to become familiar with them. For admission to hospice, Medicare requires a prognosis that the patient has six months or less to live. A patient can go to an in-patient hospice unit or facility if his or her prognosis is two weeks or less. The overall goal of hospice is to increase the quality of life and not do anything that would hurt

Q — Is having a sense of control important to a cancer patient?

HOSPICE CARE

Hospice care is end-of-life care provided by health professionals and volunteers. They give medical, psychological and spiritual support.

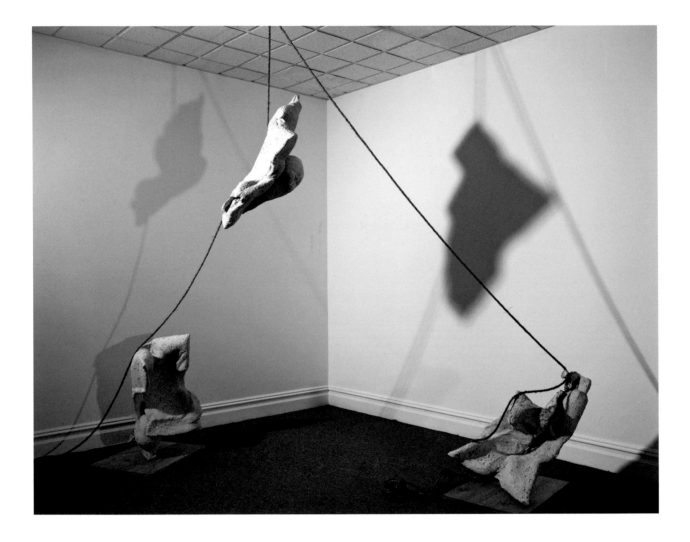

MUTUAL SUPPORT

the patient. That means no monitoring of vital signs and no drawing of blood for lab work. There are no food restrictions. The care is palliative, not curative. The only medications given are meant to alleviate suffering and to make the patient comfortable. Most insurance plans cover hospice. Again, it is important to find out exactly what one's insurance covers.

Home hospice requires dedicated caretakers, either by family members or caretakers hired by the family, because home hospice services provide only limited hours for nursing aides per day, leaving many hours of care to be given by others. Depending on the patient's needs, a hospice nurse will visit as needed to evaluate the patient, to answer questions and to give advice. Hospice provides a care kit of medications and a nurse will instruct the family on how to use these medications properly.

Oncology social workers are often part of a palliative care team or oncology team in hospitals. The best way to find an oncology social worker is through the American Cancer Society (www.cancer.org) or through CancerCare (www.cancercare.org), two national organizations that provide services for cancer patients in all fifty states. Many of their services are free of charge.

Complementary Medicine
Richard Dickens, M.S., L.C.S.W.-R.

Complementary Medicine is one of three commonly used terms to describe non-traditional practices during and following cancer treatment.

What Are Complementary, Alternative and Integrative Medicines?
Complementary Medicine is used to enhance traditional Western medicine, which is called standard of care because it has gone through rigorous clinical trials to prove its efficacy. Complementary Medicine complements standard of care by addressing quality of life issues including: reducing symptoms, managing pain and helping patients feel better and more in balance during and after treatment.

Alternative therapy implies using unproven therapies instead of the standard of care. As use of non-traditional therapies increased among cancer patients, these terms were combined and referred to as complementary and alternative medicine or CAM. In 1998 Congress established the National Center for Complementary and Alternative Medicine (NCCAM).

Today the term Integrative Medicine has become more commonly used to include CAM. Integrative Medicine takes into account the whole person, mind, body and spirit. It is often referred to as holistic treatment. Integrative Medicine, in emphasizing whole-person care, includes lifestyle, beliefs and cultural and traditional needs of patients by integrating all appropriate therapies—alternative and complementary. Most of these therapies come from centuries-old practices in Asia, as well as from indigenous peoples throughout the world.

Where Are these Practices Used?
Today most major cancer centers have Integrative Medicine or CAM departments that research these practices. Most U.S. medical schools include CAM classes in their curricula. Common CAM therapies include acupuncture, homeopathy and herbal remedies, as well as vitamin and mineral supplements. Common mind–body techniques are: meditation, guided imagery, Tai Chi, yoga and Reiki.

A Personal Experience with Integrative and Complementary-Alternative Medicine
I grew up in in the 1950s and '60s in a Christian family at a time when one was defined by his denomination, not faith. As such, faith segregated many families in worship and rituals. While I was raised Lutheran, my cousins who lived next door were Catholic. On the other side of our house were my Catholic grandmother and Masonic grandfather. In those days, spirituality was thought to be synonymous with religion. In the ensuing decades the increase in multiculturalism brought recognition that while spirituality is central to all religions, religion is not inherent in spirituality. Spirituality speaks of the life force of all matter and energy, making it a unifying reality; religion speaks of the practice and rituals individuals follow to ground themselves in the spirit.

U.S. perceptions of spirituality began to change in the 1960s when the Beatles brought the founder of Transcendental Meditation (TM), Maharishi Mahesh Yogi, to the U.S., at a time when many cultural perceptions were being challenged. During college in the 1970s, I decided to train in TM to address the stressors of college and young adulthood. This new practice, in turn, increased my awareness of other emerging mind–body–spirit practices, including ancient holistic practices of Native Americans. Little did I know that these practices would become a cornerstone of my own healing when I was diagnosed with an incurable form of non-Hodgkin lymphoma in 1991. In my twenties and thirties I had been an avid runner and nutritionally conscious, so learning that I had cancer at thirty-seven took me by surprise. My practices offered me a roadmap to tolerate the toxic treatment and to hope that my holistic care might possibly help me be cured.

While I was treated at a world-renowned cancer center, there was no CAM or Integrative Medicine Department in the early 1990s. When I told my oncologist I was running, albeit at a snail's pace due to treatment, he strongly suggested otherwise. As for my ongoing meditation practice, prayer and juicing, he implied it was a benign folly. So like many patients, I didn't stop taking some control in my treatment, I just stopped telling my doctor.

During my first recurrence in 1993, I opted for an allogeneic bone marrow transplant (BMT), thanks to having a sister who was a perfect match. A donor transplant at that time carried a lot of risk, including death or, what for me would be worse, a lifetime of chronic and possibly life-altering side effects.

It also carried the potential for a cure. I was forty years old. I didn't want to die but I also didn't want to live a debilitating life. Again, I used meditation, visualization and vibration therapy techniques during and after treatment. I never thought of them as curative, but I knew they were central to my mind–body–spirit well-being. While I was in the hospital, on her daily rounds my BMT doctor didn't know what to make of the rattles and drums beside me and often moved them to the side of the room. Through forty days in isolation and due to painful mouth sores, there were some days that these tools were the only way I could express myself and calm my mind.

My doctors weren't bad. They wanted the best outcome for me. But because the empirical science affirming the efficacy of these techniques had not yet been found, they were skeptical. Today we know that exercise is very important during and after treatment. And today, almost all, if not all, major cancer centers have CAM or Integrative Medicine departments. The 2007 National Health Interview Survey (NHIS), which included a comprehensive survey of CAM use by Americans, showed that approximately 38% of adults used CAM in the last twelve months; 83 million adults spent $33.9 million on CAM uses; and CAM costs are 11.2% of total out-of-pocket expenditures on health care. To read more, see the NCCAM website: www.nccam.nih.gov/news/camstats/costs/costdatafs.htm.

Explanations of Some Integrative Medicine Practices
Meditation was one of the earliest mind–body–spirit practices brought to Western countries, preceding CAM and Integrative Medicine. Very simply, meditation is a technique to focus the mind and bring the mind–body to a state of peace or balance. There are many types of meditation practice. The most common are: one-pointed and two-pointed meditation.

Transcendental Meditation is a type of one-pointed meditation. Like many meditation practices, it uses a mantra—a word or sound—as the point of focus to quiet the mind from its tendency to wander. This is done twice a day for twenty minutes while sitting comfortably in a quiet place. The goal in Transcendental Meditation is to transcend to the beginning of thought that is no thought. During training in Transcendental Meditation you are given a Sanskrit word. One does not need formal training to meditate. Without formal training one can use affirming words such as peace, love, hope or joy as a mantra to quiet the mind. A mantra can also be a phrase. In this way repetitive prayer can be considered a type of meditation.

A more common meditation practice is Mindfulness, sometimes referred to as two-pointed meditation. In this practice you use your breath as the point of focus. As the mind wanders and the body feels, you look at these thoughts and sensations non-judgmentally, then guide your focus back to the breath. In the West, Mindfulness has evolved into a sitting and walking meditation. The best-known teacher of Mindfulness is Jon Kabat-Zinn. He is a founding director of the Stress Reduction Clinic at the University of Massachusetts Medical School.

"Much research has been done in the area of the mind–body connection. Some studies show that what happens to the mind affects the body and vice versa. For example, if I relax my mind, my body relaxes and if I relax my body, my mind relaxes."

— Kerry Kay

There have now been twenty-five years of research in the beneficial effects of Mindfulness practice on the mind–body.

Yoga is an ancient Hindu and Buddhist practice. Like meditation, it is centered on breath, while also including a series of postures. Very simply, yoga works around seven chakras or vital energy centers of the body that are connected to major organs. Through the practice, one opens the channels so that energy can flow more naturally. There are many different types of yoga and many different schools of yoga, but no official nationwide certification guidelines for yoga instructors. However, the non-profit group Yoga Alliance specifies minimum educational standards for yoga teacher certification, which are nationally recognized and required to teach yoga in certain states. Per Yoga Alliance standards, a registered yoga teacher must have a minimum two hundred hours of formal training. To read more, see: www.livestrong.com/article/397089-what-certification-do-i-need-to-teach-yoga/#ixzz23Ss6UuAE.

Yoga continues to grow in popularity in the U.S. and might be the most common mind–body practice done in a group setting. Many gyms and community centers in the U.S. provide yoga classes by certified teachers. Because some forms of yoga can be quite strenuous, it is recommended that patients practicing yoga work with a teacher who understands the limitations of their disease and its treatment.

Tai Chi and Qigong are Chinese practices developed thousands of years ago. Tai Chi was originally a martial art practice, which evolved into a slow, meditative series of exercises to reduce stress and alleviate side effects of physical ailments by improving circulation. Qigong has roots in Chinese medicine, martial arts and philosophy. Both practices use movements to facilitate the flow of Chi (life force, also spelled Qi). The exercises involve mental concentration, visualization and graceful movements, many of which mimic animals. The goal of these practices is to cultivate balance, and encourage life force or energy flow through the body to create serenity and peace.

Training centers for Tai Chi and Qigong are usually part of a larger association such as the American Tai Chi and Qigong Association or the Institute of Integral Qigong and Tai Chi. You can also rent or purchase instructional videos. Some gyms, seniors centers and community centers provide Tai Chi and Qigong classes. There has been a lot of research, especially in Asia, on the efficacy of these practices to reduce stress, improve concentration and promote longevity.

Guided Imagery is sometimes called creative visualization or shamanic journeying. These techniques use visualizing, similar to guided daydreams, to produce a desired outcome. In creative visualization you sit quietly before an event and see it transpiring in the most positive and fruitful way. Creative visualization has a history in sports psychology, medicine and corporate environments, often done before a stressful event or meeting. Guided imagery can be literal or can include abstract images such as the four elements of life: water, air, earth and fire. These elements often represent larger ideas: water = purification; air = life force; earth = mother or womb; and fire = light or spirit.

"I determined to live a well-balanced lifestyle that included: Good nutrition and exercise, balance of rest and activity, transcendental meditation and Tai Chi."

— Sushma Prasada

You can do a guided imagery connecting to or immersing yourself in one of these elements as a healing balm to cleanse your body of illness or disease. Shamanic journeying incorporates spirit, often appearing as animal guides or plants and trees, as companions on a path to healing. Shamanic journeying can be used to cleanse yourself of negative energy (unresolved hurts) or to envision a healthy future. Many mental health practitioners as well as life coaches use guided imagery.

Acupuncture has an ancient history in Chinese medicine. Chinese medicine is based on a detailed chart of meridians, which are channels of energy throughout the body. When these channels become blocked, unease and discomfort occur. An acupuncturist inserts very fine needles into different meridians of the body to address the presenting issue and open up channels of energy to nourish the tissue. These needles are left in place for a period of time. For most people the needles elicit little or no discomfort.

Acupuncture has a 2,000-year history in China and has been used for decades by many people in the U.S. The World Health Organization recognizes the use of acupuncture in a wide range of treatments. Many cancer patients find it helpful in addressing pain, nausea, digestive and muscle disorders, as well as other treatment and side effect issues. Some insurance companies reimburse for acupuncture treatment. Acupuncture is a CAM practice that is used in conjunction with the established standard of care. Acupuncture is a licensed practice. Each state has its own guidelines so it is important that you go to a state-licensed acupuncturist for treatment.

The Future of CAM and Integrative Medicine

Many non-profit cancer organizations offer workshops in mind–body–spirit techniques. Many licensed social workers in non-profit organizations and therapists in private practice have expertise in different mind–body–spirit techniques that they incorporate into their therapy practices, sometimes under stress management.

Where I work, at CancerCare, a non-profit in New York City, we provide monthly workshops on meditation, Reiki, visualization and yoga to patients and caregivers. While I am trained in meditation, imagery and vibration therapy (using a Native American frame drum), many of my colleagues have expertise in other modalities. Oftentimes, this training is provided over the phone or Internet, since our outreach includes the whole country. More and more clients seek out this service during the stress of cancer. With recognition that for many people Integrative Medicine is part of their treatment, I have presented at many professional and layperson conferences throughout North America and in Hong Kong, as well as provided one-day workshops for oncology professionals in Cape Town, South Africa, and throughout Australia. With newer technologies, science has begun quantifying the benefits of many of these practices within the field of neuroscience. With growing proof of efficacy, doctors are involving patients more in the use of CAM and Integrative Medicine during and after treatment.

Q — How can I alleviate the initial fear, depression and/or stress that often comes with a cancer diagnosis?

Currently, most major cancer centers in the U.S. have CAM or Integrative Medicine departments and many smaller hospitals have created departments to specialize in these therapies. If you are still in treatment, these would be your best first referral resources because your medical team can coordinate holistic care with your CAM or Integrative Medicine team.

Resources
To learn more about CAM and Integrative Medicine go to:

- National Center for Complementary and Alternative Medicine (NCCAM) at 1-888-644-6226 or nccam.nih.gov
- Andrew Weil, M.D. at www.drweil.com
- LIVESTRONG Foundation at www.livestrong.com/integrative-medicine/
- The Art of Breathing at www.theartofbreathing.com
- Local gyms, health spas and YMCAs and YWCAs.

Gawain, Shakti. *Creative Visualization: Use the Power of Your Imagination to Create What You Want in Your Life*. Bantam Books/published by arrangement with Whatever Publishing, Inc. Whatever Publishing, Inc., Mill Valley, CA, 1978.

Gaynor, Mitchell L. *The Healing Power of Sound: Recovery from Life-Threatening Illness Using Sound, Voice, and Music*. Shambhala Publications, Inc., Boston, MA, 2002.

Kabat-Zinn, Jon. *Full Catastrophe Living: Using the Wisdom of Your Body and Mind to Face Stress, Pain, and Illness*. Bantam Dell, Division of Random House, Inc., NYC, NY, 1990.

Kearney, Michael. *Mortally Wounded: Stories of Soul Pain, Death, and Healing*. Spring Journal, Inc., New Orleans, LA, 1996.

Lerner, Michael. *Choices in Healing: Integrating the Best of Conventional and Complementary Approaches to Cancer*. MIT Press, Cambridge, MA, 1994.

Pert, Candace. *Molecules of Emotion: The Science Behind Mind/Body Medicine*. Touchstone, NYC, NY, 1999.

Using the Mind–Body Connection to Get Physical and Emotional Relief: *Jin Shin Jyutsu*, Gentle Self-Acupressure

Kerry Kay

What if you were told there is a form of gentle, easy treatment you can do for yourself, or someone can do for you, that will help you feel better during your journey with cancer?

While tremendous advances in cancer treatment have been made in recent years, we increasingly recognize that we are more than our bodies alone. As multidimensional creatures, we benefit greatly when we participate actively in our care and when our needs, beyond the medical ones, are met.

We have many tools to assist us in reducing the effects of a cancer diagnosis and treatment. The most basic of these tools are eating well, getting adequate sleep and finding ways to reduce stress. Beyond these basics are numerous complementary medicine or mind–body practices and therapies that provide real benefit to us.

Complementary and alternative medicine are groups of practices and therapies that are generally not taught in medical school and are usually not considered parts of conventional medicine. Complementary medicine comprises practices and therapies that are used in conjunction with conventional medicine, whereas alternative medicine is used alone, without conventional medicine.

Some of the best-known components of complementary medicine include meditation, Tai Chi, yoga, acupuncture and *Jin Shin Jyutsu*. These practices can be extremely helpful as they aid in stress reduction and increase relaxation. Several of these can even provide physical relief from symptoms experienced during cancer treatment.

Much research has been done in the area of the mind–body connection. Some studies show that what happens to the mind affects the body and vice versa. For example, if I relax my mind, my body relaxes and if I relax my body, my mind relaxes. Research shows that body and mind are constantly interacting and affecting one another.

A mind–body therapy or practice that provides real emotional and physical relief is *Jin Shin Jyutsu*. Since *Jin Shin Jyutsu* provides us with tools that we can use to help ourselves feel much better, I am describing it in detail here. I am also providing techniques or "holds" that address specific issues that one might experience during one's journey with cancer.

Jin Shin Jyutsu can be used to address perhaps innumerable symptoms and issues. In fact, in *Jin Shin Jyutsu*, we refer to symptoms and diseases as *projects*. Projects of particular relevance to people with a cancer diagnosis include fatigue, pain, anxiety, fear, worry, nausea, loss of appetite, stress, respiratory issues, insomnia, surgical complications and negative side effects of medications or treatments (e.g., anesthesia, chemotherapy, radiation and antidepressants).

A form of gentle acupressure, *Jin Shin Jyutsu* employs light touch on pressure points on the body to bring harmony to the body, mind and spirit. *Jin Shin Jyutsu* brings balance to the body's energies, thereby promoting optimal health and well-being and facilitating our own profound healing capacity. It is a valuable complement to conventional healing methods, inducing deep relaxation and reducing the effects of stress from physical, emotional and mental sources.

As with acupuncture, this healing art comes to us from the East. Its roots lie in ancient healing traditions that became lost. In Japan in the early twentieth century, Jiro Murai, close to death after leading an overindulgent life, healed himself using his knowledge of healing methods, meditation and fasting. For the rest of his life, he studied the human body, illness and healing. He incorporated this knowledge into the healing system that became *Jin Shin Jyutsu*.

Jin Shin Jyutsu can be administered by a practitioner. If you are unable to locate a practitioner in your area, relax in the knowledge that you can treat yourself. All that is required is openness to a new idea, some patience and your own two hands.

The body is wise and its aim is to be in equilibrium or harmony. By using the breath and our hands, which are like jumper cables, we can bring harmony to our systems.

"Taking classes such as Tai Chi Chih, Jin Shin Jyutsu, yoga, meditation and stretching, to benefit the whole me, opened up a new normal and a new way to deal with being a survivor."

— Mariann Linfante Jacobson

How to Self-Treat with *Jin Shin Jyutsu*:
- Look for your project. Choose a hold (see below).
- Keep your ankles and legs uncrossed.
- Breathe.
- Use a light touch.
- Be curious.
- Be comfortable—make adjustments to your body to relax any tension that you discover.
- Exhale and unburden. Inhale and breathe in abundance.
- Use the relevant hold for several minutes.
- Each hold requires both hands.
- Where more than one hold is listed under a heading, experiment to see which hold works the best for you.

Please note that you can treat another person using the holds below or someone can work on you to bring you relief. There are several holds that apply to more than one project.

There are a number of holds that can help to alleviate many of the common cancer side effects and problems listed below. When more than one hold is listed under a project, experiment to see which hold suits your temperament the best.

Chemotherapy Side Effects
- Place your right fingers at top center of the right half of your head and place the left fingers at the top center of the left half of your head.
- Hold your little fingers, one at a time.
- Place your fingertips on the lower edges of your collarbones.

Constipation
- Place your hands on your left calf towards the outside of the leg.

Depression
- Use the *Jin Shin Jyutsu* Hug: cross your arms and touch the outer edges of your shoulder blades by your underarms, placing your hands in your underarms or around the outside of your arms.
- Try holding your ring fingers (next to your little fingers), one at a time. Another option is to place the right hand on the left upper arm and place the left hand on your right elbow. Hold and then reverse your hands.

Diarrhea
- Hold your calves towards the outside of your legs.

Fatigue
- Place your hands at the base of your skull (feel the ridge).

Indigestion
- Cross your hands and hold your upper arms.
- Cross your hands and touch each inner thigh.

Insomnia
- When you can't sleep, place your hands at the base of your skull (feel the ridge).
- For another hold, place your right hand on your heart. Hold your right thumb with your left hand and always remember to breathe in and out.

Lymphatic Systems Projects
- *Jin Shin Jyutsu* Hug: cross your arms and touch the outer edges of your shoulder blades by your underarms, placing your hands in your underarms or around the outside of your arms.

Nausea
- Cross your hands and place them on your inner thighs.

Pain
- Place your right hand on the inside of your left ankle. Place your left hand on the outside of that ankle. Hold. Place your right hand on the inside of your right ankle. Place your left hand on the outside of that ankle.

Respiratory Projects
- *Jin Shin Jytusu* Hug: cross your arms and touch the outer edges of your shoulder blades by your underarms, placing your hands in your underarms or around the outside of your arms.
- Place your right hand on your left upper arm and place your left hand on your inner right thigh. Hold. Then do the reverse.

The above techniques or holds are equally good for anyone undergoing stressful situations. They are also useful to incorporate into one's daily life to provide a healthy mind–body balance. For more information on *Jin Shin Jyutsu*, see the *Jin Shin Jyutsu* website, www.jinshinjyutsu.com.

VIII

Financing Your Wellness—
Cancer and money management

Affording Cancer Treatment
Megan McQuarrie

Hearing those three words, "You have cancer," changes your life, but it does not mean that your life is over; rather a new journey has begun. Regardless of your financial situation, the next steps—how to find a doctor, where to do your treatment, which treatment to choose—can all be overwhelming. For some, another question may also be looming: "How am I going to afford treatment?"

It seems logical that those with no insurance face the greatest challenge in pursuing treatment. Surprisingly, it is those with health insurance and/or some form of income that may have the most difficulty affording care. As the Executive Director of the Elixir Fund, a non-profit dedicated to improving the comfort and support of cancer patients and their caregivers, I receive calls and emails almost daily from people looking for financial support, who have failed to qualify for assistance because they have some form of health insurance and/or some income—not enough to pay for treatment or the additional added expenses, but too much to qualify for aid programs. One woman wrote to say that she found that you had to be "essentially homeless" to receive support.

> I am writing on behalf of a 25-year-old girl battling stage 4 breast cancer. I am currently holding fundraising efforts to help offset the out-of-pocket costs for her treatment. She is covered by COBRA but it does not cover most of the treatment she needs.

> My mother was just diagnosed with stage 4 breast cancer and, very unfortunately, did not have health insurance as she was laid off of her job about six months ago. We are now scrambling to get her the care she needs and tests done (some have been done, but they are incomplete as she cannot pay for the others). Your organization came up as someone who might be able to point us in the right direction. We tried our state health plan but apparently the $1,500 in social security/disability checks she now receives to sustain her are too much money to qualify her for assistance. We have also looked at moving her to my home state but she would have to be here for six months or more before she qualified for assistance. Finally we are now applying for financial needs help from a local Academic Health Care Center but they admit that the wait list is long and it could be awhile—if ever—before she can get help.

So what programs are available for those with limited insurance and/or limited income? Unfortunately, there are no simple answers but there are places that you can turn to for help. Whether or not you have insurance, the first step is the same. A good place to start is with the social services department at the

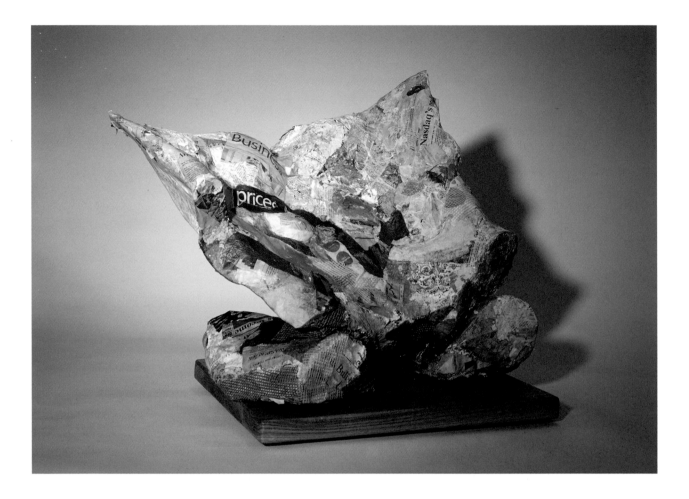

THE PRICE IS HIGH

hospital where you are doing your testing or treatment. If your care is being managed by your doctor's office, then ask if you can talk with the social services department at the hospital with which your doctor is affiliated. Some hospitals even have a social worker who specializes in working with oncology patients. The programs and resources available to cancer patients vary greatly from state to state. The hospital social services department is usually well versed in the available state programs and resources as well as the necessary applications.

If you have some capital, such as a house or investments, or even a life insurance policy, you should sit down with a financial planner to discuss ways to pay for your care and the associated costs. There is life after cancer, and while it may be difficult to think long-term and beyond cancer treatment, it is important to do so; not only for yourself, but for your family as well. So often the reaction to hearing, "You have cancer" is, "I (or we) will do whatever it takes." What happens if "whatever it takes" drains all of your financial resources? You could survive cancer only to find that you are faced with a race against creditors or a fight to save your financial future. A financial planner should be able to advise you on the best ways to utilize your existing resources without accruing additional costs or draining all of your funds. If you are not already working with a financial advisor, then ask around and find one with whom you can talk.

It is also important to be open and honest with your doctor and your health care providers about your financial situation when discussing your treatment options. There may be ways to reduce the costs of your treatment or you may be able to set up a payment plan with the billing office at the hospital and/or your doctor's office. Being honest about your financial situation does not mean that you have to sacrifice quality care.

There are non-profit organizations that provide assistance to help with co-payments or out-of-pocket expenses associated with your treatment. These organizations will help to cover the costs of your prescribed treatment (chemotherapy drugs), but not necessarily for medications that help to manage side effects. A few of these organizations are listed below.

"The Cancer Support Community (CSC), the largest cancer support organization in the U.S., is dedicated to providing free services to anyone living with cancer, along with their families and friends."

— Ellen Levine, M.S.W.

CancerCare Co-Pay Foundation provides co-payment assistance for chemotherapy. More information is provided on their website about the specific cancers that they cover. Visit www.cancercarecopay.org or call (866) 552-6729.

Patient Access Network (PAN) provides assistance for specific medications. You must be insured and your insurance must cover the medication for which you need assistance. For more information, including the medications they cover, visit www.panfoundation.org or call (866) 316-7263 on weekdays.

Chronic Disease Fund's Good Days Program assists patients in getting the prescription medications they need and also helps patients comply with the treatment plan through a free online tracking tool. For more information, visit www.gooddaysfromcdf.org or call (877) 968-7233 on weekdays.

Patient Advocate Foundation's (PAF) Co-Pay Relief Program offers financial assistance for pharmaceutical co-payments to those who have insurance. To learn more, or to apply, visit www.copays.org, or call (866) 512-3861.

"The program provides outreach, education, screening and treatment for no or low cost for women and men in our community."

— Aretha Hill-Forte, M.P.H.

If you are having difficulty with access to care, maintaining your job, or debt issues related to treatment, the Patient Advocate Foundation also offers a Case Management program. This program does not offer direct financial support; however, the PAF will mediate between the patient and the insurer, employer and/or creditors to help resolve such issues. Visit their website for more information at www.patientadvocate.org, or call (800) 532-5274.

There are also additional costs associated with cancer treatment that can cause a financial strain: transportation to and from appointments, whether you need to rely on public transportation or just the added costs of gas; time off from work for you and/or your caregiver; childcare; medications; nutritional supplements; the list goes on. These costs, in addition to the cost of your medical care, may make it difficult for you to afford your other monthly expenses such as housing costs and utilities. There are state and local programs that provide support. You can also talk with your utility companies about setting up a payment plan. Again, these are good questions for the social services department at your hospital. The Patient Advocate Foundation's website also offers a list of potential support services by state. Visit their site at www.patientadvocate.org and look under Resources–Financial Resources to conduct a state search.

The Elixir Fund is available to help you track down potential support services in your area. We recognize how taxing, both emotionally and potentially physically, cancer treatment can be. Our programs are designed to give patients and caregivers a break from cancer so they may live full and rich lives during treatment, better preparing them for life after treatment. If you or a loved one is diagnosed with cancer, we can help. We do not offer financial support, but we are available to conduct a search and narrow down the list of support services and programs that meet your needs. We have also compiled tips and suggestions from patients and caregivers that will help to make your journey with cancer a little easier. You can contact us through our website, www.elixirfund.org, or by calling (800) 494-9228.

A diagnosis of cancer impacts your life in many ways. The associated stress of whether or not you can afford treatment should not be one of them. There is help available.

Additional Resources
CancerCare: They require an application but do offer assistance for transportation, home care, childcare and pain medication (in some states). They also have additional information on their website based on your diagnosis and have support groups. www.cancercare.org

Susan G. Komen: Your local Komen affiliate may also be able to offer assistance for medical treatment or medications. Their Linking A.R.M.S. program is a partnership with CancerCare and their Co-Pay Relief is a partnership with the Patient Advocate Foundation. To find out more about these and other possible programs, you may call the national Komen number at (877) 465-6636.

Medical Insurance
Stuart Van Winkle, C.F.P.®

The world of medical insurance is evolving rapidly towards positive change for individuals seeking treatment for cancer. Traditionally, medical insurance in the U.S. was regulated by each of the fifty states individually, setting forth rules for companies that operate in their jurisdictions. This, however, is changing. The reform is taking place in the form of the Patient Protection and Affordable Care Act (PPACA), which was signed into law in March 2010, and was deemed constitutional by the U.S. Supreme Court in June 2012. The provisions go into place on a timetable that concludes January 1, 2014. PPACA is the most comprehensive medical insurance reform in decades.

Many of the positive provisions of PPACA will improve the insurance benefits for cancer patients; most notably, the ban on pre-existing conditions and the guarantee of issuance of a policy providing coverage.

Q — Can the Patient Protection and Affordable Care Act (PPACA) help you?

How is medical insurance provided? Typically, in one of three ways: (1) it can be purchased individually from an insurance company, (2) it can be purchased by an employer for the respective employees or, (3) in the case of individuals over the age of sixty-five or disabled, purchased from or made available by the government (known as Medicare or Medicaid). Often, people over the age of sixty-five, who are covered for medical insurance by Medicare A and B, will also obtain either a Medicare Advantage Plan (Medicare C) or a Medicare Supplement. Both the Advantage Plan and Supplements are sold by private insurance companies and are designed to cover the expenses not covered by Medicare A and B. Prescription drug coverage is typically provided with a medical insurance plan, and in the case of Medicare, is referred to as Medicare D.

There are four types of health insurance plans: (1) Managed Care (HMO), (2) Fee for Service (POS), (3) High Deductible Plans, which can and ought to be combined with a Health Savings Account or Health Reimbursement Account (HSA or HRA), and (4) Employee Retirement Income Security (ERISA) Plans.

The terms managed care and HMO are used interchangeably. HMOs are a way for health insurers to help control costs. Managed care influences how much health care you use. Almost all health insurance plans have some sort of managed care program to help control health care costs. This is achieved by requiring the patient to use a specific network of doctors and medical facilities, such as a particular hospital or hospital group. The network of doctors and facilities are contracted to charge specific rates for specific procedures and treatments, thus allowing the insurance companies to know what their costs will be. With most HMOs, you either are assigned or you choose one doctor to serve as your primary care doctor. This doctor monitors your health and administers most of your medical care, referring you to specialists and other health care professionals as needed. With a referred plan you would get a referral from your primary care doctor, who is expected to manage the health care you receive, to a specialist who is also in the network. Over the past few years the trend has been to remove the referral process, which many considered too onerous. This newer plan would be called an open access HMO. Essentially, with managed care HMOs, you agree to use a particular network in return for lower premiums and fewer out-of-pocket costs.

Fee-for-Service (POS) Health Plans are the traditional kind of health care policy, combined with an HMO Option. An insured person may choose at the time or "point of service" whether to go "in network," with the HMO, or "out of network" (which costs more). Health insurance companies pay fees for the services received by the insured people covered by the policy. This type of health insurance offers the most choices of doctors and hospitals. You can choose any doctor you wish and change doctors any time. You can go to any hospital in any part of the country. With fee-for-service health plans, the insurer pays only part of your doctor and hospital charges.

A certain amount of money each year, known as the deductible, is paid for by you before the health insurance payments begin. The deductible requirement applies each year of the health insurance policy. Also, not all health expenses you have count towards your deductible. Only those covered by the health insurance policy do. For instance, chemotherapy is typically covered under the prescription provisions of the plan and would not accrue towards the deductible. You need to check your health insurance policy to find out which expenses are covered. After you have paid your deductible amount for the year, you share the bill with the health insurance company. For example, you might pay 20% while the health insurer pays 80%. Your portion is called co-insurance, and when your deductible and co-insurance reach a certain maximum (MOOP—Maximum out of Pocket) then the insurance company pays 100%.

While this will all change with PPACA legislation, in some states there is only comprehensive coverage and in other states there are two kinds of fee-for-service health coverage: basic and major medical. Basic protection pays towards the costs of a hospital room and health care while you are in the hospital. It covers some hospital services and supplies, such as X-rays and prescribed medications. Basic coverage also pays towards the cost of surgery, whether it is performed in or out of the hospital, and for some doctor visits. Major medical insurance takes over where your basic coverage leaves off. It covers the cost of long, high-cost illnesses or injuries.

High deductible plans have been gaining much traction recently as a means to control health care costs, and, at the same time, empower the insured to take a more active role in the treatment they receive. Essentially, a high deductible plan is more up-front cost to the insured with the tradeoff being lower premiums. A high deductible medical plan, which could be either an HMO or a POS, could have, for example, a $2,500 individual and $5,000 family deductible that must be met by the insured before any plan benefits are paid by the insurance company. The concept is that the premium savings, which often can be 35 to 50% of the premium, can be contributed towards an HSA/HRA account that is then used to pay the deductible and coinsurance (if any) on a tax-favored basis.

ERISA plans, while not technically a medical plan design, are medical plans offered by an employer that currently are controlled by Federal ERISA laws and not state laws. The plan design could be any of the three types previously mentioned. It is important to know if the medical plan offered by your employer is an ERISA plan, because ERISA plans are often exempt from many of the state mandates on what coverage and benefits must be provided, such as coverage for routine clinical testing.

While COBRA (Consolidated Omnibus Budget Reconciliation Act) will become less relevant under PPACA, COBRA is a provision that permits employees to continue their medical insurance uninterrupted for eighteen months following a termination of employment. This applies to employer-sponsored plans, and the COBRA premium (which is the same as the sum of the prior employer's contribution and that of the employee). It is paid by the individual. COBRA was, and in some states still is, valuable to prevent an interruption in coverage when a medical condition, such as cancer, exists.

Lastly, and this is often the nature of cancer treatment, experimental care or treatment can fall outside the contractual terms and conditions of the medical insurance policy regardless of the plan. This is very important to know ahead of time in order to work with the insurance company to see if a solution can be identified. To sum up the current state of insurance as it applies to cancer treatment, the situation is looking brighter than ever: the removal of pre-existing conditions restrictions and guaranteed issue plans will be required in all states by January 1, 2014. This means that, for employees covered by a plan at work, they will no longer be confined to a job because of the fear of losing coverage if they change employers. Additionally, those purchasing individual policies will have the comfort of knowing that they can get coverage without the chance of being denied or restricted.

"We find that the patients in most need of help are those recently diagnosed with cancer."

— Wanda Diak

The Road to Financial Wellness

Richard A. Fontana, Financial Advisor, C.F.P.®

Receiving a cancer diagnosis can be overwhelming, and naturally, your first thoughts will focus on medical treatment. Your next thoughts may be to wonder how you are going to pay for your treatment. Health care insurance may or may not provide coverage for all your costs, and you may have to turn to your own financial assets.

If you're like many women, this is where things can become challenging. Regardless of your comfort level with managing your finances, health concerns are a new complication.

A significant life event, such as an illness, often forces us to take charge of our finances, if we haven't already. It also offers an opportunity for you to discuss finances with any adult children. These conversations may be difficult, but they can also be empowering. You are choosing to take control of your assets and to allocate them according to your values and wishes. You are also enabling your children to make decisions without guilt, and without wondering about your choices.

You may choose to meet with a certified financial planner to assist you with this process, but there are steps that you can take on your own. The first step is to review your assets and determine where you stand. Do you know where your money is?

This may sound simplistic, but many people don't have a clear picture of where they stand financially. How much cash do you have on hand? Where are your investments? By organizing your records and making a list of your assets, you will have taken the first step to controlling your finances.

You will have also taken an important step in dealing with the financial fears that accompany any life-altering situation. Many people avoid gathering this information because they're afraid that whatever the amount they have, it won't be enough. Once all your financial information is complete, you may find that you are in a more secure position than you had thought.

You may also find that you want more control over your spending, especially if you want to maintain a strong cash reserve. You can start by keeping a record of all the money you spend in a week. This can be an eye-opening experience because of the Latte Factor—a term coined by David Bach in his book *Smart Women Finish Rich* to describe the miscellaneous spending we do every day, like buying a latte or stopping at your favorite store because there's a sale and buying something you didn't really need.

The point is that all of us spend money on items every day without really thinking about how it impacts our budget. By saving even pennies per day, you can build your short-term and long-term finances. Most importantly, you can determine whether or not you're spending money on your priorities. Again, you're taking control and empowering yourself.

"When it comes to your personal health, it is critical not to overlook any possible resources."

— Christine Bonney

Finally, this is the time to make certain that your legal documents are in order, and that they're updated and valid. Even if you have a will or a living trust, you should check it to make certain that it is current (no more than five years old) and that your beneficiaries are up to date. Your family should know where your will is, and they should be able to access it if it is needed. You may also wish to delegate power of attorney for your finances and health directives.

This is also the time to review all of your insurance coverage: health insurance, life insurance, disability and long-term care. Having insurance coverage is not the same as understanding it. You will need to know what is covered and how the benefits are accessed. If you don't have health insurance, you can get information about your options from hospital social workers and organizations like the American Cancer Society.

If you don't have life insurance, the cancer diagnosis may make it challenging to obtain, but it's not impossible. Your options will vary depending on the type of cancer you have, the stage and grade of the cancer and possibly the treatment you'll receive and the cure rate for your cancer.

Because this may be a difficult time emotionally, you'll want to be especially careful to deal with a reputable life insurance company. An independent insurance broker can help you review plans from many companies with various options.

Taking control of your finances isn't simple, but it may be easier than you had imagined. By taking steps toward financial wellness, you can focus your energy on your physical health and start your journey to recovery.

Richard A. Fontana, C.F.P.®
Portfolio Manager
Senior Vice President – Investments
Financial Advisor
CA Insurance Lic. # 0D02832
Raymond James & Associates, Inc.
www.fontanawealthmanagement.com
For more information on FA Fontana, refer to the bio section.

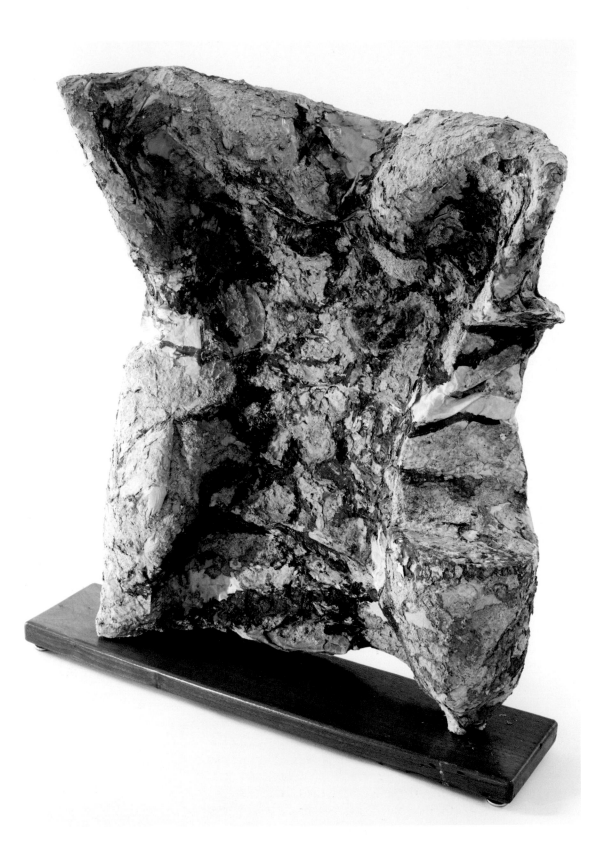

LIGHT COMING THROUGH BLUE

Essential Help from the
Women's Health & Counseling Center

Christine Bonney

Help comes in many forms. One that is irreplaceable in Somerset County, New Jersey, serves as an example. As of the writing of this article, Women's Health & Counseling Center (WHCC) has provided health services to the uninsured (and underinsured) residents of Somerset County and beyond for thirty-nine years.

In the early days, this award-winning agency provided services to all ages and genders. Later, the agency focused more on services to women. Today, WHCC offers full primary care services for women and some services for men, including reproductive health screenings and vital cancer screenings.

Where cancer is involved, a patient's need for help comes in a variety of forms. One of the common comments is: "I should have been more willing to ask for help." Usually this refers to everyday activities. However, women and men in our society, as well as in so many disadvantaged countries, are all too often unable to get financial and medical assistance.

Early cancer prevention and detection saves lives. A variety of national and regional organizations corroborate this. WHCC is an excellent example of a community-based agency that offers a unique program and access to free cancer screening. This service comes through Cancer Education and Early Detection (CEED), a program that promotes the early detection and treatment of breast, cervical, prostate and colorectal cancers with support from New Jersey's CEED program at the N.J. Department of Health and Senior Services.

WHCC offers screening services for the early detection of cancer in women including breast exams, pap smears, pelvic exams, mammograms and colon cancer screenings. For men, screening includes colorectal exams and prostate screenings. Knowing that the best way to fight breast, cervical, colorectal and prostate cancer is to detect it early, when it is most treatable, WHCC works with a broad array of community organizations and faith-based institutions to bring these free cancer screening programs to area residents.

WHCC is the local access point for one county, which is part of a state-wide program. In all, there are twenty-one CEED centers in New Jersey. The number of centers varies in different states, as do the funds allotted to each center.

For the record, during 2011 alone, WHCC provided medical and counseling services to 3,031 clients through 5,853 sessions and provided educational programs to 7,244 women, men and adolescents, serving 10,275 individuals overall. For more information, visit www.womenandhealth.org.

When it comes to your personal health, it is critical not to overlook any possible resources. With respect to clients with cancer-related concerns, the best insight sometimes comes from personal experience. The following is an excerpt

"Federal CDC (Centers for Disease Control) created a framework called the National Breast and Cervical Cancer Early Detection Program, which provides a Medicaid option for the individual states… Indian Health Service and tribal organizations."

— Omri Behr, Ph.D., J.D.

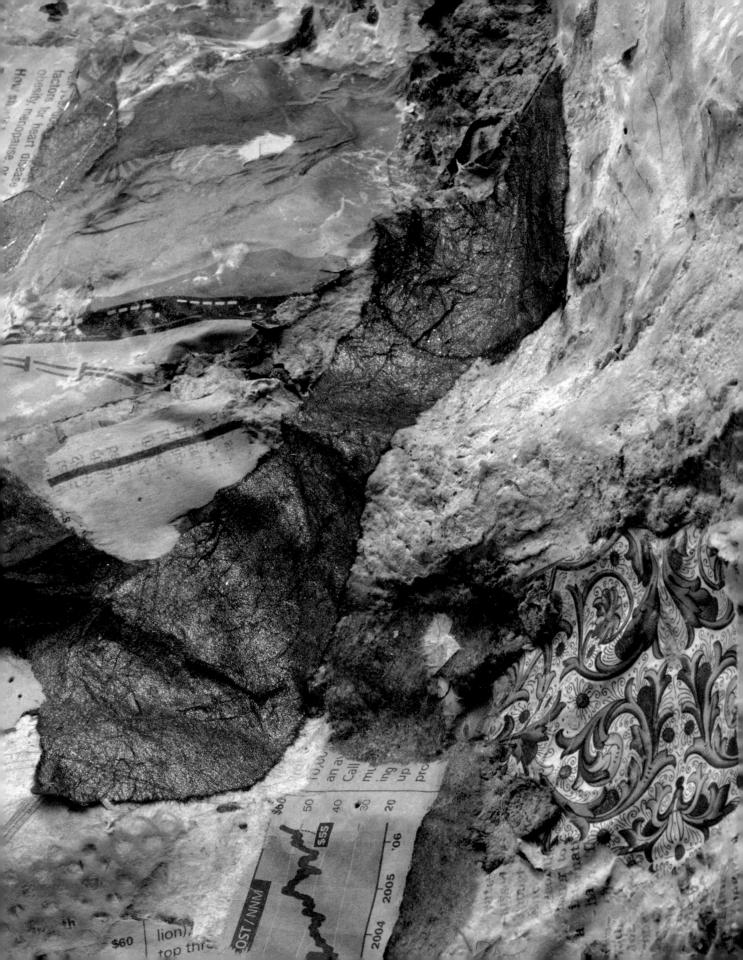

from a letter sent to WHCC that serves as an example of just how vital early detection can be:

> *My husband told me about the Women's Health & Counseling Center (WHCC) and suggested I should start going there. My thought was, "that's not a place for someone like me."*
>
> *Over the years, as I went without annual mammograms and ignored most of my health issues, he quietly prompted me to call WHCC and again, my thought was, "that's not a place for someone like me."*
>
> *Then, just about this time nearly two years ago—I found a lump.*
>
> *Without a moment of hesitation, I called WHCC. And that is where my story begins. They made sure I saw a doctor right away and I quickly realized this was actually the perfect place for me. They could see the worry on my face about the lump and sensed my concern for the potential financial burden that would be a result of needed tests and possible surgery. Comfort came with learning that I was eligible for the Cancer Education and Early Detection (CEED) program which would cover the costs for the vital tests coming up.*
>
> *Despite the hope we had that my extensive tests would come back negative, that was not the case. Had I not called WHCC that day, the cancer would have no doubt taken over my body, and more than likely it would have taken me.*
>
> *The continued support from all the caring professionals who have touched my life has been amazing. From a helping hand, to a reassuring smile and a box of tissues, the doctor and staff at WHCC have made it known that I'm not just a time slot...not just another file number, rather I'm part of their family. And, when you find a lump and your whole world is rocked to its very core, feeling comfortable in a doctor's office is not something you take lightly. I am so much further down my road to recovery because of the access to care provided by WHCC. Slowly but surely I have fought the good fight and will continue to seek health care services through WHCC. They are family now. They want the best for someone like me.*

WHCC has expanded its services to include men and children. Medicare, Medicaid and certain other insurances are now accepted. Currently, WHCC operates as Zufall Health, Somerville.

(COBRA) Consolidated Omnibus Budget Reconciliation Act: Health Insurance after Job Termination

Omri Behr, Ph.D., J.D.

The Consolidated Omnibus Budget Reconciliation Act of 1986 included an insurance-continuation provision, which has come to be known as COBRA. COBRA is not a health care insurance system. Rather, it provides to employees and their dependents a limited right to continue a health insurance group plan coverage when the person who is the main beneficiary of a policy paid by an employer loses that coverage.

COBRA requires that a person who would otherwise lose coverage but who is entitled to continuation of coverage, pay the employee's as well as the employer's share of the premium, plus a 2% administrative cost. The expense may, then, be substantially more than the insured is used to paying, as the employer's share of the insurance premium is usually substantially the larger share, possibly as much as two or three times larger. The continuation can extend for at least eighteen months. Thus while the right to continuation appears to be attractive, it is very frequently much more expensive than a recently terminated worker can afford.

The conditions for eligibility under the act are rather detailed and complex and will only be dealt with in outline. Anyone who thinks they might qualify is advised to consult a very informative U.S. Department of Labor webpage at www.dol.gov/ebsa/publications/cobraemployee.html. The Patient Protection and Affordable Care Act (PPACA), sometimes called "Obamacare," did not change the rules applicable to COBRA, although it does provide alternative avenues of coverage for people who lose group coverage.

The advantages provided by COBRA depend on a number of prior conditions. There is no legal requirement that an employer provide any group health care coverage at all. COBRA extension rights do apply, however, to group health plans provided by employers that had twenty or more employees on more than 50% of the working days in the previous calendar year.

Termination of coverage usually occurs when the termination of the main beneficiary was not for cause, but rather when work hours were reduced, or when the employee was terminated through a general reduction in workforce. While the trigger is usually due to action by an employer, an employee may also become ineligible for the basic company plan through voluntary reduction in work hours or even self-termination. Prior to 2014, an employee who secures new employment that provides health insurance coverage could continue to be eligible for COBRA continuation coverage if the new coverage has a period of pre-existing condition exclusion. Beginning in 2014, however, the PPACA prohibits pre-existing conditions exclusions.

Spouses and children who are affected by a termination may receive benefits under COBRA. For example, a spouse whose covered partner separates by reason of divorce, judicial separation or death may also benefit for thirty-six months, as can a dependent child. Interestingly that extension is also available where an employee becomes Medicare eligible, of course that assumes the policy in question is more generous than Medicare to justify the substantial additional cost.

The extension privilege due to termination is not limited to a COBRA extension of the initial group plan of the terminated beneficiary. It may be advantageous to choose coverage under another group plan, provided that group plan was available when COBRA extension was declined by the potential beneficiary. Under HIPAA (Health Insurance Portability and Accountability Act), coverage may be sought in a different plan of a spouse or for a dependent child of a different parent. In this case the usual need to wait for the next normal enrollment period is waived.

In this entire procedure there are notice and filing time requirements for everyone. An employer must notify a new employee as to whether the company plan qualifies under COBRA within a set time period. Equally, notice must be given by the employer to the insurer within thirty days of a triggering event. An employee must also give notice of changes in qualification situations within a given time period.

In sum, COBRA is a valuable interim measure for those who can afford it. Its specific rules for availability of its benefits require strict attention but are not overly burdensome. When the Patient Protection and Affordable Care Act ("Obamacare") comes into full operation and insurance exchanges are available, reliance on COBRA, even as an interim measure, may not be desirable if individual coverage through the new Health Insurance Exchanges is less expensive. As of this writing, however, COBRA continuation coverage will continue to be available, and eligible persons should continue to evaluate its costs and benefits.

The author thanks Professor J.V. Jacobs of Seton Hall School of Law for his assistance.

(NBCCEDP) National Breast and Cervical Cancer Early Detection Program: A Path for Patients without Insurance or Funds

Omri Behr, Ph.D., J.D.

Is there help for uninsured women and men who suspect, but don't know, that they may have cancer? Yes there is, with some limitations. The federal government has created a program intended to serve those individuals who have not been covered for screening by insurance and about 90% of those who will still not be insured for screening even after the full operation of the Patient Protection and Affordable Care Act (PPACA or "Obamacare"). However, the PPACA will provide insurance coverage to most people in America.

The screening solution comes through a Medicaid option framework that has been established by the Federal Centers for Disease Control (CDC) called the National Breast and Cervical Cancer Early Detection Program (NBCCEDP). Since 2001 these provisions also apply to the Indian Health Service and tribal organizations.

The NBCCEDP provides funding to all fifty states, the District of Columbia, five U.S. territories and twelve American Indian organizations. The purpose of this funding is to make certain that diagnostic services are available to many low-income, uninsured and underinsured people. Since this is a Medicaid option, the actual extent to which these services are available depends on how much additional funding can be obtained from the appropriate non-federal governmental entities responsible for Medicaid.

The funded services include breast examination, mammograms, Pap tests, pelvic examination and diagnostic testing, if results are abnormal. Men may receive tests for prostate and colorectal cancer and, if symptomatic, for breast cancer. The program does not cover treatment should this be required. It will, however, make referrals for treatment, and the treating location may have funding to treat low-income individuals, or other organizations may cover those costs. Federal guidelines for NBCCEDP require that income levels (for single applicants or those in families) should be at or below 250% of the federal poverty level, and there are age limitations for certain procedures.

The services rendered by individual state entities may exceed screening and may also include education, outreach, case management tracking, follow-up and help for finding and financing treatment. The extent of these services depends on the degree that the federal funding is further supported by the state or by private donations. The number of such screening centers varies by state. In some states there are centers in most counties, but in others only in some. The one drawback to this excellent system is that it will only enroll women who have not already had a mammogram screening.

"Don't allow fear to delay you, or prevent you from getting the care that may very well save your life. Early detection does save lives. It saved mine."

— Kathi Edelson Wolder

For most women, after the Patient Protection and Affordable Care Act comes into force, screening coverage will result from their employment or from the purchase of other group or individual insurance. In the case of purchasing other individual insurance, this could become subsidized by the federal government to some extent, depending on family size and level of income compared to the federal poverty level. Those who are insured are assured of a certain level of testing for cancer because the provisions of PPACA require insurance providers to cover such testing, and prohibit them from blocking coverage due to pre-existing conditions.

While NBCCEDP is not as extensive as would be desirable, the results are nonetheless impressive.[1]

Women receiving an NBCCEDP-funded mammogram from Jan. 2007 to Dec. 2011

Breast Results and Outcomes

Mammograms provided	1,617,110
Mammograms with abnormal results [1]	231, 282
Percentage of mammograms with abnormal results	14.3
Breast cancers detected [2]	16,922
Rate of breast cancers detected per 1,000 mammograms	10.5

1: Abnormal results include mammogram results of: suspicious abnormality, highly suggestive of malignancy and assessment incomplete (further imaging studies or film comparisons required).
2: Breast cancers include invasive breast cancer, ductal carcinoma in situ (DCIS), and other in situ excluding lobular carcinoma in situ (LCIS).

Note: Approximate ethnic breakdown of women in the program by percent: African-American 18.2, Hispanic 23.4, Caucasian 7.1, balance other minorities.

A substantial amount of research on the applicability and effectiveness of this program has been carried out and published. Recent publications may be found on the CDC website.[2]

Although Obamacare will provide health insurance and preventive care to many, it did not eliminate the NBCCEDP, as many women will continue to need these services. The continuation of the program is, of course, subject to funding from Congress and non-federal governmental entities.

The author thanks Professor J.V. Jacobs of Seton Hall School of Law for his assistance.

1. www.cdc.gov/cancer/nbccedp/data/summaries/national_aggregate.htm
2. www.cdc.gov/cancer/nbccedp/index.htm

IX

Finding Community and Compassion—
Interactions between cancer support organizations and survivors

My Cancer Story
Mariann Linfante Jacobson

I went into the field of sign language interpreting and education because my parents are Deaf. I love my work and the language and culture in which I grew up. The highlight of my interpreting career, which has included working with presidents, politicians, authors and celebrities, was interpreting for the Dalai Lama. At that time, I was being treated for breast cancer. Going through chemotherapy was rough. I was pretty sick a lot of the time, lost my hair everywhere (no need to shave my legs that summer) and was always fatigued. When chemo was completed, I started to get a little peach fuzz but was still wearing scarves and hats. Months earlier, although already sick, I'd agreed to interpret for the Dalai Lama when he would be in New Jersey. I had no idea what shape I'd be in but really wanted to do this assignment. On the day of the event, when the planner was deciding where to place me, I wondered if the sun would be facing me and whether I should keep my scarf on my head for protection (and some vanity). I asked the planner what to do. "Let me see how much hair you have under the scarf," she said. When I showed her, she pointed to a wonderful picture on the wall of the Dalai Lama's followers—monks and nuns who looked just like me with their shaved heads. The scarf never went back on my head after that meeting.

My work experiences give me the opportunity to travel and meet extraordinary people. Being in private practice allows me to set my own schedule and to do different kinds of interpreting, often in the field of medicine. It is never boring. My schedule was so intense for a while that my husband urged me to slow down. Well, I did; I had to.

When first hearing the word cancer assigned to me, I was stunned and scared. My work at the Cancer Institute with Deaf patients showed me what clients go through. My personal experiences were with two people who had died—my father from lung cancer and a cousin of my husband from breast cancer. Those were the people who immediately came to mind. Any wonder I was stunned and scared? It was not easy hearing the "C" word.

In early 2005, my tumor was detected by an annual mammogram, which had been delayed by two months due to a new standard instituted by radiology groups insisting on double readings of all mammograms. Not a bad idea. But my usual birthday mammogram would have been preferable, instead of two months later. Having cystic breasts nearly my entire adult life, I was used to having an ultrasound after the mammogram. It was no big deal, that is, until the technician went over the same area several times then left the room. When she returned and brought the radiologist with her, it suddenly didn't feel like a little deal. The radiologist performed the ultrasound herself and asked a few questions. What was she seeing? She said it was a mass that looked like cancer

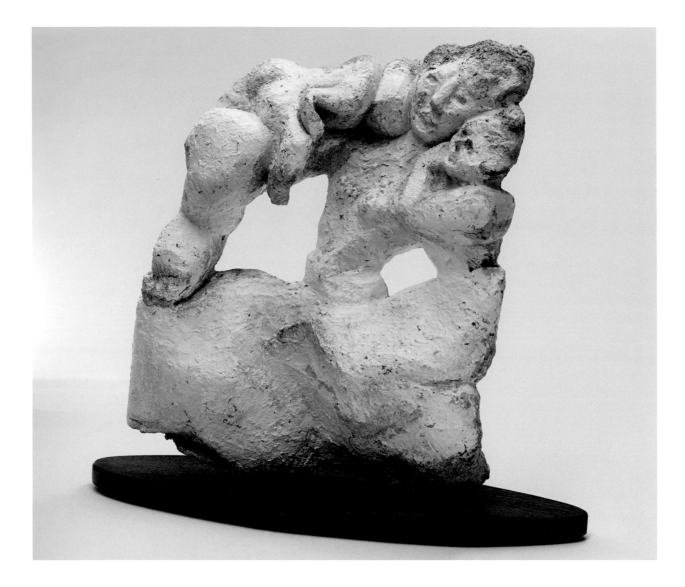

and should immediately be seen by a breast surgeon. I could hardly believe my ears. How could this be when I was so good about going for annual checkups and doing self-exams? Although dazed, I was aware that the staff was neither consoling nor comforting. They saw my distress, but let me leave without making sure I was all right. Somehow I got into my car and called to make an appointment with the breast surgeon, an excellent doctor who had removed cysts of mine before. She is at the top of her field; I would be in good hands. The appointment was set for ten days later. Having done something constructive and positive about my disease, I was ready to call my husband. He tried to get clear information from me so he would know how to respond. He told me to calm down and drive straight home.

As soon as we talked, his clear thinking helped me see that we were going to do what we needed to take care of this tumor. Within hours the doctor's office changed the appointment to Sunday, just a few days away, instead of ten. (Yes, she has hours on weekends—this helps her help all the women she can.)

Within two weeks I had a lumpectomy and some lymph nodes removed and was on the road to recovery. Then I contacted the top oncologist in my area, who prescribed chemotherapy, radiation and a year of Herceptin for my estrogen negative, progesterone negative and HER2 positive breast cancer. That year, I found out more about breast cancer than anyone needs to know—I hadn't even known there were different kinds, thinking "breast cancer is breast cancer." That year, I focused on fighting the cancer by doing everything possible to be a survivor.

Although I continued to work—limiting the kinds in order not to expose myself while my immune system was being compromised—the cancer still surrounded me. As it happened, during my five months of chemotherapy, I interpreted for a patient going through his own cancer. This turned out to be a step in my recovery as well.

The opportunity to interpret for the Dalai Lama, an inspirational leader and proponent of peace and love, was a once-in-a-lifetime dream. That day was memorable as my symbol of healing and of freedom from the disease. Although I was not able to have a personal conversation with him—he was very well-protected and, at that time, some political things were going on so there was no extra time for one-on-one meetings—I definitely felt something, an inner peace. He blessed all of us on stage and in the audience.

I needed to be enveloped by all that this man of peace and harmony represented. It was truly inspirational. My husband, who was in the audience, said he felt the tranquil feeling in the bleachers. Can you imagine, with so many people in the Rutgers University outdoor stadium, to be encompassed by that serene umbrella? It was a very personal feeling for me and my husband. I don't really know if it was cancer-related, but it was in the midst of my treatment and gave me a new perspective on my disease.

A strong support system—my husband, daughter and son, sister and friends—surrounded me. They were there when I needed them, and even when

I didn't know or think I needed them. Because they were so strong for me, it never occurred to me to go to a support group or for counseling or to seek out resources and contacts for cancer survivors. I felt being around those who loved and cared for me, and going to regular follow-up exams and procedures, was enough... Until the second shoe dropped.

Three and a half years later, once again, through a routine mammogram, a tumor showed up on the same breast in nearly the same area. I was shocked; the doctors were shocked. How could this be? Why did it happen? Not one to wallow, I made appointments and had every test known to modern science. The decision was definitely a mastectomy, but the choice of a bilateral mastectomy was up to me. It was a no-brainer. I could not imagine waiting my whole life for that third shoe to drop—after all, we only have two feet!

My mind could not wrap around being hit twice with breast cancer. But I was lucky to have outstanding professionals on my team. This time I sought counselors to help me with my fears and got the help of The Wellness Community (TWC) and Gilda's Club (which have joined to become Cancer Support Community) and the Breast Cancer Resource Center. Taking classes such as Tai Chi Chih, *Jin Shin Jyutsu*, yoga, meditation and stretching, to benefit the whole me, opened up a new normal and a new way to deal with being a survivor. My wish is that every survivor takes advantage of additional ways on the road to healing.

While writing this article, I felt so enmeshed in my healing in this extraordinary way, participating in Cancer Support Community (CSC). It was an opportunity to be with people who were going through similar experiences. Yet it turned into much more. It enabled me to express myself through complementary ways of looking at my healing. I'd always thought I had a creative side but I see myself differently in my creativity now. CSC has been a lifeline for me and is truly a community of caring, sensitive and professional people. It allows survivors and caregivers the rarest opportunity: to share their time, experience and friendship with each other. By being part of CSC, I have taken control of my healing and of my survivorship.

> *"Currently, most major cancer centers in the U.S. have CAM or Integrative Medicine departments and many smaller hospitals have created departments to specialize in these therapies."*
>
> — Richard Dickens, M.S.

Cancer Support Community
Ellen Levine, M.S.W., A.C.S.W., L.C.S.W., O.S.W.-C.

As a social worker, I have always been drawn to the health field and, early in my career, worked with people with chronic illnesses, both adults and children. I wasn't specifically looking for a job in the field of oncology, but when the opportunity came along to work at The Cancer Institute of New Jersey, affiliated with the University of Medicine and Dentistry of New Jersey, it was a good fit. As an oncology social worker and member of the Association of

Oncology Social Workers, I was familiar with The Wellness Community (TWC), a national cancer support organization that impressed me because of how well its programs complemented the care offered in medical settings. When the director of the Cancer Institute asked me to sit in on a meeting with a group of women who wanted to start a Wellness Community locally, I found my interest in the mission and the work of the organization compelling. The Wellness Community, unlike most national organizations that set up local affiliates, was designed to have groups bubble up from grassroots efforts—a big undertaking.

The Wellness Community was founded in 1982 in Santa Monica, California, by Dr. Harold Benjamin in response to his wife's experience with breast cancer. He wanted to create an environment for people with cancer to participate in their fight for recovery, convinced that those who actively worked with their health care team would improve the quality of their lives and even enhance the possibility of recovery.

In 2009, The Wellness Community and Gilda's Club (a similar organization founded in 1992) merged to become Cancer Support Community (CSC), the largest cancer support organization in the U.S. dedicated to providing free services to anyone living with cancer, along with their families and friends.

The organization's mission is to ensure that all people impacted by cancer are empowered by knowledge, strengthened by action and sustained by community. CSC is comprised worldwide of nearly fifty local affiliates and over one hundred off-site and satellite locations.

The Cancer Support Community Central New Jersey (CSC-CNJ), which was chartered as the Wellness Community of Central New Jersey in 2002, opened its doors in a home-like setting in Bedminster in 2005. The heart of our program is ongoing professionally facilitated support groups for people with cancer, caregivers and children or bereaved loved ones. Data show that such groups decrease distress and improve quality of life. Group members come together to gain support and learn from one another.

For example, we have weekly participant groups for adults who have been diagnosed with cancer and are involved in the day-to-day journey with the disease. The participants can attend these groups until they are cancer-free or have no treatment side effects for eighteen months after the end of their treatment. These groups greatly decrease stress. As one participant told me, "I am so grateful for the support that I have received from the group. It is a safe spot where I can feel free to talk, laugh and cry with others who are on the same emotional roller coaster."

We also have biweekly Family and Friends' Support Groups for adult family members or friends of the person with cancer. The cancer patient does not have to be a CSC participant for a family member to join a group.

We have several other groups that give participants and caregivers an opportunity to connect with others coping with the same type of cancer, or a similar issue. These include: Advanced Breast Cancer, Men's Cancers, Life after Cancer and Kids Connect/Parents Connect. We also offer Bereavement Groups

"...participating in the Cancer Support Community provided an opportunity to be with people who were going through similar experiences. Yet it turned into much more."

— Mariann Linfante Jacobson

for family members or friends who have recently experienced the death of a loved one from cancer. Separate bereavement groups are held for adults, parents and children. These groups are small, with a maximum of twelve participants.

Then there are the Healthy Living programs that provide a variety of ways to manage the mind's and body's responses to living with cancer. These include several gentle exercise and movement classes, and relaxation and energy techniques to help our participants learn ways of coping with the stress associated with a cancer diagnosis.

In addition to ongoing groups and activities, we have an array of educational programs, all free of charge, such as "Everything You Wanted to Know about Diagnostic Imaging Procedures," "Frankly Speaking about Cancer Treatment," "Nutrition: Smart Snacking" and "Genetic Counseling and Testing: What Is It and How Do I Know if I Need It?" led by experts on the specific topic.

One woman, interested in nutrition during her chemotherapy, stated that our program with area nutritionists "increased my awareness of the best foods to eat and spices to use" and inspired her to make healthier meals for her family.

At CSC-CNJ we have four full-time and three part-time staff members, along with six licensed mental health clinicians, who facilitate the support groups. Other specialists lead weekly groups such as yoga, wellness workout, and relaxation/visualization. The staff is rounded out with many volunteers.

Our educational programs are held at the CSC-CNJ house, as well as in the community. The goal is to reach all community members, including those who are underserved, through these programs. One such program, the showing of a relevant movie for young adults between twenty and forty years old who have cancer, was held at the Morris Museum. Another program was for educators about strengthening the school's response when a child's parent has cancer or when children have cancer. This one-day conference reached some two hundred educators. A virtual wellness community was established in 2002 and currently there are at least five online support groups that meet weekly.

The value of CSC-CNJ is perhaps best illustrated by one of the participants, who observed, "overall, coming here has been a total uplifting experience. CSC-CNJ has taught me that even in my town, there are wonderful caring people, in a cozy setting, to help me move forward in this difficult, life-changing journey."

For more information, see our website, www.cancersupportcnj.org, or call (908) 658-5400.

The Most Painful Trial of My Life

Lucinda (Cindy) Newsome

I grew up in a Christian home with five sisters and four brothers, sailing along with my life, always attempting to tie everything up in a neat little package and make everyone happy. My belief was that if I followed Jesus' example toward others, life would be great most of the time. "Do unto others as you would have them do unto you" was my mantra. I am married with two children and four grandchildren. Writing is my passion and I became a published author in 2006 with the release of *Hobbstown: The Forgotten Legacy of a Unique African-American Community*.

I'll never forget the day I was diagnosed with breast cancer and ultimately experienced the most painful trial of my life. It began in August 2007, with my yearly ob-gyn checkup. My doctor, of fifteen years, performed the usual Pap test and breast exam. We played catch-up about our families, and suddenly in the midst of examining my left breast, he asked, "Can you feel that?" My heart went cold. "No," I replied, as the knot of fear grew larger in my throat. He guided my hand to the area of concern in my breast and there was a lump that felt hard to my touch. I was overwhelmed with fear that it was breast cancer. I had come to the appointment alone since it was just a routine yearly exam. The doctor explained that I needed a mammogram as quickly as possible, although he "didn't feel too concerned about the lump."

I wondered why I had not previously felt the mass, since I had faithfully performed breast self-exams; yet I had missed it. A digital mammogram and biopsy confirmed my worst fears. Breast cancer. My daughter was with me during the mammogram confirmation and my husband was with me during the biopsy findings. They were both very supportive. I had a good support system of family and friends who prayed for me and walked with me through surgery and chemotherapy.

Between chemo treatments, I determined to better educate myself about the disease. I obtained information from my oncologist's office and the Internet, and joined an African-American breast cancer support organization, Sisters Network of Central New Jersey. All of this was very helpful, but major strength came from talking to other survivors at Your Sister's House, by listening to their journeys and sharing mine. Sharing information is a valuable tool that may benefit any cancer survivor. Somehow, it made me feel that I was not alone in this fight because it is a very solitary illness. Unless someone has experienced this life-threatening disease, try as they may, they do not understand how debilitating it can be. It took over my life for a time, as everything revolved around treatments and getting myself healthy again. In the beginning, a myriad of emotions caused depression. I felt shame (I must have done something wrong), anger (because I followed the preventive guidelines) and fear (that I

"Having this additional time with a nurse navigator helps to reduce anxieties, as well as provide the patient and family members with the opportunity to review and reflect on the patient care plan."

— Sherry Melinyshyn, P.H.C.N.P.

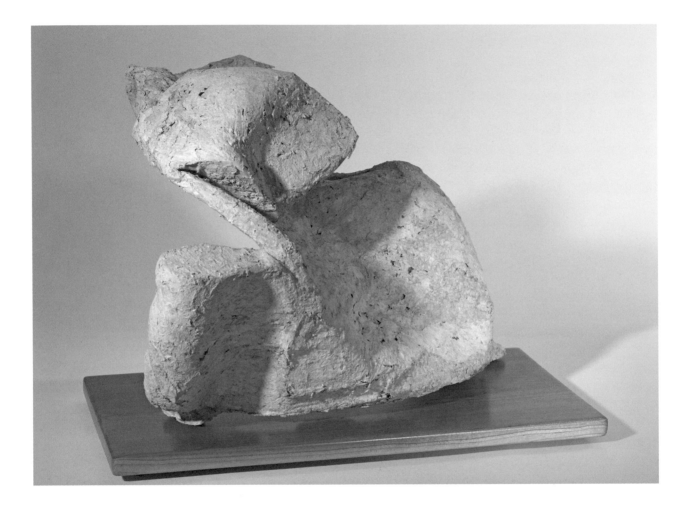

was dying). However, through speaking with other survivors and guest health experts at the support group, I came to the realization that I could do many things to limit my chances for recurrence. I already belonged to a gym and increased my workout time. I also changed my eating habits and began to eat more of the foods that are good for the body, green vegetables and fruits. I added organic foods and cut down on white foods, like bread and rice. My best advice to others is to look and listen to your body, sometimes the signs of illness are there, but we are so busy with our daily lives that we miss them.

It's 2013, and I'm almost a six-year survivor! I got my life back and, through prayer and thanksgiving, God has increased my creativity and my love of writing. I thank God every day for allowing me to be here to continue in love with the beautiful family that He has given me.

Sisters Network: Founding a Chapter
Dorothy Reed

I began a closer walk with God when I was diagnosed with breast cancer in 1998, at the age of forty-five. I had found a lump in my breast during a breast self-exam. My first thought was that I was going to die, and I was afraid I had not done what God wanted me to do on earth. Attend church—yes; work on ministries—yes; I was very busy in the church, but was it for my enjoyment or God's Will? I found myself praying for extra years so that I could listen to God and do the Will of God.

After a mastectomy, chemotherapy and radiation treatments, I began a mission to spread the gospel of early detection in the African-American community. Statistics show that African-American women have the highest death rate and shortest survival rate of any racial and ethnic group in the U.S.

God gave me a vision and a mission to support women, particularly African-American women, as they battle the devastating disease of breast cancer. I had awesome support from my church family, immediate family and friends. Deacons and ministers came to visit me. Prayers from the prayer ministry came to the hospital too. I felt every woman should have this type of support.

It took me ten months to get through surgery and treatments. I was sick, lost my hair, eyebrows, appetite and weight, and I spent a lot of time in bed. My blood cells stayed low so I had to get weekly Procrit shots and give myself Neupogen shots ten days out of the month. One time I looked at myself in the mirror and asked, "Am I going to beat this thing called cancer?" I recited daily Psalm 118:17, *"I shall not die but live and declare the works of the Lord."*

In the Central New Jersey area, I found no support and a lack of culturally sensitive material for African-American women dealing with breast cancer. My own experiences helped me to bring a complete, personalized and objective

"During this journey my oncologist referred me to the Sisters Network ...which played a very supportive role in helping me deal with my breast cancer."

— Keshia D. Hammond-Merriman

perspective of the pain, sorrow, medical disparities and lack of sensitivity suffered by African-American women fighting to live. So in 2000, I became the co-founder and president of Sisters Network of Central New Jersey (SNCNJ). SNCNJ provides education, awareness, meals, food vouchers, prosthetics, monthly support meetings, events and special programs for seniors and teens. Under my leadership SNCNJ has grown from four breast cancer survivors to fifty-four and has over two hundred volunteers. I was featured in a commercial and many magazines, spoke on television and radio, and have lobbied in Washington, D.C., concerning the devastating disease of breast cancer.

In the past ten years, twenty-two women from SNCNJ have succumbed to this dreaded disease, nine have experienced recurrences and many who are diagnosed are under forty. I am determined to advocate until African-American women no longer have the highest death and shortest survival rates. I thank God every day for the extra years, and I am always reminded of the message of St. Francis of Assisi, "Preach the Gospel at all times. When necessary use words."

When Life Pulls Out the Carpet from Beneath Us ... Do Flips!

Pamela Schwartz

It was just three months after my son's bar mitzvah when a physiatrist got to the bottom of my migraine headaches. His phone call on that Saturday afternoon stopped me in my tracks when he said, "highly suspicious lymphoma." The next six months can be summarized by three events: chemotherapy, radiation and, thank goodness, graduate school.

I was just beginning my second semester when my health situation put my life into autopilot mode. My family and friends were there every step of the way. Their help took the form of taking me to treatments, helping with carpools and dropping off dinners for my family on days when I had treatments. There were times when I did not have the strength to lift laundry baskets or straighten up around the house. My two children rose to the occasion and did the heavy lifting that I was not able to do. During those very somber and private moments when I needed someone to wipe away my tears and soothe my deepest fears, my husband, Jack, was always there with a strong shoulder and soft tissue for me. The army of support that I had was immeasurable, and I was the recipient of absolute unconditional love!

Graduate school was a saving grace—lending focus and direction during a time in my life that was uncharted. Homework, tests and internships gave me very little time to cry and say, "Why me?" In retrospect, I am so thankful that I was able to focus on my professional goals. Becoming a guidance counselor required six hundred hours of fieldwork. During my internship at the

Plainview-Old Bethpage Middle School, I was introduced to Mrs. Aviva Sala, the district's middle school social worker.

What a dynamic lady Aviva is! Aviva, for the two years prior to my meeting her, was the event chair for American Cancer Society's Relay for Life fundraising event. Aviva had brought Relay for Life to Plainview after losing her father to cancer. She took a painful experience in her life and turned it into something meaningful for her family, friends and community. She put together a committee and over seven years has helped raise more than $750,000 for a charity that is so near and dear to her heart. What finer tribute could be paid to her dad?

For community members, Relay for Life is a place to gather, share, celebrate, reflect and remember all those touched by cancer. When I understood what she was involved in, I asked if I could help and she immediately put me to work. I was appreciative that my condition was now in remission and I was ready to do something for the cause. Aviva sent me around town soliciting donations from local banks, bagel shops and friends. My soliciting was just a small part, and Aviva continued to invite me to the meetings, allowing me to learn about the various components of the event.

As the event drew near, I was invited to be one of the keynote speakers at the survivor dinner. Could I speak publicly about something so private? What could I say to a room filled with others who have experienced cancer either directly or as caregivers? I wondered how I might get through a speech without crying, sharing feelings that were private to me, and whether others would understand. With twisted emotions, I accepted the invitation and began writing my speech. I rewrote it at least a half dozen times because it just did not seem relevant. When I finally had something that I thought was worth sharing, I gave it to my husband. Jack is a great editor and brutally honest. He came back to me with tear-filled eyes saying, "It's good the way it is, don't change it," and it dawned on me that because everyone in the room had shared a similar experience, anything that I had to share was relevant. I was able to stand in front of a crowded room and signify hope. No other message could speak louder. During my first public speaking engagement as a cancer survivor, I was able to laugh a little, cry a little and give my first public speech about battling non-Hodgkin's lymphoma. *Little did I know where this would take me.*

My family and close friends formed a team for the Plainview Relay for Life. We walked the track, talked, ate, drank and celebrated life that night. By 11:00 p.m., many had gone home, leaving my immediate family, a few friends of my children and a friend from grad school to stay the night. Relay is typically an overnight event that finishes when the sun comes up the next morning. The event ends with a closing ceremony and final lap around the track. By 3:00 a.m., the weather had turned cold, but the spirit of the event kept on going until it was time to go home.

We were determined to stay. As Jack and I shivered into the wee hours of morning, we talked about what an unbelievably meaningful event Relay for Life was for so many community members, and that maybe Relay would be nice to

"Many people told me how pleased they were to be asked for their help. It made them feel good to know that they could do something and I learned how important it is to ask."

— Evie Hammerman, M.S.W.

have in our own school district, Half Hollow Hills. Jack told me he would support my efforts a hundred percent. *Little did we know where this would take us.*

Two weeks later, with a Relay for Life marketing video in hand, I had an appointment to meet with my school district superintendent. I explained that Relay was a way to bring out our entire community—who today does not know someone whose life has been touched by cancer? After the hour-long meeting, my school district superintendent, Dr. Karnilow, had enough information to speak with the school board of trustees for their approval to host such an event and promised to be in touch with me after he did. During the last week of August in 2006, the call came that the school board of trustees approved bringing American Cancer Society's Relay for Life to Half Hollow Hills. With Dr. Karnittow's unwavering support, it was now time to ready a committee and find a co-chair to get this project off the ground. The more immediate task was finding someone willing to share the responsibility of running the event with me. Initially, I thought working with another cancer survivor would bring the same passion and commitment to chairing the event. What I actually learned is not everyone's cancer experience makes people feel the same way. After approaching a friend in the community, she explained it would put her family back to a very tumultuous time and make them feel as though they were going through the experience again. She was happy to support the event, but in her own quiet way. I was still in need of a co-chair.

Debbie Picker and I had known each other for close to eleven years. We had worked on numerous PTA committees and fundraising events for our sons' school over the years. When I explained the project I was about to embark on, Debbie was ready to jump in and roll up her sleeves. We called everyone who we had worked with on committees in the past and invited them to be part of our committee and journey. We managed to rally twenty-four other volunteers to round out the committee and we were off and running for a June 2007 event.

Our goal, as a committee, was to evangelize this new event so that we could get high community participation and fundraising. In years past, first-time events typically generated $30,000–$40,000. Although we never shared a fundraising goal with the community, we were all hoping that we could raise at least $100,000 our first year.

Even though this was a volunteer role, Debbie and I took it on with the vigor of a full-time job. It was not your typical two hours of volunteer activity for the week. For us to be truly successful, we set out to share information about the new upcoming event that would take place in June with over 10,000 students and staff members in the school district and the community at large. From September to June, we spoke in schools, religious organizations, local businesses, town libraries, PTA meetings and clubs to explain Relay. Conversations continued with local politicians and newspapers to help spread the word, too. Everyone on the committee brought something special to the event. From survivor dinner, raffle baskets, children's activities, logistics, security, sponsorships, luminary ceremony and entertainment, everyone felt a sense of ownership for their areas and shared our excitement. Relay for all of us was truly a labor of love!

June came, the weather was perfect, and more people than we ever could have imagined came out for Relay. Over 2,000 attendees and more than $250,000 was raised for our first year event! We were recognized by the American Cancer Society as the #1 Rookie Event for the Year in 2007 in the nation. What an honor!

For the following two years, Debbie and I continued to chair Relay, with our families helping in many capacities and a committee that grew in number and support. In three years, we can proudly say that the Half Hollow Hills community has raised over $600,000 for the American Cancer Society, added an annual event to our community calendar, and made a difference in the lives of many.

In April of 2010, I celebrated a major milestone in the life of a cancer survivor—five years well. I continue to count my blessings every day, trying not to sweat the small stuff and treasuring the gifts that each day brings. I will continue to support the work of the American Cancer Society so that more people will celebrate birthdays in the future. Life can pull out the carpet from underneath us sometimes… but I say, do flips!

Seventeen-Year Breast Cancer Survivor

Kathi Edelson Wolder

I was fifteen years old when I first learned about breast self-exam. It was late at night; I was reading a magazine. It was 1968—long before people talked openly, comfortably, matter-of-factly about breast cancer. I ran my hand over my breasts and discovered a lump. In tears and panic, I knocked on the door to my parents' bedroom. A trip to my mother's gynecologist, a lumpectomy (it was benign), and my journey had begun.

As I grew into a woman, I came to understand that I had densely fibrocystic breasts and that regular, diligent monitoring was the key to tracking what was normal and what was not. I had no idea just how diligent, until I moved from Massachusetts to New Jersey in 1991 and asked for my medical records to be sent. When they arrived, I read them. And what I read was (I'm paraphrasing), "this patient's breasts are so dense that it is impossible to tell a suspicious lump from an innocent one." It was a rude awakening. How would they know, then, if I *did* have breast cancer? I called Mount Sinai Hospital in New York and connected to a breast specialist there. We assembled a team, and every six months I saw "the team." A visit to the breast specialist, a mammogram and a sonogram, an extreme regimen perhaps, but it ultimately saved my life.

In 1992, another lump was found, another lumpectomy performed. I held my breath for days until I got the call from my doctor that it was benign. Phew.

FIBROCYSTIC BREASTS

Fibrocystic breasts are composed of tissue that feels lumpy or rope-like in texture. Doctors call this nodular or glandular breast tissue. It's not at all uncommon to have fibrocystic breasts. www.mayoclinic.org

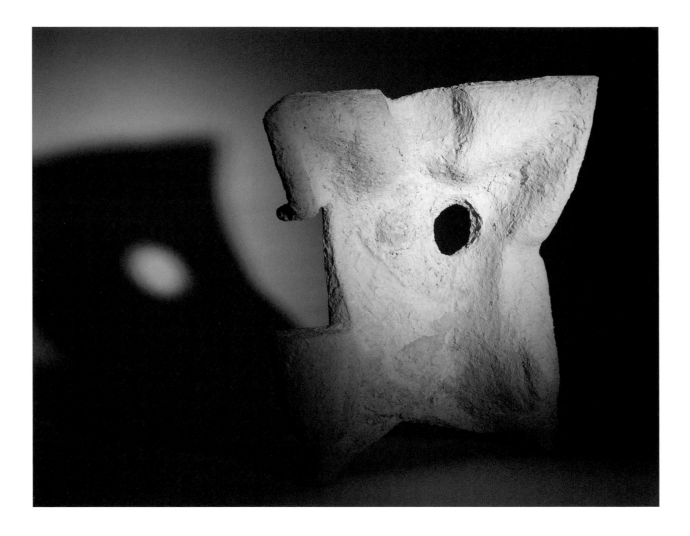

But four years later, I was not to be so lucky. At a routine exam, the sonogram revealed something unusual. Further investigation and a deep tissue biopsy of my right breast revealed that I had ductal carcinoma *in situ* (DCIS), a non-invasive, microscopic form of breast cancer that infiltrates the milk ducts. But that wasn't all. In my left breast, there were microcalcifications that might be a sign of more breast cancer to come. And, with DCIS in the right breast, there was, statistically, a 60% chance of occurrence in the other breast. Back then, the recommended treatment protocol for DCIS was a mastectomy—no chemotherapy, no radiation. The cure rate with a mastectomy, I was assured, was 99%. I had decisions to make, but I wasn't ready to think about it. I packed it all safely away in a corner of my brain, sent my parents home, left the doctor's office and went back to my job at a major arts organization to attend a patron event.

Later that night, I worked hard to keep the fear at bay and sat down at my computer. My father used to say that if you have difficulty making a decision, chances are you don't have enough information. And I didn't. So I pored over everything I could find online about DCIS, about mastectomies and about the various options for reconstruction. By dawn, I had reached an educated, but deeply soul-searched, decision. I was weary of the years and years of monitoring, tired of the find a lump, get an exam, wait a week in a panic for the results routine. I was not going to live the rest of my life waiting for the other shoe to drop. I would have a mastectomy.

For days, one giant thought kept churning through my brain: I have breast cancer; now I don't know how long I am going to live. I thought this over and over again until I was jolted by a profound revelation: I didn't know how long I was going to live *before* I knew I had breast cancer. Sounds simple, but it was a genuine eureka moment. The fear began to give way to a bubbling over stream of consciousness: *I am not about breasts.* They don't define who I am, and I am not going to let breast cancer define me either. Life is precious. Live it wisely. From now on. Never miss an opportunity to tell the people you care about that you love them. And when you come through this, remember to share what you know and what you've learned. Pay it forward.

Two months after my initial surgery in the right breast, I had a prophylactic mastectomy of the left breast, followed by reconstruction. I am free, I thought, from worrying about this forevermore. It was time to give back. In the fall of that same year, I shyly stepped up to a registration table for the Susan G. Komen® New York Race and was captivated—rescued, really—by the love and support of two Komen volunteers. Carol and Gail were both breast cancer survivors. They reached across the Survivor Registration Table, hugged me close in a three-way-embrace, and said: "you're not alone; we're here for you." They shared their stories. They listened to mine. They welcomed me; they recruited me into the remarkable sisterhood of survivors that permeates the Susan G. Komen organization. I became, at that defining moment, a tireless crusader for breast cancer awareness. I volunteered for their Speakers' Bureau and was sent out to speak to women's groups all over the metropolitan area about breast health and

"...I had to make a decision myself because ultimately it is the patient's responsibility, not the doctor's nor the spouse's."

— Sondra Schoenfeld

breast cancer awareness. I wanted to be that figurative poster child for breast cancer survival, a living, breathing early detection example to others. But I also wanted to tell women what I had learned: Know your own body. Take charge of your own breast health. Doctors are human, not demi-gods. Get educated—learn as much as you can, so that *you* are an active participant in your medical decisions. And don't allow fear to delay you, or prevent you from getting the care that may very well save your life. Early detection *does* save lives. It saved mine.

My journey, unfortunately, was not yet over. In 1998, I had a serendipitous event. While carrying a small, hard box, I slipped and fell. The corner of the box ruptured my right implant, and when I went to the plastic surgeon for a consultation, he discovered a very tiny lump just under the skin. He and my breast surgeon were quite sure that it was scar tissue. A biopsy revealed that it was not scar tissue, but rather a malignant invasive second occurrence. I was that mystical, impossible 1% recurrence, which was so rare and unusual, it became a case study at Mount Sinai. This time, however, I chose a bright young oncologist at Sloan-Kettering for my treatment who was, I was told, always on the cutting edge of the latest clinical trials. (If I ever needed one, I wanted to be sure my doctor knew about them.) We would break out all the guns this time— six months of chemotherapy followed by six weeks of radiation, and then five years on Tamoxifen.

This was a real test of survival, but I was not about to lose my poster child status. Soon into chemotherapy, I bought a treadmill for my apartment so that I could continue with my exercise regime. I bought a wig that perfectly matched my hairstyle, and later bought a second, cheaper wig just to wear to the gym. I set up a "salon" in my dining room and learned to style the wigs like a pro. I learned makeup techniques to mask my missing eyebrows and lashes, and continued in my job as a public relations director for a renowned crystal company, struggling with fatigue through evening events, but otherwise carrying on without skipping a beat. I had a fax machine and a laptop computer and worked at home during the five days I took off, every three weeks, for my chemotherapy sessions. I passed on Sloan-Kettering's suggestion that I participate in group sessions, but found comfort in the extraordinary network of support provided by my parents, my extended family at Komen, my friends and my work colleagues. Like a corps of personal cheerleaders, on my worst days, they reassured me that I was still beautiful and would survive this ordeal; at my best moments, they applauded me for my courage and perseverance.

Life is never the same after breast cancer; anyone who has taken the journey will attest to that. But what you learn along the way can be cathartic: There *is* life after breast cancer. Your hair and your sense of self grow back. Love is still a possibility—I married a wonderful man in 2004 and learned to love more deeply than I had ever imagined I could. And I learned from my fellow survivor volunteers at Komen that sometimes the best way to rekindle your spirit is to share a part of it with someone else who needs it.

Formation of a Chapter for the
Susan G. Komen® Organization

Kathi Edelson Wolder

The Susan G. Komen organization was founded on a heartfelt promise made by Nancy G. Brinker to her dying sister, Susie, that she would do everything in her power to end breast cancer forever. In that defining moment, a global breast cancer awareness movement began. Over the next thirty years, Affiliates in communities across the U.S. rose up to spread the word that early detection saves lives and to bring that mission to millions of underserved and uninsured women in their respective neighborhoods. The Susan G. Komen North Jersey Affiliate in Summit, New Jersey, is one of these powerful, passionate local armies. It was also founded on a promise—a promise made by Deborah Q. Belfatto to a ten-year-old girl who had just lost her mother to breast cancer.

It was 1988 and, as Deb would say, life was good. She was thirty-three years old and had been married to a wonderful man for five years. She had a beautiful little girl just two years old and owned her own children's clothing store—three of them, actually. Life was very, very good. Then she discovered a lump in her breast. Life was about to change for Deb in more ways than she'd ever imagined. She went to her gynecologist, a rather cavalier physician who reported that she had nothing to worry about because she was so young. "Nothing to worry about?" she thought. She pushed onward, positive that she did have something to worry about. When nothing showed up on a mammogram or a needle biopsy, she turned to her personal network to find a general surgeon who could and would help her get to the truth (breast specialists were extremely rare in her state in those days). A surgical biopsy confirmed that it was cancer and Deb was scheduled for a mastectomy. Following her instincts, she took control of her own health and body in a way that was unconventional for the time, and forged ahead to get a second opinion. She networked with family and friends to find a resource she felt she could trust with her life and headed to the University of Pennsylvania Hospital, renowned at the time for their multi-disciplinary approach to treating the disease. Though the team of doctors there had little experience developing treatment protocols for young women with breast cancer, they decided on a course for her that was fairly aggressive, but would spare her breast—a lumpectomy followed by chemotherapy and radiation.

All through what Deb describes as a very surreal time in her life, it became amazingly clear that because of her resources, her connections and her relationships, she had been able to seek out, and secure, the best medical care available; but what about the women who don't have this access to quality medical care? What about the women who don't have the network, the family, the friends and the support that Deb had? All of a sudden, breast cancer, already a presence in her life, became a driving force. She knew that she had to do something to make a difference for all those women in New Jersey for whom life-saving breast health care, screening and treatment services are out of reach geographically, financially, mentally and emotionally.

Then she met Jackie B., another young mother who had been diagnosed and was surviving. Her initial diagnosis was stage 1, but there was involvement of one lymph node and, five years later, Jackie lost her battle with breast cancer. Deb made a solemn promise to Jackie's ten-year-old daughter (the same age as Deb's own daughter) that she was going to do everything she could so that no little girl would ever have to face those fears, or lose her mommy, again.

That promise was to become a lifelong crusade for Deb. In 1996, after long hours of research, Deb, along with her two co-founders, Kathleen Hubert-McKenna and Lisa Herschli, traveled to Dallas and petitioned the national office of Susan G. Komen to bring Susan G. Komen to northern New Jersey. On June 17, 1997, after a year of arduous work with their organizing committee, Susan G. Komen North Jersey was born. It started in Deb's basement, grew into a small space and then finally moved into the famous pink-shuttered Komen House in Summit, New Jersey. More than an office, the headquarters quickly became known as a safe haven, a place where women (and men) could walk through the door and feel protected, supported and cared for.

It all began with "the power of one," the power of one courageous "can do/ will do" breast cancer survivor determined to make a difference. Today, Susan G. Komen North Jersey, our Affiliate, remains true to its original mission: to provide life-saving screening and treatment support services to women and men who cannot afford to pay for them, to educate people about breast health awareness and the importance of early detection, and to reach for a world where breast cancer will no longer touch the lives of so many North Jersey residents and their families.

Our Affiliate is just one of the one hundred and twenty local Komen Affiliates that are saving lives in cities and communities throughout the U.S. Through the Race for the Cure and other local events and activities, each Affiliate mobilizes and educates thousands of community members while raising funds to support community-based breast cancer programs. To date, this nationwide network of Affiliates—working in concert with more than 2,000 local organizations—has awarded more than $1.3 billion in local, needs-based community grants. Susan G. Komen is now the largest and most progressive grassroots organization in the world committed to ending breast cancer. Susan G. Komen North Jersey and all the organization's Affiliates are driven by an extraordinary passion for the cause: to provide access to quality breast health care education, screening and treatment to those who need it most; and to fund the most cutting-edge research to find better and more effective treatment options and hopefully, in our lifetime, a cure for breast cancer.

"In The Pink was established in 1999 with funds from the Susan G. Komen for the Cure North Jersey Affiliate."

— Aretha Hill-Forte

Cancer Hope Network Volunteer
Linda Kendler

Life takes the strangest twists and turns. Last week Cancer Hope Network sent me a thank-you note for seven years of volunteer service. Part of it read, "We could never say enough about what your kind words, thoughtful deeds and shared understanding have brought to those you have been matched with…" However, I did understand because, prior to my volunteering, I had used the Network's service to get help during my bout with thyroid cancer.

The chance to speak with someone who has gone through a similar experience and therefore can identify with common fears and questions makes a big difference for one's state of well-being.

I was terrified of my thyroid cancer, didn't know where to turn and believed in getting every possible bit of information available. When I called, my match listened to me carefully and thereby helped to alleviate much of my stress. Having cancer is difficult enough without having the stress factor pull one down even more. Now, I'm able to give back through Cancer Hope Network.

One year must pass before a survivor can be trained as a volunteer. Once trained, volunteers wait to be matched with callers who have a similar condition. If someone at the agency comes up with a match, they call. Knowing how terrible waiting for help can be, whenever possible, I call back the same day.

When someone calling through the Cancer Hope Network wants advice, I state that because something has worked for me, it isn't necessarily the answer for someone else. Then I listen. The most important factor is for each person to be comfortable with her individual choice. Personalities are different.

I have been matched with and spoken to over fifty patients experiencing either thyroid cancer or lobular carcinoma *in situ* (LCIS), in which the growth of abnormal cells increases a woman's chance of developing breast cancer later on in life.

In 1994 a doctor told me I had LCIS and promptly advised a lumpectomy. However, when my radiologist stated that because I had dense breasts, there might be a chance that it would not be possible to catch everything, I decided to have a double prophylactic mastectomy because I find stress is impossible to handle. It makes me crazy. LCIS was a danger signal for me.

I called hospitals in New York and New Jersey and proceeded to collect recommendations as well as information about various doctors. My ultimate choice was made in part based on the doctor having an office close to my home. Then my main concern was to get an appointment quickly. Waiting was not for me. When I arrived at the doctor's office, it became clear that my appointment would have to be altered due to an emergency. Upon realizing how serious my anxiety was, the receptionist made sure to have me come back later that afternoon.

"Breast cancers are an extremely diverse group of diseases that are treated very differently depending on their type. Therefore, proper diagnosis is essential."

— Christine Rizk, M.D.

The doctor was excellent. She referred me to someone who provided a relaxation tape to quiet me prior to the operation. This relaxation method was beneficial. I never regretted my decision to have a double mastectomy. My checkup was six months later and everything was fine.

A number of years after the initial cancer scare, my husband and I were enjoying a three-day holiday at the beach. It was in August 2002; the ocean was perfect. We went out on a friend's boat and on the last day went to a picnic. One of the other guests was being treated for non-Hodgkin's lymphoma. I remember thinking: "Thank heavens it's not me." On the following Monday I felt a pain in the right side of my neck. There was a lump there;. I examined it in the mirror every day; it was easy to detect and wasn't going away.

Maybe I had strained my neck while jumping in the waves or turned it the wrong way at the picnic? Cancer never entered my mind. Just to be sure there was no problem, I went to my primary care doctor for his opinion.

I had an MRI and was told there was a mass in my neck, so I found an ear, nose and throat surgeon from a list in a magazine of the best doctors. The doctor said he was not sure if I had cancer. He saw how nervous I was and explained it would be necessary to operate to find out what was going on. He found that I had an aggressive variant of papillary thyroid cancer that was also wrapped around my vocal cords.

I was worried, scared and confused because after the surgery it was necessary to go on a low iodine diet and go off my thyroid hormone to induce temporary hypothyroidism in order to get ready for the radioactive iodine treatment that kills off any residual thyroid cancer and thyroid tissue. Although my husband, other family members and friends were very supportive, I needed to speak to people who had gone through a similar experience.

It was then that I spoke with members of Cancer Hope Network and THYCA (Thyroid Cancer Survivors Association). These were people who had gone through similar situations and I felt so much better after speaking to them. They gave me encouragement, hope and support. What a difference they made for me!

Now it is nine years later and I get so much satisfaction from giving others support.

Cancer Hope Network: All About Hope

Joe Wojtowicz

Cancer Hope Network is an organization that is all about its middle name—hope. The national non-profit group was founded in 1981 by Diane Byrnes-Paul, an oncology nurse whose uncle had cancer. After undergoing treatment he told his niece that his anguish and emotional pain would have been greatly reduced if only he could have spoken to someone who had been through a similar cancer experience and had survived. It was a lament that Diane had heard before—from many of the cancer patients to whom she administered chemotherapy on a daily basis. She came to realize that those who had survived the same cancer, treatment and side effects were uniquely able to offer hope and support to despairing cancer patients.

Her idea has evolved into the Cancer Hope Network. This New Jersey-based national organization provides one-on-one support to cancer patients, and their families, on a free and confidential basis through a group of over three hundred and fifty trained support volunteers, all of whom are cancer survivors. Wanda Diak, CHN's Managing Director (and a survivor herself), notes: "We find that the patients in most need of help are those recently diagnosed with cancer. At that point many people are overwhelmed by a wide range of emotions and concerns. The combination of fear, anxiety, uncertainty and side effects causes many to despair."

Cancer Hope Network provides customized patient support at this critical time. When a patient calls the toll-free number, he or she is interviewed by a member of CHN's Patient Services Team and a patient profile is created. This profile is then matched against Cancer Hope Network's database of cancer survivors based on:

- the type of cancer the patient has;
- the treatment program the patient is undergoing;
- the side effects the patient is experiencing;
- the stage of the cancer; and
- various psychosocial factors, which include age, gender, marital status, whether children are involved, as well as the patient's level of understanding of the cancer experience.

Also included is the immediate major concern or need of the patient. This factor is virtually unlimited in its diversity.

The support volunteer most closely matched against the patient's profile and immediate concerns is then asked to contact the patient by telephone. If the match works well for the patient, additional support calls from the support volunteer can be requested by calling the Patient Services Team and they again notify the support volunteer.

The initial trauma of a malignant diagnosis is undoubtedly one of life's worst experiences and will remain so until a cure for cancer is found. Until then, Cancer Hope Network offers unique one-on-one support to help patients through this unknown and fearful experience. Through their internal and external resources, CHN shares the successful experiences of cancer survivors, dispelling fears, myths and uncertainty, and replacing those with a much better feeling—the feeling of hope.

Cancer Hope Network is non-sectarian, non-denominational and is not affiliated with any religious, political or commercial entity. It is funded totally

"...prior to my volunteering, I had used the Network's service to get help during my bout with thyroid cancer."

— Linda Kendler

by its own fundraising efforts. Cancer Hope Network's support volunteers do not endorse or recommend treatments, facilities or physicians. In addition to emotional support and encouragement, they provide practical information, helpful hints and methods for coping with diagnosis and treatment.

For more information about Cancer Hope Network and its support services, call toll-free (877) HOPENET or visit the website at www.cancerhopenetwork.org.

In The Pink:
Early Cancer Detection and Education Program
Aretha Hill-Forte, M.P.H.

In The Pink is a program at Saint Michael's Medical Center. The program's goal is to eradicate cancer as a life-threatening disease in our community. Saint Michael's Medical Center's mission is to provide excellence in health care to the communities we serve, integrating principles of inclusion, educating the next generation of care providers in the Franciscan tradition of compassion, dignity, respect and commitment to poor and marginalized persons. In The Pink is just one example of an education- and outreach-based program focused on early detection— imagine the benefits nationwide if every community had a similar program.

About the Program
The program provides outreach, education, screening and treatment for no or low cost for women and men. In The Pink Cancer Early Detection and Education Program promotes healthy behavior among underserved persons of the Essex County community.

In The Pink's primary focus is to increase the proportion of age-appropriate men and women who are screened for breast, cervical, colorectal and prostate cancer by:

> *"I turned forty years old recently. There was a time I didn't believe I could make it to forty."*
>
> — Meera Bagle

- decreasing barriers to screening and follow-up services;
- reaching out to engage high-risk men and women for screening services;
- educating the community about the value of cancer screening;
- increasing knowledge of cancer screening protocols among health professionals; and
- providing comprehensive navigation/case management services before, during and after the diagnosis of cancer.

In The Pink was established in 1999 with funds from the Susan G. Komen for the Cure North Jersey Affiliate. In 2001 the program became a Lead Agency for the Department of Health and Senior Services, New Jersey Cancer Education and Early Detection Program (NJCEED).

In The Pink has:

- educated over 40,000 women and men;
- funded more than 17,000 screening tests;
- developed and implemented innovative strategies to overcome barriers to screening;
- developed partnerships with key stakeholders to promote early detection.

For more information, call (973) 877-2989. To schedule a screening appointment,* call (973) 465-2792.

*Patients must meet eligibility criteria to receive free screenings.

Why?

Jeanette Joyce

It all started on a beautiful morning in May 1998. I was working as a mammography technologist. It was just before lunch and the radiologist had left for the day. I asked my co-worker if she would do a quick mammogram for me since it was time for my routine screening exam.

I had no reason to be anxious. At forty-two years of age, I had no family history of breast cancer and was in excellent health. I collected my films from the processor and looked at them on the view boxes. This was the turning point, since I knew at that moment that my life would never be the same again.

I could just hear what the radiologist's interpretation would be—multiple microcalcifications present, involving over a quarter of the breast, arranged in a branching pattern, pleomorphic, highly suspicious for malignancy, recommend biopsy.

This couldn't be happening. I pulled down a film and checked the patient identification. They were my films. There was no mistaking it. I had breast cancer. My God, please help me! How could this be happening? I have small children at home and they need their mother! I felt betrayed. Working in mammography for years, I never could have imagined this scene.

The next several months were a blur. Modified radical mastectomy to be followed by five years of hormonal therapy (Tamoxifen). The axillary lymph node dissection resulted in limited motion to my arm and shoulder so I made regular visits to a physical therapist. The thought of returning to work nearly paralyzed me and I gave much thought to changing occupations. A friend suggested that I sell Beanie Babies on the Internet. It was 1998 and they were all the rage at that time. Crazy suggestion.

The questions continued to nag me. Why was I diagnosed with breast cancer and what could be the cause? I tested negative for BRCA1 and BRCA2 genetic mutations, which meant it was not hereditary. I spent time researching all the possible risk factors and nothing made sense until I read more about reproductive factors. What I read both scared and angered me, resulting in insult upon injury and more pain. The choices I had made as a teenager may have resulted in my breast cancer.

My physician specialists refused to discuss it with me. They told me there was not enough evidence to support the studies. One doctor told me I had enough to worry about and shouldn't burden myself with the information. Another told me the subject was too explosive to even suggest!

There are studies that go back to 1957 that link abortion to breast cancer. Those first pregnancies that occur during the teen years ending in an abortion pose the highest risk of future breast cancer. What? Abortions are legal and we've been assured that they are safe procedures. It doesn't matter what your views are regarding abortion because this is a women's health issue! It is all about informed consent. If there is any increased risk of breast cancer in women choosing abortion, they have the right to this information so they can make an informed decision based on the evidence available.

> *"(In previous years) not many women knew that smoking not only increased their lung cancer risk, but their breast cancer risk by several hundred percent."*
>
> — Breast Cancer Prevention Institute

Oral contraceptives manufactured before 1975 exposed women to extremely high doses of hormones, and they too caused an increased risk of future breast cancer. But more recently, in 2002, the National Institute of Environmental Health Sciences labeled steroidal estrogen a "known carcinogen," which is the same estrogen present in birth control pills and hormone replacement therapy.[1,2]

More federal studies are needed in order to better understand how these hormones work and the effects they have on our bodies. Until that information becomes available, we must concentrate on the early detection of breast cancer by mammography. Breast cancer detected early is often curable. The only tool available to catch early *in situ* breast cancer, before it becomes palpable, is routine annual mammography beginning at the age of forty.

I am alive today because I decided to have a screening mammogram when I was forty-two years old. We must do all we can to convince other women that this valuable screening tool could save their lives. I am in a wonderful position now. As a breast cancer survivor, mammography technologist and breast health educator, my passion is to make a difference in women's lives. When a woman receives a diagnosis of breast cancer, I am there to walk beside her and help her to stay focused on the future. And for as long as I can, I will continue saving women's lives, one mammogram at a time!

1. http://ntp.niehs.nih.gov/ntp/roc/twelfth/profiles/EstrogensSteroidal.pdf
2. World Health Organization IARC monographs (2007) 91 pg 169 #5.2, pg 175 #5.5

Breast Cancer Prevention Institute

Angela Lanfranchi, M.D., F.A.C.S.

In 1999 the Breast Cancer Prevention Institute, a 501(c)3 charitable corporation, was started by three physicians and a professor of endocrinology. The incidence of non-invasive breast cancer had risen over 400% and the incidence of invasive breast cancers had risen 40% in young women. My three colleagues and I agreed that, while there were many organizations concerned with cancer victims and looking for a cure, there were none looking at ways that would help women prevent breast cancer.

In 2001 the Breast Cancer Prevention Institute presented results from a research project, supported by a grant from the Susan G. Komen Foundation, at the San Antonio Breast Cancer Symposium. Despite that success, we did not reach the women who needed to know how to accurately assess their risks for breast cancer and what they could do to reduce their risk. The Breast Cancer Prevention website was created in 2002. The website was soon followed by the first edition of our booklet titled *Breast Cancer Risks and Prevention*. That booklet explained the biology and physiology of the breast so that women could understand why some things they were exposed to increased their risk and why other things could decrease their risk. The booklet made sense of the increase in women with breast cancer by discussing the changes in the average woman's life over the last thirty-five years. Many women did not know that smoking both increased their lung and breast cancer risk by several hundred percent. Within a few short years, after searching the words "breast cancer prevention," our website appeared on the first page of search results. The Breast Cancer Prevention Institute became a national and international source of information for women and medical professionals. The booklet was placed online with all the references.

The Breast Cancer Prevention Institute continues to be at the forefront of prevention. We informed women that hormone replacement therapy (HRT) was a risk for breast cancer three years before it became more widely known through the publicity surrounding the publication of the Women's Health Initiative Study. We also made women aware that the same drugs that were in HRT were in the oral contraceptives that premenopausal women took, except that they were in much higher doses in oral contraceptives. Most women are still unaware of this, despite oral contraceptives being classified as a Group 1 carcinogen, the same group as cigarettes, by the World Health Organization.[1] We tell women about the healthy and natural ways they can control their fertility through natural family planning techniques. On our website are the papers published by our board members, in journals and brochures, which highlight lesser known risk and preventive factors. Women are made aware that reproductive factors can either decrease or increase their risk of breast cancer.

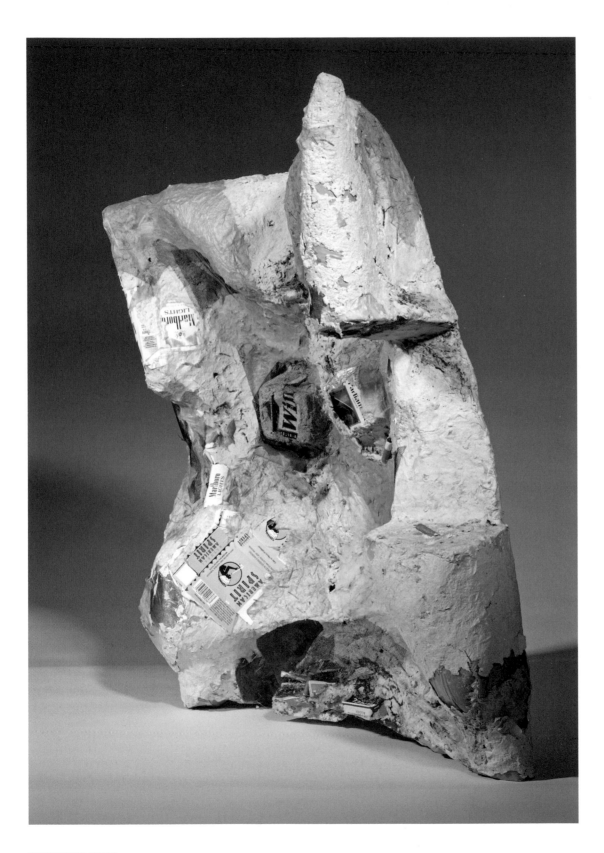

QUITTING TIME

Women should know that early full-term pregnancy lowers breast cancer risk and delaying pregnancy into their thirties and beyond may not be optimal for breast health.[2]

Clear explanations and diagrams with supporting references make this lesser known information easy to understand, giving women information they need to consider when making important decisions.

My mission, as President of the Breast Cancer Institute and as a breast cancer surgeon, is to see fewer women suffer through treatments for breast cancer. Through speaking engagements and articles I have been able to keep both professionals and the public informed about the progress made in the prevention and treatment of breast cancer. My audiences have included the United Nations' Commission on the Status of Women and Children, government personnel in the U.S., Canada, Australia and New Zealand, and medical schools in South Africa and India and the U.S. My articles have appeared in medical and bioethics journals in the U.S. and Europe.

In order to support the Institute's educational mission, all of our informational materials are free and available for download on our website, www.bcpinstitute.org. There are no membership dues but we are supported in our mission by the donations of those who have found our work valuable. All of our officers and professionals on our board are unpaid volunteers.

We want to continue to grow as an organization so we can make our materials more widely available to and known by the public. We know how much we've been appreciated by the letters of thanks and support that we receive by those who have used our website or have had their questions answered. We have been encouraged to continue as an organization because of the national and international interest we have received.

We can be reached through our toll-free number, 1-86-NO-CANCER (1-866-622-6237), or our website, www.bcpinstitute.org.

1. World Health Organization IARC monographs (2007) 91 pg 169 #5.2, pg 175 #5.5
2. Lord et al., Cancer Epidemiological Biomarkers Prev. Breast Cancer Risk etc. (2008) 17 (7) 1723–30

Searching for Answers—
*Two perspectives on research and
programs that look to the future*

Growth Hormone-Releasing Hormone and Its Analogs in Cancer

Andrew V. Schally, Ph.D., Nobel Prize Laureate

Among the avenues of research that doctors hope will one day lead to a cure for cancer, very important work has been done in isolating factors that can halt the growth of tumors. GHRH antagonists inhibit the growth of a variety of human cancers and thus appear to provide an exciting alternative to chemotherapy.

There is a universal agreement that the present methods of cancer treatment must be improved. This short overview deals with a new class of anti-tumor compounds called GHRH antagonists, which are related to a natural peptide hormone found in the brain known as growth hormone-releasing hormone (GHRH). Antagonists are compounds that act against the effect of the named material while agonists, on the contrary, act to enhance it. GHRH antagonists show great promise, free of side effects in experimental studies, as an effective therapy for various cancers.

In the years 1954–73 I was deeply committed to pioneering work on the demonstration of the existence of hormones in the hypothalamic[1] region of the brain. After revealing their biological activities, this undertaking involved the purification, structural identification and chemical synthesis of several neurohormones from this region of the brain including TRH[2] (*thyrotropin-releasing hormone*), LH-RH[3] (*luteinizing-hormone-releasing hormone*) and somatostatin.[4] Among the hormonal activities we demonstrated in 1965 was GHRH, but because GHRH was present in microscopic quantities, no structural work could be undertaken. The successful work on TRH and LHRH eventually led to my being awarded the Nobel Prize in Physiology and Medicine in 1977. The Nobel Prize made it possible for me to meet with top medical leaders in various countries and become acquainted with international health problems, among them cancer. As early as 1971 we began to make synthetic modifications of the structures of hypothalamic hormones in order to make more potent agonistic analogs, or conversely their antagonists to nullify their effects.

Our approach to treating cancer was based on the synthesis of novel peptides (a chain of different amino acids linked together). I was profoundly influenced by the enormous activity of these analogs in normal subjects, as well as in patients with various malignancies. I thought that we should take advantage of the high activity of both agonistic and antagonistic analogs of hypothalamic hormones, and after 1975 I became more and more interested in their therapeutic applications in the cancer field.

Consequently, I decided to switch my field from neuroendocrinology to endocrine oncology and focus my work on cancer therapy. We concentrated our early efforts on prostate cancer and in 1979–82 we developed a new method for treatment of hormone-dependent prostate cancer based on LHRH analogs, which is still the preferred therapeutic approach today. In 1981 the production of GHRH, occurring in abnormal locations, was demonstrated in carcinoid and pancreatic tumors. In 1982 this allowed two independent groups to isolate and characterize GHRH extracted from pancreatic tumors that had caused enlargement of bones of the head. Two forms of GHRH, consisting of 44- and 40-amino acids, respectively, were structurally identified in these tumors but their full intrinsic biological activity was only present in that segment of GHRH which contained the first 29 amino acids [GHRH (1-29)NH$_2$]. Subsequently, GHRH was isolated from human and animal hypothalami. Later, various groups, including my own, started to synthesize analogs of GHRH (1-29)NH$_2$ for clinical and veterinary applications. We also became involved in clinical trials with GHRH.

In the following decade, diverse experimental and clinical studies were conducted. In 1993 we began the development of antagonists. We felt that GHRH antagonists could offer distinctive advantages over other classes of prospective anti-tumor agents. Therapy with GHRH antagonists would not cause the severe side effects typical of chemotherapy. Since IGF-1 and IGF-2 (insulin-like growth factors) are potent growth factors for many cancers, a suppression of their production would inhibit tumor growth. GHRH antagonists could also be used for the suppression of tumors that do not show the presence of receptors for somatostatin (SST), such as human bone cancers, or those that contain only low levels of SST receptors, such as pancreatic cancers. Several series of antagonistic analogs of GHRH have been synthesized in our laboratory in the past seventeen years. We have shown that GHRH antagonists inhibit the growth of diverse human cancers such as pancreatic, colorectal, prostatic, breast, renal, glioblastomas (aggressive brain tumors), small and large cell lung cancer, ovarian and endometrial cancers, osteosarcomas and non-Hodgkin's lymphomas.

The production of GHRH in the tissue and the presence of mRNA (messenger RNA) for the gene of GHRH was demonstrated in cell lines of prostatic, breast, ovarian and endometrial cancers, small cell lung cancer, osteosarcomas, and specimens of human prostatic, breast, ovarian and endometrial cancers. Thus, GHRH is present in various human cancers and appears to function as a growth factor on the cells which generated it. Early GHRH antagonists have been tested clinically and shown to exert inhibitory effects on GH secretion.

Further development of GHRH antagonists should lead to potential therapeutic agents for various cancers. Recent findings also reveal that GHRH agonists, after lying unexploited for some seventeen years, may find important applications in cardiology, diabetes and wound healing. I hope that the discovery of GHRH will lead to practical clinical use of its analogs in the field of cancer treatment and to other applications.

"Meera is the sister of my heart and together we share the same reason for walking— so our daughters will not have to."

— Tracy Redling

Glossary
1. The hypothalamus controls certain metabolic processes and other activities of the autonomic nervous system. It synthesizes and secretes neurohormones, often called hypothalamic-releasing hormones. These hypothalamic-releasing hormones control and regulate the secretion of pituitary hormones. www.news-medical.net
2. Thyroid-releasing hormone (TRH) (also known as TRF or thyrotropin-releasing factor) is a byproduct of the hypothalamus and serves to stimulate the pituitary gland to produce the thyroid-stimulating hormone (TSH). www.biology-online.org
3. Luteinizing-hormone-releasing-hormone (LH-RH) is produced in the hypothalamus and regulates the release of luteinizing hormone by the pituitary gland. http://dictionary.reference.com/browse/Lhrh
4. Somatostatin is a hormone that is widely distributed throughout the body, especially in the hypothalamus and pancreas, that acts as an important regulator of endocrine and nervous system function by inhibiting the secretion of several other hormones such as growth hormone, insulin and gastrin. www.MedicineNet.com

Good Treatment and Good Science
Richard Margolese, M.D., C.M., F.R.C.S.(C.)

The key to good treatment is good science. Good clinical trials provide evidence that the chosen treatment offers the best chance for success. Some of the most confusing aspects of cancer treatment are alternative therapies, prevention issues and second opinions.

No sooner does someone receive a diagnosis of cancer than they are swamped with recommendations for treatments from well-meaning friends and relatives. Although many of these suggestions appear to be very attractive, especially when viewed against the fears and anxieties accompanying a cancer diagnosis, they too often represent unproven and worthless treatments.

Alternative Therapies
There are many ways to help cancer patients outside of specific treatments. "Alternative" suggests a choice of one or the other, so a better description might be "additional" therapies. These encompass all of the support mechanisms: nursing, social services, psychological support and best efforts of friends and family to help one go through the trials and difficulties of cancer treatments, and they can be very helpful. They do not involve unproven therapies such as massage, naturopathy, homeopathy, acupuncture, touch therapy, QiGong, and unusual diets, all of which fall under the heading commonly known as alternative therapies. The best definition of an alternative therapy is: "it doesn't work." If it did work it would be mainstream medicine, not alternative. All of these alternatives have been carefully tested by good scientific methods, and when they are, they are shown to be useless in treating cancer.

Prevention Issues

The best treatment for cancer is prevention. We know we can prevent most lung cancers and many G.I. tract cancers by not smoking. It is an indication of how resistant people are to good ideas that so many people continue to smoke. This is similar to the success of unproven therapies despite evidence that they are useless.

For prevention of other common cancers, the situation is complex. Unfortunately, the concept of prevention is somewhat oversold and we cannot do as well as we would like with the tools we have. There are many books and articles urging better eating and exercising. Of course we should all eat a prudent diet, and yet many people who do will still develop cancer. The problem is that cancers (and other common diseases like heart disease) are very common and have complex causes so that there is no simple pathway to prevention. Many studies show a benefit from a good diet, but the effect is small—sort of like driving on the highway at a slightly slower speed—safer, but not by much.

Contrary to common perception, we are not in the midst of a cancer epidemic. Most of the increase in cancer in recent decades is explained by the increasing number of elderly people. While cancer too often does happen in younger people, it is essentially a disease of aging and the failure of normal defense mechanisms, which protect us when we are younger. To date, despite loudly trumpeted claims to the contrary, there is little settled evidence that any diet or food additive will prevent cancer.

That leaves us with a few bright spots that we can exploit. Colonoscopy can discover precancerous polyps, which can be removed before they turn into an invasive cancer. If we could apply this intervention universally, we could possibly eliminate almost all deaths from colon cancer. Some breast cancers can be prevented in high-risk women with an anti-estrogen drug like Tamoxifen. Important clinical trials have shown that, among high risk-women, the incidence of cancer is reduced by 50% with very few serious side effects. The normal risk for a forty-year-old woman is only 4% so this intervention is reserved for high-risk women.

Second Opinions

Second opinions can sometimes be worthwhile but can also be confusing if the two opinions don't agree, and the patient must become the referee. If your doctor is patient and calming and provides understandable information with explanations and answers to questions, a second opinion may not contribute much. Many cancers have more than one acceptable treatment, which can cause confusion and anxiety in patients.

We never have symposiums on how to treat appendicitis—that is a settled issue—but because cancer is not always cured, different therapies are tried and evaluated, often without major differences in outcome. This does not mean doctors are confused, just that differences exist and this must be understood and accepted. For example, Tamoxifen and Arimidex are two anti-estrogen type treatments given after surgery. They both help prevent the recurrence of cancer, almost equally, and it can be difficult to say that one is preferable. Doctors often choose by the side effects, which differ more noticeably, although both are very safe. Often, a calm discussion between patient and doctor can bring out a clear view of possible alternatives and lead to a comfortable choice for that patient.

Progress in Research and Clinical Trials

In the last few decades we have seen real progress. Breast surgery has changed from very radical procedures to breast conserving treatments. The use of anti-estrogens and chemotherapies as adjuncts to surgery has led to improved survival rates. Unfortunately, not everyone is helped by the chemotherapy. Further research is now ongoing to find those tumor characteristics associated with better responses to specific treatments. The hope is to tailor the treatment more specifically to each patient's personal tumor characteristics. Some women with breast cancer may be treated with chemotherapy before surgery in order to be able to observe the response of the tumor and to improve outcomes. Treating patients in different ways is usually done in a carefully controlled scientific program called a clinical trial. Participation in a clinical trial often provides access to new treatments before they become standard. Since all progress is made in this fashion, it is clearly worthwhile for patients to enroll in clinical trials when they can. The clinical trial process has helped us improve survival outcomes by comparing treatments. The old treatment is compared against the new and if the new treatment is found to be superior, this treatment becomes the new standard. Then, this newfound treatment is later compared against the next new hopeful idea. Clinical trials have also taught us which treatments can be avoided because they are not helpful or are actually harmful. Clinical trials are the main tool guiding us in evaluating the world of all medical advancement.

"…I heard of a study being conducted by some doctors in Montreal hospitals about early diagnosis of breast cancer. I wanted to help…and volunteered as a subject."

— Sushma Prasada

Summing It All Up—
Inspiration and information

A Relay for Life
Alicia Rockmore

It is Monday morning and I am reflecting on what an incredible three days I just experienced. Yes, I am tired and sore and the pouring rain was not pleasant, but it was an experience of a lifetime and none of it would have been possible without the support of everyone involved. As a matter of fact, on Saturday when I would have loved to get in a shuttle and be driven back to camp, it was everyone on the relay that kept me motivated and going to get it done.

I cannot put into words how moving the experience was, but let me say when you see thousands of people coming out to cheer you on, multiple times each and every day (rain or shine), because they have been touched by this disease, it is overwhelming. I saw kids coming out to walk for lost moms, husbands who have lost wives, friends who have lost their "breast friend" and survivors (both very young and old) at every turn. They were cheering us on, making us laugh (the "melon men" are a personal favorite) and giving us everything from candy, to Kleenex, to margaritas and French toast. Then I realized why this was so important.

The third day had lots of rain and wind, but as we got four blocks from the finish line we stopped off for a celebratory lunch: pizza, beer, french fries and sliders. The food just kept coming! We were joined by some family and friends (my daughter, Lucy, and my husband, Adam, were there) and then walked (in the sunshine) the last four blocks through a sea of cheers and many familiar faces from the three-day journey. Lucy walked with me, holding my hand, and got a glimpse of why this was worth mommy's time and effort. As I crossed the finish line she was crying. I thought maybe the crowds were scaring her, but instead she just hugged me and said, "I am so proud of you Mommy and I love you."

The walk in October 2010 in San Diego, CA, with 4,000 women, raised almost $11 million dollars!

> *"Two years later, when I participated in a walk for breast cancer awareness, there was a sign-up table for routine mammograms at the local hospital. I decided it was time to submit to one and stop being foolish about it."*
>
> — Lori Cohen

What Kept Me Going
Lori Cohen

When I sat down to write about my experience with breast cancer, I began to think about what kept me going. Two years prior to having a mammogram, I had brain surgery for a cavernoma, which is a cluster of blood vessels. I learned that many people have them and live their lives without ever knowing it. In my case, it began to bleed, and that was the start of the problem. Needless to

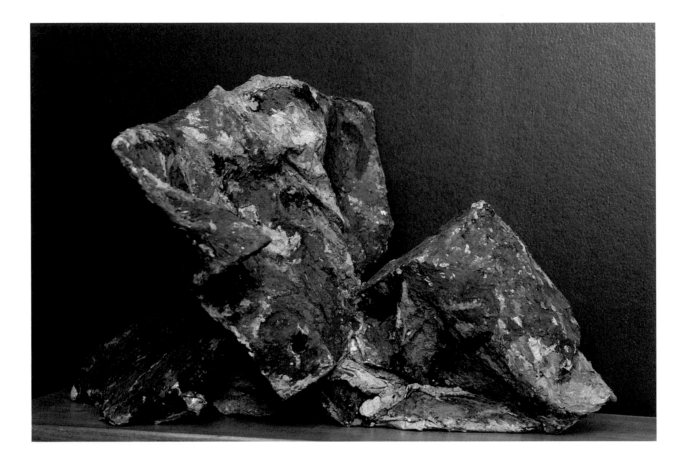

DETERMINATION

say, after that experience, I wasn't anxious to have a routine mammogram the following year.

Two years later, when I participated in a walk for breast cancer awareness, there was a sign-up table for routine mammograms at the local hospital. I decided it was time to submit to one and stop being foolish about it.

During the mammogram the technician saw something suspicious and proceeded to do further tests and, ultimately, a needle biopsy. A week later I got the call we all hope never comes. It was cancer. After the tears and the "why me?" I looked up the credentials of several breast surgeons and called three of the best for consultations.

Once the surgery was done, I met with oncologists for the proposed treatment. I was not convinced, after hearing the statistics, that the regimens they recommended would make that much of a difference. Only after I spoke to two survivors did I realize how important it was to know you did everything necessary to fight the cancer.

My son, at the time, was twelve and I needed to be strong and persevere. My husband was amazingly supportive. He sat by my side each time I went for chemotherapy and told me how beautiful I was without my hair.

A year later my son was a Bar-Mitzvah. His speech was about how proud he was of me and my fight against breast cancer. Needless to say, there wasn't a dry eye in the synagogue.

In the last five years, I have volunteered with Breast Friends and Gilda's Club, two organizations that provide cancer support. It is so important to be able to provide encouragement to others who are experiencing the fears we have encountered ourselves.

"It is normal to feel anxious and scared."

— Evie Hammerman, M.S.W.

Avon Walk
Tracy Redling

I suppose it wasn't until the mid-to-late 1980s that I remember breast cancer really surfacing and causing people to become concerned. Pink ribbons were ubiquitous and women were being diagnosed. Organizations and corporations clamored to become involved; fundraising for the cause seemed to take off overnight. Looking back, I was in my early twenties and about to attend my first of many charitable events for breast cancer. It was the Boca Raton Women's Council of Realtors Bachelor Auction, whereby I contributed to the cause by purchasing a wonderful man who eventually became my husband. Little did I know that breast cancer was not going away any time soon.

I firmly believe that as citizens of the planet we each need to pick a few charities and support them to the best of our ability. Of the several causes near and dear to me, finding the cure for breast cancer is one of them. Although breast cancer has not affected me directly, it has affected dozens of people in my life. Unfortunately, today, one would be hard-pressed to find a person who didn't know of someone diagnosed with this dreadful disease.

The Avon Walk for Breast Cancer entered my radar screen around ten years ago, when a friend of mine who lives in New York City told me that she would be "walking" in October. I'll never forget how her face lit up when she talked about "the walk." At the time I didn't understand how one person among 5,000 other walkers could possibly make a difference.

A few years later I became friends with Meera, who happened to be a breast cancer survivor. Diagnosed at thirty-one years old in 2000, not long after giving birth to her daughter, Meera battled breast cancer with surgery, chemotherapy, radiation, five years of Tamoxifen and is now a ten-year survivor. Meera is the sister of my heart and together we share the same reason for walking—so our daughters will not have to.

In October 2005, Meera and I, along with our dear husbands, each decided to raise the mandatory $1,800 and participate in the New York City Avon Walk for Breast Cancer. We subsequently walked the next five years, having recently completed our sixth walk in April 2011 in Washington, DC. Each walk is special and significant for one reason or another, but we all agree that that very first walk was the best.

I never really understood why people walked for causes until I did it myself. There is something extremely empowering about standing among 5,000 strangers who have gathered together over a weekend for one common cause. In this case, ending breast cancer. There is an enormous sea of people in pink pounding the pavement of New York City for two days. This is certainly not going to go unnoticed.

The Walk takes place on Saturday and Sunday on different weekends in nine cities across the country. On Event Eve walkers check in at the host hotel and take care of any last-minute details. Along with the various sponsor booths, there is a table covered with 12"x10" white pieces of coated paper with "I'm Walking For:" across the top. The purpose here is to write the names of the people for whom we are walking and pin it to the back of one's shirt. These little "bibs" (the same ones used in marathons) serve not only as inspiration to each individual walker but to all of the other participants along the route since they seem to initiate conversation as well as inspire and energize walkers, especially during those last miles of each day.

Opening ceremonies usually begin by about 6:30 on Saturday morning. Music is blasting as everyone steadily streams in through the cool, crisp air. The sun isn't even up, yet the walkers are jazzed up and ready to go. There are welcoming remarks and the crowd revs up. A few minutes pass, some last-minute stretching and we are off.

I can tell you that walkers come in all shapes and sizes, colors and socio-economic backgrounds. Sixteen is the minimum age to participate. Most of the people are probably in their thirties and forties. Many people walk in teams

"When you see thousands of people coming out to cheer you on, multiple times each and every day (rain or shine), because they have been touched by this disease, it is overwhelming."

— Alicia Rockmore

for a mutual friend, family member, neighbor or co-worker. There was one story about a man who pushed his wife in her wheelchair the entire distance because she was undergoing treatment. There are many women walking who are undergoing treatment. Survivors also walk. Most participants are women and the cheering stations go wild when they spot an occasional man in the crowd. There are always people who walk alone. One year we met a man whose mom had recently lost her battle to the disease and he decided to walk in her honor. I suspect it was his way of grieving. Not all are fit as a fiddle to walk thirty-nine miles over two days or are able to easily write a check for $1,800. But they do it. In fact, most are the complete antithesis because it is not about that. It's not an athletic competition or about who has the biggest bank account. It's about coming together with others to raise awareness and put an end to breast cancer.

I hate asking people for money. It's pretty much my least favorite thing to do among my friends and family. But I do it anyway. To make a significant difference with regards to supporting ongoing research, make early detection an option for the uninsured, provide screening, support and treatment, money is needed... and a lot of it! From my perspective, the Avon Walk is extremely well organized. I can only guess how many countless hours go into planning and executing such an event. Rest stops, snacks, meals, toilets and medical care are just a few of the things that have to be well planned to make the walk a successful one. It simply would not be worth the effort to coordinate such an event without netting millions of dollars.

I walk regularly for exercise throughout the year so walking twenty-plus miles in one day is not that hard. The critical thing is to put miles on your feet. If your feet are in shape, you are good to go. One year we walked thirty miles the first day and I can tell you that was not fun at all. Everyone was in a great mood for the first twenty or so miles and then the pain set in and people were cranky. I would never do that many miles in one day again. Personally, I don't think it's necessary to walk yourself into extreme pain and discomfort. Fewer people will not be diagnosed with breast cancer by walking until you can't stand up. There are other walkers who want to feel the pain. Good for them. You will not save any more lives by walking until you feel like your feet will fall off.

The overwhelming highlight of completing the Avon Walk is the closing ceremonies. As much as people are jazzed up and ready to go during the opening ceremonies, it is the closing ceremonies when the emotion comes crashing down like a ton of bricks. Particularly in New York City, the feeling in the air is exhilarating, palpable and downright electrifying. Thousands of people gather to cheer the walkers and to bring the weekend to a close. Usually around the last half mile or so, friends and family members meet up to cross the finish line with their loved ones who have just spent the past two days walking. Approaching the finish line, the scene is always the same, and this is usually the precise moment when the tears cannot be held back any longer—the kids. It really hits home seeing so many little kids lined up with their dads anxiously waiting to see their moms come through the finish line, many of whom are survivors. It is an in-your-face type of reminder that so many women are diagnosed shortly after giving birth. Here at the finish line is proof of that. I have no idea what the statistics are but it is a very emotional scene witnessing little kids cheering and waiting for their moms. This scene is etched in my mind and is the reason I continue to walk.

Inspiring Hope
Angela Lanfranchi, M.D., F.A.C.S.

The narrations and artwork in this book are intended to inspire hope, both in women with breast cancer and in their loved ones. After all, cancer, especially when associated with the breast, can strike fear in the hearts of the most resourceful and resilient of women.

Breast cancer not only affects a woman. It affects her spouse, family, friends and can be especially hard on children. The narrations are by women who rose to the challenge. What better way to conquer fear than with the grace of hope? Hope in a cure. Hope in prevention. Hope that whatever the challenge is, they will be able to surmount it and live their lives to the fullest each day into their survivorship.

Every October during Breast Cancer Awareness Month, we all hear that one in eight women, or 12.5% of women, will develop breast cancer in their lifetime. That is the cumulative lifetime risk for breast cancer, which is a statistically derived number that assumes all women will live to the age of eighty-two and not die of something else first. Many times, women hear that number one in eight and they look about the room and start counting off, one, two, three… they believe that someone in that room will get breast cancer if there are more than eight present.

But we also need to know that if a women has *no* risks for breast cancer (other than that she is a woman, living in this country and getting older) her risk of getting breast cancer is only 3.3%. Unfortunately, few women have no risk factors but even if a woman has a factor that increases her risk 100%, or doubles her breast cancer risk, that is now only 6.6%. That's a lot different from one in eight. We also need to hear that a woman's chance of dying from breast cancer in this country is one in thirty-five, or less than 3%.[1]

So can we really hope for a cure?
Most women are unaware that it's already happening. Lots of women are being cured without great fanfare. One is only officially cured of breast cancer when one dies of something else first, like a heart attack in old age. That's just how statistics are done and reported. We hear about five- and ten-year survival rates. Maybe some ten-year survivors will have a relapse of cancer. So we have to wait until they die of something else first before we say they were cured.

But what about women who have stage 0 breast cancer, also known as ductal carcinoma *in situ* or DCIS? With a partial mastectomy and radiation, they have a 97% cure rate. With mastectomy they have a 99.9% cure rate. No chemotherapy is needed to cure them. According to the American Cancer Society, there were 62,280 women diagnosed with *in situ* breast cancer in 2009. We can expect that a *minimum* of 60,411 will be cured!

What about women with stage 1 invasive breast cancers? Those are the women with small tumors, less than three quarters of an inch, which have not spread to the lymph nodes under the arm. Those women have a 95% cure rate. At the hospital where I work, 53% of all patients who are found to have cancer just because they went for a screening mammogram (nobody thought they had cancer when they were screened), 53%, or over half, were stage 0 and stage 1. That's why mammograms are so important. They give women excellent odds for a cure. No bookie would take a bet against them. Based upon data when treatment wasn't as sophisticated and effective as it is now, the five-year survival rate for tumors up to two inches and which had already spread to local lymph nodes, or stage 2 breast cancers, is 86%. So I do believe there will be even higher cure rates in the future.

We know for sure that there is hope for prevention
Look at what happened in 2002 after the Women's Health Initiative Study[2] became known to the public because it made the news. Women found out that Pempro® (conjugated estrogens and medroxyprogesterone) hormone-replacement therapy (HRT) increased breast cancer risk by 26%. That summer 15 million, or half of the 30 million women that were on HRT, abruptly stopped. As one of my patients said, "I'd rather have hot flashes than cancer." Just a few years later in 2007, it was reported that there was an 11% decline in breast cancer rates in women over fifty with estrogen receptor positive cancers. After much scientific debate, those in the medical field conceded that the decline in rates was attributable to the reduction in the use of HRT.

Information that these hormones could cause breast cancer was in the medical literature for over twenty years. But when that knowledge was put in the hands of women who needed and considered it, many acted upon it and breast cancer rates fell.

What do you think will happen when women learn that these same hormones are in oral contraceptives but in much higher doses? Will half of the 75% of premenopausal women in the U.S. who take hormonal contraceptives stop these hormones like their mothers did after menopause? What if they learn that in 2005 the UN's World Health Organization listed oral contraceptives as Group 1 carcinogens,[3] the same group that contains asbestos and cigarettes?

As acknowledged in an authoritative text,[4] each full-term pregnancy is associated with a 3% reduction in premenopausal breast cancer risk and a 12% reduction in risk of postmenopausal breast cancer.

Let's be more than aware in Breast Cancer Awareness Month. You'd have to be deaf, dumb and blind not to be aware that breast cancer exists and is a threat

"I am a very lucky seventy-four-year-old woman who has had two cancers in the past five years. The first was breast cancer and then, two years later, colorectal cancer. Early detection was the key to discovering the equivalent of a cure in both cases."

— Evie Hammerman, M.S.W.

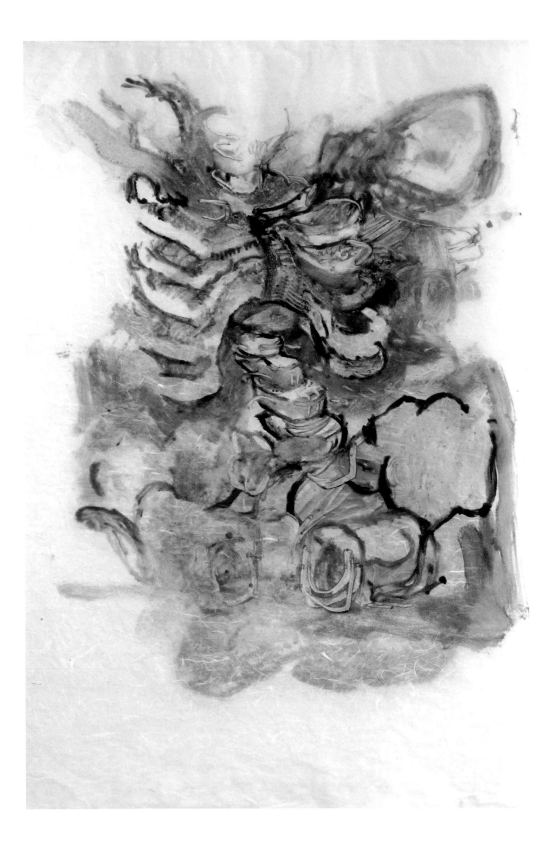

IMAGE EARLY

to many women. It's on the TV news and cable channels, radio, the Internet, magazines, newspapers and even the shopping channel. As a patient once told me, "You can't even go to the grocery store in October without being faced with pink ribbons on food containers to benefit one organization or another."

Let's be proactive and not just aware that breast cancer is curable in many cases if not in at least half of those diagnosed with screening mammograms. We already know a great deal about what causes breast cancer and what can increase a woman's risk. Breast cancer is not the fickle finger of fate randomly pointed at women. There are many other avoidable risks. We can hope and expect to reduce breast cancer rates with prevention.

Hope in survivorship

There are 2.5 million survivors of breast cancer in our country right now. It would be a shame if they worried every day that their cancer might come back, waiting for the other shoe to drop, not able to enjoy life to the fullest and not knowing how to reduce the risk of it coming back. They need to know that there are a number of wonderful national survivorship programs with branches throughout the U.S., programs that help women to overcome the challenges of survivorship.

1. Susan Love M.D., Breast Book 2nd ed., Addison Wesley (1995) pg 146.
2. Writing Group for the Women's Health Initiative Investigators. Risks and Benefits of Estrogen Plus Progestin in Healthy Postmenopausal Women JAMA (2002); 288:321–333.
3. World Health Organization IARC monographs (2007) 91 pg 169 #5.2, pg 175 #5.5.
4. Bland and Copeland, The Breast, 4th ed., Saunders (2009) (Page 336) Chapter 19.

Mammogram Math

Lora Weiselberg, M.D.
Chief of the Breast Cancer Service Monter Cancer Center

- *Annual incidence of breast cancer in the U.S. = 207,090*
- *About 5–12% of cancers are diagnosed by mammography = lives saved*
- *About 4,000–18,000* lives per year are saved by screening mammograms*
  (Does not account for reduced morbidity of treatment with earlier diagnosis)

* Ruth Dugan, Gilda's Club NJ NY Times 10.29.11

The Beginning...

Below are the six individuals who were on the panel discussion at what is now known as The Center for Contemporary Art in Bedminster, New Jersey.

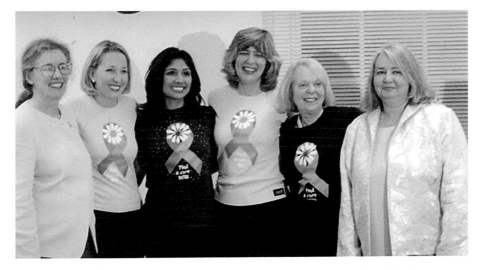

In order from left to right: Dr. Toomey, Pam Adams, Meera Bagle, Cheryl Hardy, Marion Behr and Dr. Lanfranchi.

Out of four presenters, one was in her twenties, one in her thirties, one in her forties and one just seventy years old. Their narrations, and the information given by the two doctors present, inspired me enough to compile this book. *Surviving Cancer: Our Voices and Choices* has been an act of determination and love for humanity on the part of everyone involved.

Here, at last, is our finished product that we hope will benefit all the women who feel frightened the way we did on first hearing, "You have cancer."

Information and Resources for Cancer Patients

American Cancer Society
Dedicated to helping persons who face cancer. Supports research, patient services, early detection, treatment and education.
www.cancer.org

American Psychosocial Oncology Society
The American Psychosocial Oncology Society (APOS) fosters multidisciplinary activities that relate to the subspecialty of psychosocial oncology and the psychosocial dimensions of cancer treatment.
www.apos-society.org

Angel Flight America — Free Transportation for Those in Need
A group of pilots throughout the U.S. who use their private planes for more than weekend pleasure trips. Angel Flight America has a mission with a purpose: they "arrange free flights of hope and healing by transporting patients and their families in private planes to hospitals for medical treatment."
www.angelflight.com

Breastcancer.org
A non-profit organization dedicated to providing information and community to those touched by this disease.
www.breastcancer.org

Breast Cancer Prevention Institute
BCPI is an organization which educates health care professionals and the general public through research, publications, lectures and the Internet on ways to reduce breast cancer incidence.
www.bcpinstitute.org

CancerCare: Professional Support for People Affected by Cancer
CancerCare is a national non-profit organization that provides free, professional support services for anyone affected by cancer.
www.cancercare.org

Cancer Clinical Trials — Coalition of Cancer Cooperative Groups
Provides the most up-to-date source of cancer clinical trial information for cancer patients, health care providers and advocates. It is run by a non-profit coalition working to improve physician and patient access to cancer clinical trials through education, outreach, advocacy and research.
www.cancertrialshelp.org

Cancer Hope Network
Cancer Hope Network is a non-profit organization that provides free and confidential one-on-one support to cancer patients and their families. They match cancer patients or family members with trained volunteers who have themselves undergone and recovered from a similar cancer experience.
www.cancerhopenetwork.org

NCI's Cancer Information Service (CIS) — National Cancer Institute
The National Cancer Institute's Cancer Information Service (CIS) provides the latest and most accurate cancer information to patients and their families.
www.cancer.gov

Cancer Support Community
International non-profit organization dedicated to providing support, education and hope to people with cancer. CSC offers a menu of free personalized services so that: "no one should have to face cancer alone."
www.cancersupportcommunity.org

CCR Clinical Trials at NIH
The clinical trials conducted by the Center for Cancer Research (CCR) on the NIH campus represent the core of the NCI's intramural research program.
bethesdatrials.cancer.gov

Centers for Disease Control and Prevention
The CDC maintains several departments concerned with occupational safety and health.
www.cdc.gov

Centers for Medicare
& Medicaid Services
U.S. federal agency that administers
Medicare, Medicaid and the Children's
Health Insurance Program. Provides
information for health professionals.
www.cms.gov

Corporate Angel Network
Matches cancer patients in need of travel
with private corporate jet schedules.
Information for patients and potential
corporate sponsors.
www.corpangelnetwork.org

Emerging Med
Provides matching and referral service for
cancer patients to clinical trial services.
Includes contact details.
www.emergingmed.com

FCA: Family Caregiver
Alliance Home
A clearinghouse on caregiver assistance
and long-term care public policy.
www.caregiver.org

Group Loop Home
Provides online support for teens with
cancer and their parents.
www.grouploop.org

The Inflammatory Breast Cancer
Research Foundation
Dedicated to the advancement and research
of the condition. Located in Hermosa
Beach, California.
www.ibcresearch.org

Intercultural Cancer Council
Promotes policies, programs, partnerships
and research to eliminate the unequal
burden of cancer among racial and ethnic
minorities. Based in Houston, Texas.
www.iccnetwork.org

Joan's Legacy
Joan Scarangello Foundation to conquer
lung cancer is committed to fight lung
cancer by searching for a cure and focusing
greater attention on lung cancer prevention.
www.unitedagainstlungcancer.org

LIVESTRONG Foundation
The LIVESTRONG Foundation unites,
inspires and empowers people affected
by cancer.
www.livestrong.org

Living Beyond Breast Cancer
Dedicated to empowering all affected
by this disease. Includes a newsletter,
transcripts and an email list. Headquartered
in Ardmore, Pennsylvania.
www.lbbc.org

Look Good Feel Better
Dedicated to improving the self-esteem
and quality of life of people undergoing
treatment for cancer.
www.lookgoodfeelbetter.org

Men Against Breast Cancer —
Caring About the Women We Love
For men supporting the women they love.
Located in Rockville, Maryland.
www.menagainstbreastcancer.org

MetaCancer. Foundation Resources
and Support for Metastatic Cancer
Provides resources and support for, as well
as encourages dialog among, metastatic
cancer survivors and their caregivers.
www.metacancer.org

Native American Cancer Research
Native American Cancer Research
(NACR) is dedicated to helping improve
the lives of Native American cancer
patients and survivors.
www.natamcancer.org

NCCS National Coalition
for Cancer Survivorship
NCCS advocates for quality cancer
care for all people touched by cancer
and provides tools that empower people
to advocate for themselves.
www.canceradvocacy.org

NeedyMeds
NeedyMeds is a 501(c)(3) non-profit
information resource devoted to helping
people in need find assistance programs
to help them afford their medications and
costs related to health care. The NeedyMeds
Brochure is available to organizations that
assist people who need help paying for
their medicine.
www.needymeds.org

Office of Cancer Survivorship
The mission of the Office of Cancer
Survivorship (OCS) is to enhance the
quality and length of survival of all persons
diagnosed with cancer and to minimize or
stabilize adverse effects experienced during
cancer survivorship. Supports research that
both examines and addresses the long-
and short-term physical, psychological,
social and economic effects of cancer and
its treatment among pediatric and adult
survivors of cancer and their families.
www.cancercontrol.cancer.gov/ocs/

The Office of Minority Health
The Office is dedicated to improving
the health of racial and ethnic minority
populations through the development of
health policies and programs that will help
eliminate health disparities.
minorityhealth.hhs.gov

OncoLink
OncoLink provides comprehensive
cancer information on treatments,
research advances and continuing
medical education.
www.oncolink.org

Partnership for
Prescription Assistance
The Partnership for Prescription
Assistance helps qualifying patients
without prescription drug coverage get the
medicines they need through the program
that is right for them. Many will get their
medications free or nearly free.
www.pparx.org

Patient Advocate Foundation

Patient Advocate Foundation's Patient Services provide patients with arbitration, mediation and negotiation to settle issues with access to care, medical debt and job retention related to their illness.
www.patientadvocate.org

The Patient/Partner Project

The Patient/Partner Project is a multifaceted, long-term program focused on helping cancer patients by helping their partners.
www.thepatientpartnerproject.org

The Rosalynn Carter Institute for Caregiving — Caregiver Resources

The Rosalynn Carter Institute establishes local, state and national partnerships committed to building quality long-term, home and community-based services.
www.rosalynncarter.org

Sisters Network Inc.: A National African-American Breast Cancer Network

Sisters Network® Inc. is committed to increasing local and national attention to the devastating impact that breast cancer has in the African-American community.
www.sistersnetworkinc.org

60-Mile Men

60-Mile Men, Inc. was founded in 2006. The idea originated while walking the 2006 Michigan Breast Cancer 3-Day. Since then, 60-Mile Men has produced six calendars and welcomed seventy-two men into the fraternity of 60-Mile Calendar Men! Their efforts to eradicate breast cancer and all cancers are dedicated to everyone that has battled breast cancer and all cancers.
www.60milemen.org

Stupid Cancer

A non-profit organization that empowers young adults affected by cancer through innovative and award-winning programs and services.
www.stupidcancer.org

Susan G. Komen for the Cure

Susan G. Komen® is committed to ending breast cancer forever by energizing science to find the cures and ensuring quality care for all people, everywhere.
ww5.komen.org

The Ulman Cancer Fund for Young Adults

A leading voice in the young adult cancer movement is working at a grassroots level to support, educate, connect and empower young adult cancer survivors.
www.ulmanfund.org

Vital Options International

Vital Options International is a non-profit cancer communications, support and advocacy organization with a mission to facilitate a global cancer dialogue.
www.vitaloptions.org

Y-ME National Breast Cancer Organization

Providing emotional support and information to people concerned about breast cancer. The Y-ME Hotline connects to peer counselors who are also breast cancer survivors.
www.abcdbreastcancersupport.org

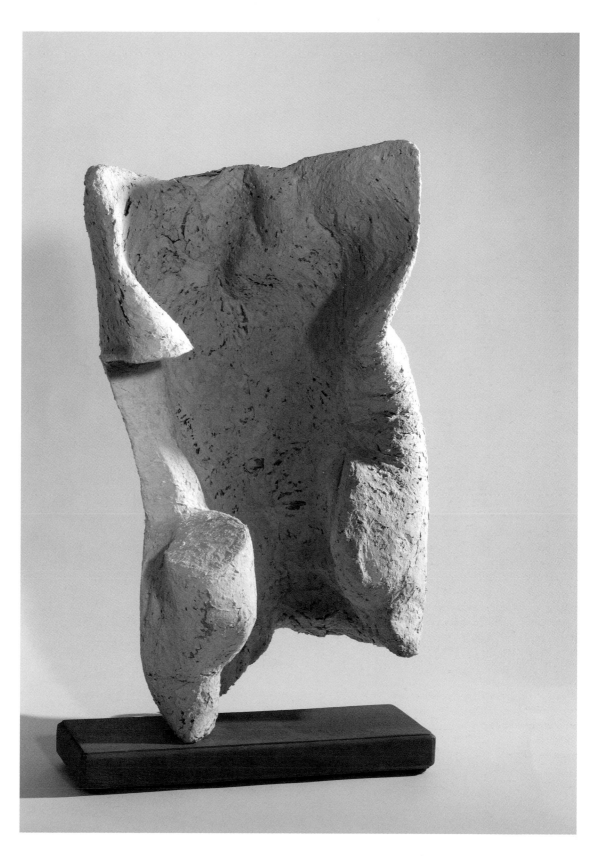

JUMPING FOR JOY (THE TREATMENT IS OVER!)

Contributor Biographies

Pamela Adams

Theatrical general manager. Passionate about supporting and fundraising for breast cancer awareness and has walked over 150 miles and raised over $10,000 under the team name "For Our Future." Holds a bachelor's degree in business and theater management from the University of the Pacific. Her father, Thomas Adams, died of lung cancer in 2006; the BRCA1 gene runs on his side of the family. Her sister, Sarah Adams, made the courageous choice to have a prophylactic mastectomy.

Meera Bagle

Previously worked in product marketing and management roles at various companies including ADP, Nabisco and Dow Jones. Holds a B.S. in marketing and philosophy from Rutgers University. Now is a stay-at-home mom to three amazing children and a beloved dog. She is proud of her participation in breast cancer walks and will continue taking steps until a cure is found.

Myra F. Barginear, M.D.

Medical oncologist at the Monter Cancer Center of the North Shore-LIJ Cancer Institute and Assistant Professor of Medicine at the Hofstra-North Shore LIJ School of Medicine. Published over thirty peer-reviewed articles, review articles, invited commentaries and book chapters. Research focuses on the prevention of breast cancer, the prevention of recurrence after surgery and the treatment of recurrences. Involved in clinical and translational studies that aim to develop better hormone therapies and improved chemotherapy drugs. Board certified in internal medicine and medical oncology, member of the New York Metropolitan Breast Cancer Group, the American Society of Clinical Oncology and the American College of Physicians. On the Committee on Advocacy, Research Communications and Ethics at ALLIANCE, a National Cancer Institute-sponsored clinical trials network.

Monica Becker

Artist, curator and educator. InterFaith Hospitality Network volunteer (2006–11), Women's Bible Study Leader (1994–2004), ceramic workshop assistant to Paul Soldner (1998–2002) and United Methodist Women Co-Vice President of Special Events (1993–2002). Event Coordinator for the American Cancer Society (2005) and was responsible for all aspects of a luminaria and survivor dinner. Organized *Sadako and the Thousand Paper Cranes* traveling exhibit (1997–2000) in libraries, children's hospitals, schools and EEC, ultimately adding a thousand more cranes and sending them to Hiroshima Peace Park by August 2000. Curator and participant of the Somerset County Park Commission Environmental Education Center exhibit titled "Nature of Women" (1997). Lord Stirling Archaeological Dig supervisor (1988). Studied at Douglass College in New Brunswick, N.J., and at the Somerset County College (now RVCC) under Ann Tsubota.

Marion Behr

Artist, writer, publisher, inventor and activist for women, as well as the compiler and illustrator of this book. For the past thirty years her paintings, sculptures, drawings and etchings have appeared in solo and group shows in the U.S. and internationally and are in major collections including ICPNA Miraflores Gallery, Lima, Peru; Centro de los Artes, San Agustin Etla, Mexico; Newark Public Library, Newark, N.J.; Ben Shahn Gallery, Wayne, N.J.; the United States Embassy, Berlin, Germany; Druckwerkstatt Bethanien, Berlin, Germany; Smithsonian Institution, Washington, D.C.; Royal Thai Art Collection, Bangkok, Thailand; Jane Voohees Zimmerli Art Museum, New Brunswick, N.J.; and Social Science Research Council for Corporate Collection, New York, N.Y.

Originated the concept of "homebased business" and co-founded The National Alliance of Home-based Business Women in the 1970s, of which she was the first President. Formed the Women Working Home Inc. publishing house in 1980, which published two editions of *Women Working Home: The Homebased Business Guide and Directory*, which she co-authored. Named New Jersey Women in Business Advocate of the Year (National Runner-up) U.S.SBA (1984), Woman of the Year in Business and Industry, Middlesex County Chamber of Commerce in New Jersey (1985) and appointed Personal Delegate by President Reagan to the White House Conference on Small Business (1986). Together with her husband, Omri Behr, invented an acid-free mode of art etching of copper and zinc (Electroetch) that was named Patent of the Week in the *New York Times* (05/02/92). Her articles on the subject have been published in *Printmaking Today*, *Chemtech* and *Leonardo*. In conjunction with this work, she was a Charles E. Lindbergh Fund: Arts and Humanities Grantee for Arts and Humanities in 1993.

    B.F.A. and M.F.A. from Syracuse University. Studied printmaking with Mohammed Khallil at Parsons School of Design, New York, N.Y. Married to Dr. Omri Marc Behr, has three children: Dr. Dawn Behr-Ventura, Darrin Behr and Dana Behr, and five grandchildren: Ilana, Elias, Ariella, Eitan and Kiran.

Omri Behr, Ph.D., J.D.

Fellow of the Royal Society of Chemistry, licensed as an attorney, before the Federal Courts and the U.S. Patent Office. Practiced intellectual property law in his own firm for almost fifty years, specializing in pharmaceutical, biological and foreign patent law, representing U.S. academic and industrial clients, as well as foreign corporations. Was an elected New Jersey delegate to a White House Conference on Small Business. Co-invented Electroetch, an acid-free mode of art etching on zinc and copper with wife, Marion. Published articles on patent protection of non-U.S. micro-organisms, on trademarks and the first article on copyright infringement via satellite transmission, shortly after the first communication satellites were in orbit.

Kelsey Blackwell

In 2006 formed Studio:Blackwell, a graphic design studio practice dedicated to the planning, design and production of creative communications projects. The flexible structure of the studio considers the unique needs of clients, building collaborative teams that work to understand and interpret a client's objective into effective, articulate tools for communication. These tools have taken the form of strategies, programming, visual identities, environmental graphics, websites, content development, books and more. www.studioblackwell.com

Christine Bonney

Planning and communications strategist with expertise in both the for-profit and non-profit sectors. Director of Development and Communications at the Women's Health & Counseling Center. Past President and Founder of Bonney Marketing Communications, a Chicago-based consultancy firm, and was an officer and member of the Corporate Public Relations team at MetLife. Her prior corporate experience includes Fortune 100 companies: Bank of America, McDonnell Douglas/ Boeing and Exxon. Recipient of Public Relations Society of America Silver Anvil Award of Excellence. On the Advisory Board of *GRAND* magazine. Recognition through the New Jersey Blood Service's Diamond Award and the City of Tampa's Mayoral Citation to civic welfare for commitment to service to non-profit organizations. B.A. from Los Angeles Valley College and M.B.A. from the University of California at Los Angeles.

Michele Capossela

Director of Patient Navigation Program Development, Eastern Division, of the American Cancer Society. On the Advisory Board of the Cancer Support Community. Married to Christopher for twenty-three years and has a son, Michael.

Michael Carr

Michael Carr lives and writes in Mendham, N.J. In 1996, he was diagnosed with Ewing's sarcoma. After one year of chemo and surgery, Carr was cleared of his illness. The cancer ended his sports career at an early age and because of this, he looked to stay involved with athletics in whatever capacity he could. He trained as an EMT and volunteered on the medical staff all through high school. He is still an active EMT with the Mendham Borough First Aid Squad. Carr graduated from Boston University in 2005 and then from Middlebury College's Bread Loaf School of English in 2010 with a Master's degree. He is the founder and President of the East Africa Ambulance Project, a non-profit group charged with outfitting rural health clinics with ambulances and basic medical supplies. Carr also published a novel called *The Viking Pawn* and will be working on various film projects in the coming months. He and his wife Chelsey had their first child in 2013. Visit www.michaelcarrprojects.com for more information on Carr's work.

Lori Cohen
Owner of A Glass Act, specializing in handmade stained glass belt buckles and other types of stone and glass accessories. Member of Therapy Dogs Inc.; she visits nursing homes and other facilities with her labradoodle. Participated in a house rebuild for a family who lost their home during Hurricane Katrina. Coordinated a Play for Pink golf tournament in 2011 that raised $3,000 for Susan G. Komen and a Golfing for Gildas golf tournament in 2012 that raised $1,800 for Gilda's Club of Northern New Jersey. Bachelor of Arts degree from Fairleigh Dickinson University.

Karen Connelly, R.D., C.S.O.
Certified Specialist in Oncology Nutrition (CSO), she works as an oncology registered dietitian at Somerset Medical Center in New Jersey. Discovered a passion and desire to assist those making their way through the life-altering journey of a cancer diagnosis after members of her family were diagnosed with cancer. Provides nutritional care to oncology patients through a variety of educational methods such as cooking classes and group nutrition classes. Membership in the Academy of Nutrition and Dietetics and the Oncology Nutrition Practice Group. Dietetic internship at the University of North Carolina at Greensboro. Bachelor of Science in Nutrition and Dietetics from the University of Delaware.

Pam Cooper
Artist, curator and corporate consultant. B.F.A. from the Pratt Institute, 1994, and B.Sc (Hons.) in pharmacy, 1970. She has five grandsons.

Naov Davin
Resident of Ampe Phnom village, Svay Kroavann commune, Chbar Morn town, Kompong Speu province, Cambodia. Diagnosed with breast cancer in 2009.

Annelise Stokkebro Rasmussen DeCoursin
Born in Odense, Denmark, she is a professional violinist trained at Oberlin College. Enjoys weaving, gardening, nature and bird-watching.

Richard Dickens, M.S., L.C.S.W.-R.
Clinical supervisor, blood cancers program coordinator and developer of CancerCare's Blood Cancer Program and the Mind–Body Project. Two-time non-Hodgkin's lymphoma survivor and allogenic bone marrow transplant survivor. Taught in post-graduate certificate programs at Smith College School of Social Work and Hunter College, mentor in the post-graduate Zelda Foster Leadership Program at New York University School of Social Work and the founder of The Cistern Fund at West End Collegiate Church to support volunteer work in impoverished world environments. Named Distinguished Practitioner in Social Work by the National Academies of Practice, Washington, D.C. Board member of The Collegiate Church Corporation and Intersections International.

Has published in *Guidepost's Coping* and the *Journal of Psychosocial Oncology*, and has co-authored chapters in two oncology books. Presentation titled "When Words Are Not Possible: Mindful Techniques for Creative Communication" received an Outstanding Abstract Award at The 5th International Social Work Conference On Health and Mental Health in Hong Kong (2006). Presented in North America, China, Australia, Ireland and South Africa on numerous psychosocial issues confronting the cancer population, which include: survivorship, psychosocial needs of older patients, integrative medicine, using metaphor in clinical practice, working in developing countries and stress management. Graduate of the Columbia University School of Social Work and has trained in Transcendental and Vipassana meditation techniques, the latter at the International Vipassana Meditation Academy in Igatpuri, India.

Nomi Roth Elbert, M.Ed., Spiritual Care Provider

Spiritual care counselor at the Herzog Hospital in Jerusalem, the Hadassah Hospital on Mt. Scopus, Jerusalem, the Koby Mandell Foundation in the Bereaved Mothers' Spiritual Care Support Group, the AMCHA–Righteous Gentiles/Holocaust Survivors Within the Russian Speaking Community and the Jewish Healing Center of East Bay, San Francisco. Staff member at the Grief & Growing Bereavement Retreat. Previous positions include ATZUM/Coordinator of Program for Righteous Among the Nations, Rand Corporation, Churchill Films, Fries Entertainment and the Marianne Frostig Center of Educational Therapy. Documentary film award for the film *Choices* (1983). Bachelor of Science from the Hebrew University of Jerusalem in archaeology and art history (1975), Master of Science from Mount St. Mary's College in special education/learning disabilities (1979), and M.Ed. from the Sharei Tzedak Spiritual Care Training Program, B'Ruach. Cancer survivor. nomire@gmail.com

Paula Flory

Master of Arts in counseling psychology from New York University, Director of the Princeton Y.W.C.A. Breast Cancer Resource Center. A fitness professional, she enjoys travel, cooking, Zumba and spending time with her husband, Chuck, and two children, Matthew and Erika. Believes that the best way for a woman to accessorize a bald head is with a killer pair of heels and a huge smile. paulaflory@verizon.net

Richard Fontana, C.F.P.

Senior Vice President Investments, Raymond James & Associates, Inc.. Member of Board of Directors at Somerset County Business Partnership, Somerset County Election Board commissioner, Board of Trustees member at Community Visiting Nurse Association, Community Board member at Family and Community Services and Somerset County 4H, Advisory Board member at Middle Earth and a BPOE #68 Elks Member. Awarded Citizen of the Year by Somerset County Business Partnership (2011), Public Servant of the Year Award by New Jersey Parks & Recreation Association (2006), Leadership Award for NACO Building Disaster-Resistant Communities (2001), Diversity Award–Government by Somerset County Cultural Diversity Coalition (2005), Freeholder of the Year Award by Marconi Foundation (2006) and Excellence in Leadership Award by Leadership Somerset (2009). Bachelor of Arts in political science from William Paterson University and C.F.P. (Certified Financial Planner) certification from Fairleigh Dickinson University. www.fontanawealthmanagement.com

Hanna Fox

Writer, editor and teacher of writing for most of her adult life. During her employment in the New Jersey Department of Human Services, she was Program Director of the Children's Trust Fund to Prevent Child Abuse and Neglect. Founded a small independent press after retiring. Her short stories, essays, poems and excerpts from novels have appeared in regional and national publications. Her dramatic works have had staged readings and workshop productions in Princeton and New York. Completed her first screenplay recently and is working on another. Received her B.A. from Smith College and M.A. from Tufts University.

Evie Hammerman, M.S.W.

Retired psychiatric social worker for Community Mental Health Center of Chicago and then in private practice in the Chicago area. Runs hospice bereavement groups and is in charge of the Lake Host program on her pond, which aims to prevent invasive aquatic plants from being transmitted from one body of water to another. Holds a B.S. from Cornell University and M.S.W. from the Jane Adams School of Social Work at the University of Illinois. Her mother survived a breast cancer diagnosis at seventy-nine years old and lived to eighty-seven. homeonpond@earthlink.net

Keshia D. Hammond-Merriman

Trust administrator and member of the Sisters Network of Central New Jersey, student member of the IMA and student member of the AICPA. Hopes to become a C.P.A and loves to bowl. Married in 2009 to Oyango Merriman. mskdh@aol.com

Tom Heller
Fine art photographer specializing in studio, portrait and landscape photography. Attended University of Dayton and Newark College of Engineering. His father was diagnosed with throat and lung cancers and was cured after surgery and radiation and stayed cancer free for over ten years until his death in 2011. behindtomslens@gmail.com

Amy Hick
Freelance editor and writer based in Toronto, Canada, who specializes in illustrated non-fiction and educational texts. Her maternal grandmother, for whom she was named, died of breast cancer.

Aretha Hill-Forte, M.P.H.
B.S., Fairleigh Dickenson University, M.P.H., Rutgers University/University of Medicine and Dentistry of New Jersey. Public Health Practitioner, Director Cancer Screening Services.

Mariann Linfante Jacobson
Certified sign language interpreter, consultant and trainer. Winner of Spirit of Courage Award (2011) from the Cancer Support Community in Bedminster, N.J. Holds a B.S. from Rutgers University and Comprehensive Skills Certification (CSC & MCSC); she is a certified Medical Assistant-Clinical Specialty (CSC-C) and has passed both the Educational Interpreters Proficiency Assessment (Native Level) and the Sign Proficiency Instrument (SCPI-Native Level). Her father had lung cancer and her sister was recently diagnosed with melanoma. hmj628@optimum.net

Anne M. Johnston, Ph.D.
Former Director of Immunology/Serology and Corporate Assistant Vice President at Laboratory Corporation of America. Retired in 2000. Recipient of the Spirit of Courage Award in 2011 from the Cancer Hope Network for work as a volunteer breast cancer counselor. B.S. from Connecticut College, M.S. in genetic counseling and Ph.D. in zoology (human genetics) from Rutgers University. Post Doctoral Fellowship at the University of Medicine and Dentistry of New Jersey. Married forty-nine years to W. Dexter Johnston, Ph.D., and has two daughters, one a stay-at-home mom and the other a pediatric infectious disease specialist. She has a family history of cancer on her mother's side. Johnsanne@embarqmail.com

Wilbur Dexter Johnston, Ph.D.
B.S. Yale 1961, Ph.D. in physics MIT 1966. Employed at Bell Labs and Lucent for thirty-five years. After retirement in 2000, worked for a start-up company, Multiplex, Inc. for four years. Interests include nature photography, traveling, bird-watching and gardening.

Jeanette Joyce, B.F.A., R.T.(R,)(M.)
Breast imaging and breast disease educator, providing support and knowledge to mammography professionals and breast cancer survivors since 1996. Certified as a radiographer by the American Registry of Radiologic Technology (AART) with advanced certification in Mammography. Provider of self-directed, online, affordable initial mammography training and continuing education credits for mammography technologists—MQSA compliant, Category A credits accepted by the ARRT. Lives near Richmond, VA.

Julie Ann Juliano, M.D.
Twenty-five years of solo family practice at South Branch Family Practice and twenty years of membership in the Rotary Club of Branchburg, N.J. District Governor of Rotary District 7510 (2007–08) and honored with the Girl Scout Woman of Achievement Award, Thanks Badge and Thanks Badge II. Graduate of the Albert Einstein College of Medicine and certified by the American Board of Family Physicians.

Mitchell K. Karten, M.D.

Director of the Division of Radiation Oncology at Nassau University Medical Center in East Meadow, N.Y. Board certified in internal medicine, medical oncology and radiation oncology. Attended the MD six-year program at Albany Medical College of Union University in Albany, N.Y., completed medical residency and chief residency at the Thomas Jefferson University Hospital in Philadelphia, PA, as well as oncology fellowships at the Hahnemann University Hospital in Philadelphia, the Montefiore Medical Center in the Bronx, N.Y., and a radiation oncology residency at New York University Hospital in New York City.

Kerry Kay

Healer and teacher of meditation and healing methods. Studied biomathematics studies at Rutgers University and training in *Jin Shin Jyutsu*, Reiki, Hellinger's Family Constellations and Kabbalistic Healing. Her maternal grandfather died of lung cancer on Christmas Eve when her mother was a teenager. She is incredibly proud of her three children, and proud also to work with the people who, in the process of experiencing illness, invite her to participate with them as a helper or guide.

Linda Kendler

Chaplain who takes pride in listening to those who need someone to talk to and a volunteer with the Cancer Hope Network. Graduated from Montclair State College majoring in home economics, which she also taught.

Cheryl Kott

Attended Douglass College and Cornell Law School.

Angela Lanfranchi, M.D., F.A.C.S.

Breast surgical oncologist interested in breast cancer prevention. Co-director of the Steeplechase Cancer Center's Sanofi-Aventis Breast Care Program and President and Co-founder (in 1999) of the Breast Cancer Prevention Institute to educate lay and medical groups in this field. Winner of the Castle Connolly "Top Doc" in surgery annually since 2008. Has traveled nationally and internationally to Australia, Canada, China, Europe, Korea, India, New Zealand and South Africa to speak about breast cancer risks and prevention. Completed residencies in family practice and general surgery, as well as a Vascular Surgery Fellowship as post graduate training and began private practice in 1983. Board certified by the American Board of Surgery and is a Fellow of American College of Surgeons. Graduate of Georgetown University School of Medicine. Daughter of a mother who died of breast cancer, she has been married for thirty-seven years and is the mother of a daughter. info@bcpinstitute.org

Ellen R. Levine, M.S.W., A.C.S.W., L.C.S.W., O.S.W.-C.

Accomplished Licensed Clinical Social Worker, certified by the Board of Oncology Social Work. Presents publications, plans conferences and has been interviewed on radio and television and in print media on many topics related to social work, women and cancer. Program Director at the Cancer Support Community (CSC) (formerly Wellness Community) of Central New Jersey, has been the manager of the Department of Social Work at the Cancer Institute of New Jersey and has worked at the Specialized Pediatric Ambulatory Center of the Monmouth Medical Center of Long Branch, N.J., and the United Jewish Federation of MetroWest in East Orange, N.J. Was the first Vice President of the Board of Directors for the Planned Parenthood of Central Jersey, on the Advisory Board of the Dean and Betty Gallo Prostate Center, a Cultural Competency Trainer at the National Asian Women's Health Organization, on the Nursing/Psychosocial Advisory Group of the New Jersey Commission on Cancer Research, on the Board of Directors of the Sisters Network of Central New Jersey as well as on the Professional Advisory Board for the Lung Cancer Circle of Hope. Member of the National Association of Social Workers, the Academy of Certified Social Workers, the Association of Oncology Social Workers and the New Jersey Society of Social Work Leadership in Healthcare. She holds a M.S.W. from the Rutgers Graduate School of Social Work in New Brunswick, N.J.

Rich Loreti

Self-employed business owner of a landscaping company and a garbage company, both of which he started from scratch on his own. The one company, R.L Landscaping, he started at the age of seventeen. He has been married to his wife, Sandi, for eighteen years and they have two beautiful daughters. Arionna is fifteen and Alessia is ten and a half, they are the world to him! What he enjoys the most is spending countless hours with his wife, children, family and close friends, as well as summers at the Shore and vacationing. His family loves the sun, beach and warm weather and so does he.

Joyce Greenberg Lott

Retired English teacher, holds a Master's from Rutgers University. Published a book about teaching and two books of poetry. Her essays, poems and stories have appeared on public radio, in the *Journal of New Jersey Poets*, *Kalliope*, *Ms.* magazine, *The Paterson Literary Review*, the *New York Times* and other publications. She enjoys playing tennis, swimming and walking along the towpath near her house.

Nora Macdonald

Financial assistant for a foundation. Conducts monthly workshops with members of her garden club to make flower arrangements for outpatients at the Carol Simon Cancer Center in Morristown, N.J. Her mother died of breast cancer in 1955.

Richard Margolese, M.D., C.M., F.R.C.S.(C.)

Director Emeritus of the Department of Oncology at McGill University's Jewish General Hospital and Herbert Black Professor of Surgical Oncology at McGill University. Research focus involves performing clinical trials in breast cancer surgery, adjuvant therapy in breast cancer and in breast cancer prevention. Executive Committee member of the National Adjuvant Breast and Bowel Project in Montreal, Canada. Honored with the Order Of Canada. Earned an A.B. from Dartmouth College and M.D., C.M. from McGill University. F.R.C.S.(C.) and certified by the American Board of Surgery.

Marcy McCaw, B.Sc.P.T., C.L.T.

Licensed physical therapist with a specialization in sports therapy. Lymphedema therapist specializing in breast cancer patients at the Holy Redeemer Women's Health Center. Traveled extensively with several national sports teams as a physical therapist. Some highlights include the 2004 Olympic Games in Athens, Commonwealth Games in Kuala Lumpur in 1998 and Manchester, England, in 2002, a significant number of Caribbean championships, as well as several stops in the International Rugby Board International 7s Series; most notably Chile and Argentina. Originally from Canada, she resides in Yardley, PA, with her husband, Brennan, and her three children. Holds a certificate in Traditional Chinese Acupuncture and Reiki Master. Breast cancer survivor.

Susan McCoy, M.D.

Board certified as OB-GYN and in a private practice in Princeton, N.J., she has worked at Martha's Vineyard Hospital. Graduate of the University of Alabama Medical School in Birmingham.

Megan McQuarrie

Executive Director and founder of the Elixir Fund. Inspired by her brother who, after almost two years of treatment, passed away from testicular cancer at the age of thirty-eight in 2003. Holds a B.S. from the University of Rhode Island and M.S. from Duke University.

Dawn Meade

Speech language pathologist, holds B.A. in speech correction and M.A. in speech language pathology from Rutgers University. Her greatest accomplishment is being a mom to her amazing eleven-year-old twin boys, Sean and Brian. She is passionate about traveling and has a strong desire to explore the world. Married for thirteen years to her husband, Patrick. Her close-knit family includes parents Catherine and Dennis. She is one of four children, including her best friend and sister, Jackie, her brothers Dennis and Thomas and all of her in-laws. She also has nineteen nieces and nephews, whom she adores.

Sherry Melinyshyn, R.N.(EC)., B.N.Sc., C.O.N.(C.), P.H.C.N.P.
Primary health care nurse practitioner and melanoma survivor. Co authored *The Role of the Nurse Navigator in the Breast Assessment Program.* Member of the Registered Nurses Association of Ontario (RNAO) and the College of Nurses of Ontario (CNO). Holds Canadian Nurses Association Certification in Oncology Nursing (CNA). Bachelor of Nursing Science from Queens University (1988) and Primary Health Care Nurse Practitioner Certificate from Queens University (2009). sherrymel@live.ca

Sedkai Meta, M.D.
This is a fictional name to preserve the anonymity of the person interviewed. Sedkai Meta means compassion in Khmer. The doctor's reflections were motivated by deep concern and a constructive commitment to improving health care for women in Cambodia.

Lucinda (Cindy) Newsome
Author of two books, *Hobbstown: The Forgotten Legacy of a Unique African-American Community* and *The Vain Girl,* and a manager for a company supporting developmentally disabled individuals. She regards her work as a hospice volunteer as a calling from God. Recipient of the 2006 Somerset County Historic Preservation and History Award from Somerset County Cultural and Heritage Commission for *Hobbstown* in 2006. Holds a B.A. in English from Caldwell College and a business degree from Raritan Valley College. lwnewsome@optonline.net

Ruth Oratz, M.D., F.A.C.P.
Clinical associate professor at the NYU School of Medicine. Board certified in internal medicine and medical oncology, specializes in treating women with breast cancer and those with genetic susceptibility to cancer. Listed in "The Best Doctors in America" and "The Best Doctors in NYC" in *New York Magazine* for many years. Established the Women's Oncology & Wellness Practice, medical consultant to CancerCare, and is on the medical advisory board of Living Beyond Breast Cancer, breastcancer.org, Cancer and Careers, Sharsheret and The New York City Metastatic Breast Cancer Network. Member of the American Society of Clinical Oncology, the American Association of Cancer Research and numerous other scientific and clinical organizations. Graduated from Radcliffe College/ Harvard University and the Albert Einstein College of Medicine as a member of Alpha Omega Alpha honor society. Post-doctoral training at the New York University School of Medicine in New York.

Meryl Marger Picard, Ph.D., M.S.W., O.T.R.
Assistant professor in the Department of Occupational Therapy at the Graduate School of Health and Medical Sciences at Seton Hall University, she has over thirty years' experience as an occupational therapist in adult rehabilitation and private practice. A practitioner and student of mind–body techniques including meditation, therapeutic touch and Reiki. Doctoral work explored the relationship between cancer-related fatigue and upper extremity functional deficits in breast cancer survivors. Other research interests include sleep, complementary medicine and developing reflection in clinical practice. Member of the American Occupational Therapy Association and the New Jersey Occupational Therapy Association. Wrote the "OT Fact Sheet: Occupational Therapy's Role in Sleep" (*American Occupational Therapy Association*, 2012). Holds a B.S. in occupational therapy and M.S.W. in social work from New York University and a Ph.D. in health sciences from Seton Hall University.

Charulata Prasada
International development professional who focuses on gender and development, women and children's rights and promoting equality through social development. Recipient of the International Gender Award from the International Development Research Center (IDRC) in Ottawa, Canada. Passionate and committed to promoting equality and social change through development, advocacy and art. Lives with husband and two children in New York City. Holds a B.A. in political science from McGill University and M.A. in gender and international development from the Faculty of Environmental Studies at York University in Toronto.

Sushma Prasada

Full-time teacher from 1978–2001 at the Summit School in Montreal, Canada, teaching developmentally delayed and emotionally disturbed students. Volunteers at Kabir Cultural Centre, building bridges between South Asian and other communities. At Kabir, she runs a book club in which fifteen to twenty people of different backgrounds attend monthly meetings to discuss and interpret various issues through different cultural prisms. In 1967 started the first nursery school on the campus of the Indian Institute of Technology, Kanpur, with a friend. Holds a B.S. in home science and B.Ed. from Lady Irwin college, Delhi University, India, and M.Ed. degree from Rutgers University. Has lived in India and the U.S., but now resides in Montreal, Canada, with husband, Biren, and their dog, Maya. Breast cancer survivor.

Barrie L. Raik, M.D.

Director of the Geriatric Fellowship Program at the Weill Cornell Division of Geriatrics and member of the Division of General Medicine at Columbia University Medical Center, where her interest in geriatrics grew out of a house calls program. Joined the Weill Cornell Division of Geriatrics as Director of the Geriatric Fellowship Program in 1999. Board certified in internal medicine and member of the American College of Physicians, the Gerontologic Society of America and the American Geriatrics Society. Spent two years teaching middle school English in rural South Korea with the Peace Corps, is an avid bird-watcher and photographer, loves camping, canoeing, and traveling. She is married and has two daughters and a son. Graduate of Harper College (now Binghamton University) and New York University School of Medicine.

Tracy Redling

Owner of A Simple Daisy—"tees you wear & feel." Her passion in life is sharing good food and wine with family and friends. B.S. in education from Florida Atlantic University in Boca Raton, FL. tracy@asimpledaisy.com

Dorothy Reed

Dedicated to spreading the gospel of early detection in the African-American community. In the absence of local support or culturally sensitive resources for African-American women diagnosed with the disease, formed and is president of Sisters Network of Central New Jersey (SNCNJ) in 2000 with three other breast cancer survivors. SNCNJ is an affiliate chapter of Sisters Network Inc., a National African-American Breast Cancer Survivorships Organization based in Houston, TX. Holds board membership on the St. Peter's Hospital Cancer Committee, the New Jersey Department of Health and Senior Services Breast Cancer work group, the Cancer Institute of New Jersey Advocacy Commission, the Cancer Institute of New Jersey Survivors Advisory Board, the Robert Wood Johnson University Hospital Community Relations Committee and is a member of the First Baptist Church of Lincoln Gardens.

On a national level, she is one of the original advocates for HR Bill 5116, the Dean and Betty Gallo Cancer Patient Compassion Act. Spent extensive time on Capitol Hill with the National Breast Cancer Coalition. An active participant in the Komen Foundation's letter-writing campaign for free mammograms. In May 2005 she was selected to participate on the Department of Defense Breast Cancer Research Program committee for the U.S. Army Medical Research Command and has received numerous honors and awards including an appearance in a 2006 National Television Commercial Campaign by Astra Zeneca, *"If you were my sister."* Selected in 2006 as one of Lifetime's breast cancer heroes. Holds a B.A. in organizational leadership from Somerset Christian College.

Elisabeth (Elsje) Reiss, M.S.W., L.C.S.W.

Licensed Clinical Social Worker. Member of the National Association of Social Workers and the Association of Oncology Social Work. Recipient of the Department of Social Work Faculty Award for Academic Excellence, the Department of Social Work Faculty Award for Outstanding Leadership, and was inducted into the Beta Rho Chapter of the Phi Alpha Honor Society at Southern Connecticut State University in New Haven. Holds degrees in French from the Université de Grenoble in France, midwifery from the School for Midwifery in Amsterdam, studied death and dying at the

University of Toledo, Toledo, B.A. in experimental psychology from Albertus Magnus College in New Haven and M.S.W. from Southern Connecticut State University in New Haven.

Christine Rizk, M.D., F.A.C.S.

Board certified breast surgeon. Assistant Professor of Surgery, SUNY Stony Brook. Recipient of Alpha Omega Alpha Bruce Hubbard Humanitarian Award. Research interests: impact of nicotine on breast carcinogenesis, impact of surgery on stage 4 metastatic breast cancer patients. Enjoys running and cooking. B.S. from the University of Buffalo and M.D. from SUNY Syracuse.

Tobias D. Robison

Retired software developer who now programs the radio show *Masterclassics with Tobias* most Tuesday mornings at WPRB FM. B.A. from Columbia College.

Alicia Rockmore

Senior Vice President of Marketing at UberMedia, holds a B.A. from Claremont McKenna College. and a C.P.A. M.B.A. from the University of Michigan.

Vilmarie Rodriguez, M.S.W., L.C.S.W.

 Oncology social worker who holds membership in the Association of Oncology Social Work (AOSW), the National Association of Social Workers and the Lance Armstrong Advisory Board. She holds B.A. in sociology from Herbert H. Lehman College.and an M.S.W. from Fordham University. Has presented at the AOSW Conference in Washington, D.C., with a poster presentation titled "Helping Hispanic Patients Find Their Voice" (2004). Her mother was diagnosed with stage 2b breast cancer and underwent a mastectomy and chemotherapy treatments; after five years of survivorship her mother continues to suffer from severe neuropathy, osteoporosis, lymphedema and vertigo due to the chemotherapy.

Men Salath

Farmer in Soken Village, So Kong commune, Kang Meas district, Kampong Cham province, Cambodia. She has four children. Diagnosed with breast cancer in 2008.

William L. Scarlett, D.O., F.A.C.S., F.A.C.O.S., F.A.A.C.S.

Associate professor of plastic surgery, Philadelphia College of Osteopathic Medicine. Medical Director of Bucks County Aesthetic Center, Bensalem, PA. Board certified plastic and reconstructive surgeon practicing outside of Philadelphia. Fellow of the American College of Surgeons, the American College of Osteopathic Specialists and the American Academy of Cosmetic Surgeons. Graduate of Dickinson College and the University of Des Moines medical school. Recipient of multiple awards and has published numerous papers in his field. He was most recently a featured speaker at the Power Symposium and the Voices for Breast Cancer Conference. Currently in private practice in Bensalem, PA, where the focus of his practice is breast reconstruction. He has patents pending on devices related to breast cancer care and is working on publishing his first book entitled *Demanding Compassion*. Developed workshops for cancer patients to help them deal with the psychosocial aspects of cancer. He is a proud father and husband and just competed in his first Olympic triathlon.

Andrew V. Schally, Ph.D.

Winner of the 1977 Nobel Prize, with Roger Guillemin and Rosalyn Yalow. Has published over eight hundred and fifty scientific papers. Conducted pioneering research concerning hormones and helped identify three brain hormones—thyrotropin-releasing hormone (TRH), corticotrophin-releasing hormone (CRH) and growth-releasing hormone (GRH)—and greatly advanced scientists' understanding of the function and interaction of the brain with the rest of the body. Findings have proven useful in the treatment of cancer, diabetes and peptic ulcers, and in the diagnosis and treatment of hormone-deficiency diseases.

Held professorial positions at the Baylor University School of Medicine and Tulane University Medical School, and was the Director of the Endocrine and Polypeptide Laboratory at the Veterans

Administration (VA) Hospital in New Orleans, LA, and presently holds the same position at Miami, FL. Additionally, is the winner of the Charles Mickle Award of the University of Toronto (1974), the Gairdner Foundation International Award (1974), the Borden Award in the Medical Sciences of the Association of American Medical Colleges (1975), the Lasker Award (1975) and the Laude Award (1975). Holds memberships in the National Academy of Sciences, the American Society of Biological Chemists, the American Physiology Society, the American Association for the Advancement of Science and the Endocrine Society. Studied at the University of London and received doctorate in biochemistry from McGill University in 1957.

Sondra Schoenfeld
Special education teacher with a B.S. in mathematics and an M.A. in special education, as well as teacher certifications in science and mathematics. She is married with two sons and four grandchildren. Enjoys playing bridge, reading, music, art and travel.

Pamela Schwartz
Board trustee at the South Huntington Jewish Center with responsibilities overseeing youth activities. A cancer survivor, she works for the American Cancer Society as a recruiter for the Making Strides Against Breast Cancer Walks on Long Island. Brought Relay for Life to her community with dear friend Debbie Picker. Enjoys spending time with family and friends, skiing, playing tennis and gardening. M.S. in education from CUNY Queens College.

Sandra Scott, R.T.(R.)(M.)
Board certified Radiologic Technologist and member of the ARRT. Conducts health fairs to educate men and women about the importance of breast, hypertension and prostate screening exams.

Kathleen Toomey, M.D.
Medical Director of the Steeplechase Cancer Center at Somerset Medical Center (SMC) in Somerville, N.J., since its opening in 2007. The first woman president of the Medical Dental Staff at SMC and a member of the board of trustees for seven years. Chairperson of the Professional Advisory Board of the Cancer Support Community of Central New Jersey since 2003. Member of the American Society of Clinical Oncology and recipient of the Wellness Community's Spirit of Hope Award and the Rotary's Paul Harris Fellow Award. Included in the "Top Physicians" issue of *New York Magazine* and in the "Top Doctors" issues of *New Jersey Monthly* for ten years. Board certified in internal medicine, hematology and oncology. Residency in internal medicine at UMDNJ-Robert Wood Johnson Medical School serving as Chief Resident. Medical degree from the University of Bologna, Italy.

Jane Tuvia, M.D.
Board certified radiologist in the field of mammography, women's imaging and nuclear medicine. Opened Madison Avenue Women's Imaging in 2001 to provide personal care to women in a timely, compassionate manner. Honored by the New York Women's Agenda (NYWA) with the Star Award for outstanding care and devotion to patients. Recipient of the On-Time Physician Award (2009), Compassionate Doctor Recognition (2009) and the Patients' Choice Award (2008–09). Holds memberships in the New York Metropolitan Breast Cancer Society, the Society of Breast Imaging, the American College of Radiology, the Radiological Society of North America and the American Roentgen Ray Society. Previously Director of Breast Imaging at North Central Bronx Hospital and Jacobi Medical Center in the Bronx, as well as an Assistant Professor of Radiology at Albert Einstein College of Medicine. Completed residency at Long Island Jewish Medical Center in New York, in both diagnostic radiology and nuclear medicine. Medical degree at Ben-Gurion University of the Negev (1983).

Stuart Van Winkle, C.F.P.®
A Certified Financial Planner who works in financial, insurance and retirement services. B.S. from Lehigh University and holds a Life and Health License, Series 6, 22, 7 as well as memberships in the N.A.H.U., N.A.I.F.A. and C.F.P. stuartvanwinkle@gmail.com

Dawn Behr-Ventura, M.D., M.P.H.

Board certified radiologist with sub-specialization in breast imaging and body imaging, as well as CAQ certification in neuroradiology. Has held appointments as the Director of Neuroradiology at South Nassau Communities Hospital in Oceanside, N.Y., neuroradiology attending at Good Samaritan Hospital in West Islip, N.Y., and neuroradiology attending at North Shore University Hospital in Manhasset, N.Y. Fellowships in body and breast imaging and neuroradiology at North Shore University Hospital, residency in radiology at Nassau University Medical Center and internship in obstetrics and gynecology at Roosevelt/St. Luke's Hospital Center. A member of the American College of Radiology, Senior Member of the American Society of Neuroradiology, and 2012–13 President of the Long Island Radiological Society.

Recipient of the Maternal Child Health Traineeship Award from the United States Department of Health and Human Services (1993), Scholarship for Research in Geriatric Pharmacology from the Hartford Foundation/AFAR (1991), Distinction in Research Program candidate honors from the State University of New York at Stony Brook School of Medicine (1989) and the John Woodruff Simpson Fellowship for Graduate Studies in Medicine from Amherst College (1988). B.A., cum laude, from Amherst College. M.D. degree with Distinction in Research from the State University of New York at Stony Brook School of Medicine (1993) and M.P.H. from Columbia University School of Public Health (1995). She is grateful to her husband, David, and four wonderful children for all their support.

Debra Walz, R.N., M.S., W.H.N.P.-BC, A.O.C.N.P., STAR/C

Board certified Women's Health Nurse Practitioner and oncology nurse practitioner. Works at the Breast Center of Faxton St. Luke's Healthcare in Utica, New York. Member of the National Association of Nurse Practitioners in Women's Health, the Oncology Nurses Society, the Nurse Practitioner Association of New York and Sigma Theta Tau-International Honor Society of Nursing. B.F.A. from Keene State College in New Hampshire, A.A.S. in nursing from Adirondack Community College in Queensbury, N.Y. and M.S. in the Women's Health and Oncology Dual Nurse Practitioner Program at Columbia University School of Nursing in New York. Received the Faculty Award for Professional Excellence in a Sub-specialty, and honored as a Rudin Oncology Scholar at Columbia University. She is STAR Clinician Certified. Mother of two and lives with her husband and children in the Utica, N.Y., area.

Lora Weiselberg, M.D.

Medical oncologist, she works with breast cancer patients at North Shore University Hospital and Long Island Jewish Medical Center. Associate Professor of Medicine at the Hofstra North Shore-LIJ School of Medicine. Certified in internal medicine, medical oncology and hematology. Residency in internal medicine at St. Joseph's Medical Center/Stamford Hospital. M.D. from New York Medical College.

Joe Wojtowicz

Outreach Director of Cancer Hope Network 2000–13 and a thyroid cancer survivor since 2006. He holds a B.S and an M.B.A.

Kathi Edelson Wolder

Public relations, marketing communications and brand image consultant. Graduate of the New England Conservatory of Music, Boston, MA, with both a Bachelor of Music and a Master of Music in Flute Performance. Received the Volunteer of the Year Angel Award in 2004 from Susan G. Komen for the Cure New York, the Certificate of Merit for Community Service (Komen) in 2004 from New York State Senator John L. Sampson and the Journey of Courage Award in 2011 from Susan G. Komen for the Cure North Jersey. She is a breast cancer survivor.

Glossary

The content of this glossary is derived directly or indirectly from numerous Internet sources. The definitions contained in it are for guidance only. For further detailed explanations, the appropriate medical professional should be consulted. Major sources of information include the following websites:

www.nih.gov
www.webmd.com
www.mayoclinic.org
www.drugs.com
medicinenet.com
www.chemocare.com
ww5.komen.org

ADJUVANT TREATMENT

A cancer treatment (chemotherapy, radiation or biological therapy) that is offered after a surgical procedure in order to improve the outcome for patients at high risk of relapse.
www.skincancer.about.com

ADRIAMYCIN

Also known as Doxorubicin, Adriamycin is an anti-cancer ("antineoplastic" or "cytotoxic") chemotherapy drug. It is classified as an anthracycline antiobiotic. Cancers treated with Adriamycin include: bladder, breast, head and neck, leukemia (some types), liver, lung, lymphomas, mesothelioma, multiple myeloma, neuroblastoma, ovary, pancreas, prostate, sarcomas, stomach, testis (germ cell), thyroid, uterus.
www.chemocare.com/chemotherapy/drug-info/adriamycin.aspx

AGONIST/ANTAGONIST

An agonist is an agent that binds to a receptor on a cell and activates that receptor in order to elicit an effect An antagonist is an agent that binds to a receptor but does not elicit the response that the neurotransmitter or an agonist would cause. The antagonist blocks the receptor and prevents activation by neurotransmitters or other drugs.
www.suboxoneassistedtreatment.org/

ALTERNATIVE MEDICINE

Encompasses healing arts not taught in traditional Western medical schools that promote options to conventional medicine.
www.medicinenet.com

ANEURYSM CLIPPING

Surgical procedure performed to treat the balloon-like bulge of an artery wall known as an aneurysm.
www.mayfieldclinic.com

ANTI-ESTROGEN

A substance that keeps cells from making or using estrogen (a hormone that plays a role in female sex characteristics, the menstrual cycle and pregnancy). Anti-estrogens may stop some cancer cells from growing and are used to prevent and treat breast cancer. They are also being studied in the treatment of other types of cancer. An anti-estrogen is a type of hormone antagonist. Also called estrogen blocker.
NCI Dictionary of Cancer Terms
www.cancer.gov

ARCHITECTURAL DISTORTION

A mammographic descriptive term in breast imaging. It may be visualized as tethering or indentation of breast tissue.
www.radiopedia.org

ARIMIDEX

Drug that lowers estrogen levels in post-menopausal women, which may slow the growth of certain types of breast tumors that need estrogen to grow in the body (generic name anastrozole). It is used to treat breast cancer in post-menopausal women.
www.drugs.com

AROMATASE INHIBITORS

Reduce the production of estrogen, while the term "anti-estrogen" is usually reserved for agents reducing the response to estrogen.
www.breastcancer.org

AXILLARY LYMPH NODES

The body has about 20 to 30 bean-shaped axillary lymph nodes located in the underarm area. These lymph nodes are responsible for draining lymph from the breasts and surrounding areas, including the neck, the upper arms, and the underarm area.
www.healthline.com/human-body-maps/axillary-lymph-nodes

B AND T CELLS

B cells and T cells are the main types of lymphocytes. B cells work chiefly by secreting substances called antibodies into the body's fluids. Antibodies ambush foreign antigens circulating in the bloodstream. They are powerless, however, to penetrate cells. The job of attacking target cells is left to T cells or other immune cells.
www.niaid.nih.gov

BENIGN CYST

Cysts are very common and rarely turn into cancers. It is extremely important to find out whether what you have is just a cyst or something else.
www.breastcancer.org

BIOIDENTICAL HORMONES

Plant-derived hormones that pharmacists prepare and label as drugs. The products claim to be biochemically similar or identical to those produced by the ovaries or body. However, the relevant chemicals (steroids) in plants are not identical to those in humans. To make products that work in humans, raw materials from the plants must be converted to human hormones synthetically. Thus, to the extent

that they are potent, the bioidentical products would pose the same risks as those of standard hormones—plus whatever problems might be introduced during compounding.
www.pharmwatch.org

BIOPSY

A medical test that involves removal of tissue in order to examine it for disease.
www.news-medical.net

BONE DENSITY SCAN

See DEXA scan.

BRCA

The BRCA gene test is a blood test that uses DNA analysis to identify harmful changes (mutations) in either one of the two breast cancer susceptibility genes—BRCA1 and BRCA2. Women who have inherited mutations in either or both genes face a much higher risk of developing breast cancer and ovarian cancer compared with the general population. A BRCA gene mutation is uncommon
www.mayoclinic.org

CA 125 TEST

A CA 125 test measures the amount of the protein CA 125 (cancer antigen 125) in your blood. Many different conditions can cause an increase in CA 125. These include uterine fibroids, endometriosis, pelvic inflammatory disease and cirrhosis, as well as pregnancy and normal menstruation. Certain cancers, including ovarian, endometrial, peritoneal and fallopian tube, also can cause CA 125 to be released into the bloodstream.
www.mayoclinic.org

125 (CA 125) is a protein found on the surface of many ovarian cancer cells and in other cancers. It is used as a tumor marker, which means the test can help show if some types of cancer are present.
www.webmd.com

CALCIFICATION

A feature that can show up on a mammogram. These calcium salt particles are not breast cancer, and they don't always mean trouble. If they cannot be readily identified as typically benign or as having a high probability of malignancy, they are labeled as being of "intermediate concern or suspicious."
www.breastcancer.org

CALCIUM DEPOSIT

Tiny accumulations of calcium salts. They can crop up in any part of the body. The causes of these deposits are baffling to many, though the list of potential culprits linked to them include deficiencies in the supply of some vitamins and emotional stress.
www.ehow.com

CANCER RADIOLOGIST

A doctor who specializes in radiology. A radiologist uses sophisticated imaging technologies (e.g., X-ray, CT scan, MRI, ultrasound, etc.) to create and interpret pictures of areas inside the body for cancer diagnosis and staging.

This is *not* the same as a radiation oncologist, who is a physician who uses radiation for treatment.
www.cancercenter.com

CANCER-RELATED FATIGUE (CRF)

Cancer-related fatigue is distinguishable from normal fatigue in that CRF symptoms are severe, distressing and unrelieved by sleep and rest.
www.medical-dictionary.the freedictionary.com/Medicine

CARCINOGEN

An agent that can cause cancer. Exposure to one or more carcinogens, including certain chemicals, radiation and certain viruses, can initiate cancer under conditions not completely understood.
www.merriam-webster.com

CHEMOTHERAPY

A drug treatment that uses powerful chemicals to kill fast-growing cells in the body. Many different chemotherapy drugs are available. They may be used alone or in combination to treat a wide variety of cancers.
www.mayoclinic.com

CHRONIC FATIGUE SYNDROME (CFS)

Severe, continued tiredness that is not relieved by rest and is not directly caused by other medical conditions. Symptoms of CFS are similar to those of the flu and other common viral infections.
www.ncbi.nlm.nih.gov

CLINICAL TRIALS

In a clinical trial (also called an interventional study), participants receive specific interventions according to the research plan or protocol created by the investigators. These interventions may be medical products, such as drugs or devices; procedures; or changes to participants' behavior, for example, diet. Clinical trials may compare a new medical approach to a standard one that is already available or to a placebo that contains no active ingredients or to no intervention.
clinicaltrials.gov/ct2/about studies/learn

COCHLEA

Part of the inner ear that converts mechanical energy (vibrations) into nerve impulses sent to the brain. It is also known as the organ of hearing.
www.medicinenet.com

COMPLEMENTARY MEDICINE

Complementary means "in addition to." Complementary medicine is treatment and medicine used in addition to a doctor's standard care. In the U.S. the National Center for Complementary and Alternative Medicine was formed within the National Institutes of Health to test the safety and effectiveness of these treatments. The center has guidelines to help choose safe treatments.
www.webmd.com

COMPRESSION

The act, process or result of compressing, especially when involving a compressing force on a body part.
www.merriam-webster.com

CT OR CAT SCAN

A computed tomography (CT) or computer axial tomography (CAT) scan is an imaging method that uses X-rays to create cross-sectional pictures of the body. Tomography is the process for generating a tomogram, a two-dimensional image of a slice or section through a three-dimensional object.
www.medicinenet.com

CYSTS IN BREASTS

Breast cysts are fluid-filled sacs within the breast—often described as round or oval lumps with distinct edges—which are usually benign (not cancerous). In texture, a breast cyst usually feels like a grape or a water-filled balloon, but sometimes feels firm.
www.mayoclinic.org

CYTOPENIA

A deficiency in numbers of the blood cell elements.
Mosby's Medical Dictionary, 8th edition. © 2009, Elsevier.

CYTOTOXIN

A substance having a specific toxic effect on certain cells.
www.thefreedictionary.com

DCIS — DUCTAL CARCINOMA IN SITU

DCIS is the most common type of non-invasive breast cancer. Ductal means that the cancer starts inside the milk ducts, carcinoma refers to any cancer that begins in the skin or other tissues (including breast tissue) that cover or line the internal organs, and *in situ* means "in its original place." DCIS is called "non-invasive" because it hasn't spread beyond the milk duct into any normal surrounding breast tissue. DCIS isn't life-threatening, but having DCIS can increase the risk of developing an invasive breast cancer later on.
www.breastcancer.org

DEFIBRILLATION

A process in which an electronic device gives an electric shock to the heart. This helps reestablish normal contraction rhythms in a heart having dangerous arrhythmia or in cardiac arrest. This may be delivered externally or internally.
www.heart.org

DEXA OR DXA SCAN

Dual X-ray absorptiometry (DXA) is the preferred technique for measuring bone mineral density (BMD). DXA has also been called dual-energy X-ray absorptiometry. DXA is relatively easy to perform and the amount of radiation exposure is low. A DXA scanner is a machine that produces two X-ray beams, each with different energy levels. One beam is high energy while the other is low energy. The amount of X-rays that pass through the bone is measured for each beam. This will vary depending on the thickness of the bone. Based on the difference between the two beams, the bone density can be measured.
www.webmd.com

DIAGNOSTIC MAMMOGRAPHY

An X-ray exam of the breasts that is performed in order to evaluate a breast complaint or abnormality detected by physical exam or routine screening mammography. Diagnostic mammography is different from screening mammography in that additional views of the breast are usually taken, as opposed to two views typically taken with screening mammography. Therefore, diagnostic mammography is usually more time-consuming and costly than screening mammography.
www.imaginis.com

DYSMENORRHEA

The medical term for pain with menstruation. Primary dysmenorrhea is common menstrual cramps that are recurrent and are not due to other diseases. Secondary dysmenorrhea is pain that is caused by a disorder in the reproductive organs, such as endometriosis, adenomyosis, uterine fibroids or infection.
my.clevelandclinic.org

ESTROGEN/PROGESTERONE POSITIVE/NEGATIVE

Breast cancer cells that are ER+ depend on estrogen to grow. Anti-estrogen hormonal therapy blocks the receptors or reduces the amount of estrogen that can get into the receptors. As a result, the cancer cells may shrink or die. If the score is Estrogen Receptor negative (ER-), then your tumor is not driven by estrogen. Similarly for progesterone (PR+ and PR-).
www.breastcancer.org
www.breastcancer.about.com

ESTROGEN RECEPTOR

Estrogens act on target tissues by binding to parts of cells called estrogen receptors. An estrogen receptor is a protein molecule found inside those cells that are targets for estrogen action. Estrogen receptors contain a specific site to which only estrogens (or closely related molecules) can bind. The target tissues affected by estrogen molecules all contain estrogen receptors; other organs and tissues in the body do not. Therefore, when estrogen molecules circulate in the bloodstream and move throughout the body, they exert effects only on cells that contain estrogen receptors.
www.cancer.gov

EXCISIONAL BIOPSY

In an excisional biopsy of the breast, the surgeon makes an incision in the skin and removes all or part of the abnormal tissue for examination under a microscope. Unlike needle biopsies, a surgical biopsy leaves a visible scar on the breast and sometimes causes a noticeable change in breast shape.
www.health.harvard.edu

FALLOPIAN TUBES

Fallopian tubes transport the egg from the ovary to the uterus (the womb).
www.medterms.com

FEMARA

An aromatase inhibitor (the generic name is letrozole), which works by reducing the amount of estrogen produced in the bodies of post-menopausal women, which may cause a decrease in bone density and increases in bone fractures and osteoporosis.
www.femara.com

FIBROADENOMA

Fibroadenoma of the breast is a non-cancerous (benign) tumor. Fibroadenomas are usually single lumps, but about 10–15% of women have several lumps that may affect both breasts.
www.nlm.nih.gov/medlineplus

FIBROIDS

Uterine fibroids are benign tumors that form on the wall of the uterus.
www.webmd.com

GENE

A short piece of DNA. Genes tell the body how to build a specific protein. There are about 30,000 genes in each cell of the human body. Together, these genes make up the blueprint for the human body and how it works.
www.nlm.nih.gov/medlineplus

GENETIC TESTING

Tests performed on blood and other tissue to find genetic disorders. There are several possible reasons for these. These include: finding out if people carry a gene for a disease and might pass it on to their children, testing for genetic diseases in adults before they cause symptoms and/or confirming a diagnosis in a person who has disease symptoms.
www.nlm.nih.gov/medlineplus/genetictesting.html

GYNECOLOGIST

A physician who specializes in the care, diagnosis and treatment of disorders of the female reproductive system.
www.thefreedictionary.com

HASHIMOTO'S DISEASE

Hashimoto's thyroiditis is a condition caused by inflammation of the thyroid gland. It is an autoimmune disease, which means that the body inappropriately attacks the thyroid gland as if it were foreign tissue.
www.medicinenet.com

HEMATOLOGY

The branch of internal medicine, physiology, pathology, clinical laboratory work and pediatrics that is concerned with the study of blood, the blood-forming organs, and blood diseases. Hematologist physicians also very frequently do further study in oncology.
www.news-medical.net

HER2

HER2 refers to a gene that helps cells grow, divide and repair themselves. When cells (including cancer cells) have too many copies of this gene, they grow faster.

Women with HER2-positive breast cancer have a more aggressive disease. They have a higher risk that the disease will return (recur) than in women who do not have this type.
www.nlm.nih.gov/medlineplus/ency/

HERCEPTIN

Herceptin (trastuzumab) is a monoclonal antibody. Antibodies are substances the body produces to help fight infection or other foreign particles. Monoclonal antibodies are made in the laboratory, and some are designed to attack specific cancer cells. Herceptin targets cancer cells that overexpress, or make too much of, a protein called HER2, which is found on the surface of some cancer cells. Herceptin attaches to the HER2 positive cancer cells and slows or stops the growth of the cells. Herceptin is used only to treat breast cancers that are HER2 positive.
www.cancer.gov

HETEROGENEOUS

Consisting of dissimilar or diverse ingredients or constituents; mixed.
www.merriam-webster.com/dictionary/heterogeneous

HOSPICE CARE

End-of-life care provided by health professionals and volunteers. They give medical, psychological and spiritual support.
www.nlm.nih.gov

HRT

Hormone replacement therapy (HRT) is used to supplement the body with either estrogen alone or estrogen and progesterone in combination during and after menopause. Estrogen and progesterone are hormones

produced by a woman's ovaries.
www.webmd.com

However, HRT can increase risk of breast cancer, heart disease and stroke. Certain types of HRT have a higher risk, and each woman's own risks can vary depending upon her health history and lifestyle.
www.nlm.nih.gov/medlineplus/

HYPOTHALAMUS

A region of the brain that controls an immense number of bodily functions. It is located in the middle of the base of the brain, and encapsulates the ventral portion of the third ventricle.
www.vivo.colostate.edu

HYPOTHYROIDISM

Hypothyroidism (underactive thyroid) is a condition in which the thyroid gland doesn't produce enough of certain important hormones. Women, especially those older than sixty years of age, are more likely to have hypothyroidism. Hypothyroidism upsets the normal balance of chemical reactions in your body. It seldom causes symptoms in the early stages, but, over time, untreated hypothyroidism can cause a number of health problems, such as obesity, joint pain, infertility and heart disease.
www.mayoclinic.org

ILEOSTOMY

A surgical procedure in which the small intestine is attached to the abdominal wall in order to bypass the large intestine; digestive waste then exits the body through an artificial opening called a stoma (from the Greek word for "mouth").
www.surgeryencyclopedia.com

IMMUNE SYSTEM

System, made up of special cells, proteins, tissues and organs, that defends against germs and micro-organisms every day. Problems with the immune system can lead to illness and infection.
www.kidshealth.org/teen/flu_center

INFUSION

The administration of medication through a needle or catheter, prescribed when a patient's condition is so severe that it cannot be treated effectively by oral medications. Typically, infusion therapy means that a drug is administered intravenously, but the term also may refer to situations where drugs are provided through other non-oral routes, such as intramuscular injections and epidural routes (into the membranes surrounding the spinal cord).
www.nhia.org

INTERSTITIAL

Occurring in the spaces between organs, tissues, etc.
Collins English Dictionary © HarperCollins Publishers 2003.

LAPAROSCOPE

A thin, lighted tube put through a cut (incision) in the belly to look at the abdominal organs or the female pelvic organs. It is used to find problems such as cysts, adhesions, fibroids and infection. Tissue samples can be taken for biopsy through the tube (laparoscope).
www.webmd.com

LCIS

Lobular carcinoma *in situ* (LCIS) is an uncommon condition in

which abnormal cells form in the lobules or milk glands in the breast. LCIS isn't cancer. Being diagnosed with LCIS indicates an increased risk of developing breast cancer. LCIS usually doesn't show up on mammograms. The condition is most often discovered as a result of a biopsy done for another reason, such as a suspicious breast lump or an abnormal mammogram.
www.mayoclinic.org

LETROZOLE

Generic name for Femara.
See Femara

LEUKEMIA

Cancer of the blood cells. It starts in the bone marrow which is the soft tissue inside most bones. Bone marrow is where blood cells are made.
www.webmd.com

LYMPH NODE

Small structures located all over the body around blood vessels and are a part of the lymph system of the body that acts as filters that can catch infectious organisms or cancerous tumor cells. *See axillary lymph nodes.*

LYMPHECTOMY

Lymphectomy, also called lymphadenectomy, is surgery to remove lymph nodes.
www.webmd.com

LYMPHEDEMA

A build-up of excess fluid in the body tissues, usually the arm, because of obstruction of lymphatic drainage back into the bloodstream. The affected limb becomes painful, swollen, distorted in shape.
www.nlm.nih.gov/medlineplus/lymphedema.html

LYMPHOMA

Lymphomas begin when a type of white blood cell, called a T cell or B cell, becomes abnormal. The cell divides again and again, making more and more abnormal cells. These abnormal cells can spread to almost any other part of the body.
www.nlm.nih.gov/medlineplus/lymphoma.html

MALIGNANT/MALIGNANCY

Refers to cancerous cells that have the ability to spread to other sites in the body (metastasize) or to invade and destroy tissues. Malignant cells tend to have fast, uncontrolled growth due to changes in their genetic makeup. Those that are resistant to treatment may return after all detectable traces of them have been removed or destroyed.
www.nlm.nih.gov/medlineplus

MAMMOGRAM

A low-dose X-ray exam of the breasts to look for changes that are not normal. The results are recorded on X-ray film or directly into a computer for a doctor called a radiologist to examine.
womenshealth.gov

MEDICAL ONCOLOGIST

A physician who is often the main health care provider for someone who has cancer.
www.cancer.gov

MEDROXY PROGESTERONE

A steroid used to treat abnormal menstruation (periods) or irregular vaginal bleeding. It is also used to bring on a normal menstrual cycle in women who menstruated normally in the past but have not menstruated for at least six months and who are not pregnant or undergoing menopause. It is also used to prevent overgrowth of the lining of the uterus (womb) and may decrease the risk of cancer of the uterus in patients who are taking estrogen.
www.ncbi.nlm.nih.gov

METASTASIS

The movement or spreading of cancer cells from one organ or tissue to another. Cancer cells usually spread through the blood or the lymph system.
www.nlm.nih.gov/medlineplus/ency/article/

MICRO-/MACRO-CALCIFICATION

Microcalcifications are specks of calcium salts found as residue in an area of rapidly dividing cells. When many are seen in a cluster, they may indicate a small cancer. About half the cancers detected appear as these clusters. In contrast, macrocalcifications are large clusters and are usually benign.
www.healthscout.com

MINIMALLY INVASIVE SURGERY

See laparoscopy.

MOLECULAR TESTING

See genetic testing.

MONITORING

Supervising activities in progress to ensure they are on-course and on-schedule in meeting the objectives and performance targets.
www.businessdictionary.com

MRI

An MRI (magnetic resonance imaging) scan is an imaging test that uses powerful magnets and radio waves to create pictures of the body. It does not use radiation (X-rays). Single MRI images are called slices. The images can be stored on a computer or printed on film. One exam produces dozens or sometimes hundreds of images.
health.nytimes.com/health/guides/

MRSA

Methicillin-resistant Staphylococcus aureus (MRSA) is a type of staph bacteria that is resistant to certain antibiotics called beta-lactams. These antibiotics include methicillin and other more common antibiotics such as oxacillin, penicillin and amoxicillin. In the community, most MRSA infections are skin infections. More severe or potentially life-threatening MRSA infections occur most frequently among patients in health care settings.
www.cdc.gov

MUTATION

A permanent change in the DNA sequence of a gene. Mutations in a gene's DNA sequence can alter the amino acid sequence of the protein encoded by the gene. Like words in a sentence where each word has a meaning, the DNA sequence of each gene determines the amino acid sequence for the protein it encodes.
www.learn.genetics.utah.edu/archives/mutations

NCCN

The National Comprehensive Cancer Network® (NCCN®) is a non-profit alliance of twenty-one of the world's leading cancer centers. It is dedicated to improving the quality and effectiveness of care provided to

patients with cancer.
www.nccn.org

NCI

The National Cancer Institute (NCI) is a division of the National Institutes of Health.
www.cancer.gov

NEUPOGEN SHOTS/ NEUPOGEN

Neupogen stimulates the production of granulocytes (a type of white blood cell) in patients undergoing therapy that will cause low white blood cell counts. It is also used to prevent infection and neutropenic (low white blood cells) fevers caused by chemotherapy. It is a support medication and does not treat cancer.
www.chemocare.com

NEUROPATHY

A collection of disorders that occurs when nerves of the peripheral nervous system (the part of the nervous system outside of the brain and spinal cord) are damaged. The condition is generally referred to as peripheral neuropathy, and it is most commonly due to damage to nerve axons.
www.medicalnewstoday.com

NON-HODGKIN'S LYMPHOMA

A type of cancer that originates in the lymphatic system. The lymphatic system is part of the body's immune system and helps fight infections and other diseases.
www.medicinenet.com

NURSE NAVIGATOR

An oncology-certified nurse who is available to guide patients through the entire process of diagnosis and treatment. The nurse navigator is a single point of contact and assists with scheduling, initial tests and consultations.
www.alegent.com

NURSE PRACTITIONER

Registered nurses (R.N.s) who are prepared, through advanced education and clinical training, to provide preventive and acute health care services to individuals of all ages. N.P.s take health histories and provide complete physical examinations, diagnose and treat many common acute and chronic problems, interpret laboratory results and X-rays, prescribe and manage medications and other therapies, provide health teaching and counseling to support healthy lifestyle behaviors and prevent illness, and refer patients to other health professionals as needed.
www.mayoclinic.org

ONCOLOGY

A branch of science that deals with tumors and cancers. The word "onco" means bulk, mass, or tumor while "-logy" means study.
www.news-medical.net

ONCOTYPE DX

A test that helps predict the chance of metastasis (when cancer spreads to other organs) for breast cancers that are lymph node-negative, estrogen receptor-positive. It may also be used in select cases of lymph node-positive, estrogen receptor-positive breast cancer.
ww5.komen.org

OSTEOPOROSIS

A condition in which the bones become thin and weak and break easily.
www.nihseniorhealth.gov

OVARIES

The reproductive glands in women. They are located in the pelvis, one on each side of the uterus. Each ovary is about the size and shape of an almond. The ovaries produce eggs (ova) and female hormones.
www.medterms.com

PACEMAKER

A small device that is placed under the skin of the chest or abdomen to help control abnormal heart rhythms. This device uses electrical pulses to prompt the heart to beat at a normal rate. Pacemakers are used to treat heart rhythms that are too slow, fast or irregular. These abnormal heart rhythms are called arrhythmias.
www.cardiosmart.org

PAPILLARY THYROID CANCER

The most common form of thyroid cancer. It most often grows in one lobe of the thyroid, though it can be present in both lobes. Treatment is surgical removal, often followed by radioactive iodine ingestion.
www.endocrineweb.com

PATHOLOGIST

A physician who identifies diseases and conditions by studying abnormal cells and tissues.
www.medterms.com

PATHOLOGY

The science of the causes and effects of diseases, especially the branch of medicine that deals with the laboratory examination of samples of body tissue for diagnostic or forensic purposes.
www.oxforddictionaries.com

PATIENT NAVIGATOR

A non-medical professional who can help guide patients through the maze of the health care system—coordinating appointments with work schedules and stressing the importance of consistent treatment and follow-up.
www.cancer.org

PEDIATRIC ONCOLOGY

The study of cancer related to children.

PEMPRO

The brand name for conjugated estrogens/medroxyprogesterone.
www.drugs.com

PET SCAN

Positron emission tomography (PET) scan is an imaging test that uses a radioactive substance called a tracer to look for disease in the body.
www.nlm.nih.gov/medlineplus/ ency/article/003827.htm

PLANTAR WARTS

Warts are usually caused by type 1 and 2 HPV (human papillomavirus). These strains are contagious and are spread from person to person via direct contact with the virus. They generally appear on the base of the foot.
www.warts.org

PLEOMORPHIC

Many-formed; a tumor may be pleomorphic.
www.medterms.com

POSITIVE ESTROGEN RECEPTORS

See estrogen receptor.

PRIMARY PHYSICIAN

Helps patients maintain overall health by focusing on preventive care.
www.ehealthinsurance.com

PROCRIT SHOTS

Procrit (epoetin alfa) is a drug given to patients who have chemotherapy-induced anemia (low red blood cell count). An injection of Procrit stimulates red blood cell production. It is a clear liquid that can be given through an intravenous infusion (IV), or as a shot. It is also known as Epogen.
Note: This drug should only be used after detailed discussion with health provider.
www.breastcancer.about.com

PROGESTERONE

A female hormone important for the regulation of ovulation and menstruation. It is used therapeutically to cause menstrual periods in women who have not yet reached menopause but are not having periods due to a lack of progesterone in the body.
www.drugs.com

PROGESTERONE POSITIVE/NEGATIVE

See estrogen positive/negative.

PROSTHETICS

The branch of medicine or surgery that deals with the production and application of artificial body parts.
www.thefreedictionary.com

RADIATION CRADLE

A thermoplastic or foam mold that supports the head, neck, back, pelvis and thighs. This mold, sometimes called a cradle, ensures accurate positioning over the course of the radiation treatments.
www.upmccancercenter.com/radonc/external.cfm

RADIATION ONCOLOGIST

Doctors who oversee radiation therapy treatments. These physicians work with the other members of the radiation therapy team to develop treatment plans and ensure that each treatment is given safely and accurately.
www.rtanswers.org

RADIATION THERAPIST

The technician who administers treatment prescribed by the radiation oncologist.

RADIOLOGY/RADIOLOGIST

Radiology is the branch or specialty of medicine that deals with the study and application of imaging technology like X-ray and radiation to diagnosing and treating disease.

Radiologists direct an array of imaging technologies (such as ultrasound, computed tomography [CT], nuclear medicine, positron emission tomography [PET] and magnetic resonance imaging [MRI]) to diagnose or treat disease. Interventional radiology is the performance of (usually minimally invasive) medical procedures with the guidance of imaging technologies. The acquisition of medical imaging is usually carried out by the radiographer or radiologic technologist.
www.news-medical.net/health/What-is-Radiology.aspx

RALOXIFENE

Raloxifene was first used to prevent osteoporosis (bone loss). In bone cells, it acts like estrogen to prevent osteoporosis in women who have gone through menopause. It is now used in women who have gone through menopause and who are at high risk for developing breast cancer. It can reduce breast cancer risk in these women, although it cannot entirely prevent it. It blocks estrogen from binding to certain cells, such as those in the breast. The cancer cells that depend on estrogen to divide stop growing and die.
www.cancer.org

R-CHOP

One of the most widely used combination chemotherapy regimens in the sphere of B cell non-Hodgkin's lymphoma since studies first began to combine the newer monoclonal antibody Rituxan with the CHOP (C= Cyclophosphamide, H= Doxorubicin Hydrochloride [Hydroxy-daunomycin], O= Vincristine Sulfate [Oncovin], P= Prednisone) regimen around 2005.
www.cancertreatment.net

RECONSTRUCTIVE SURGERY

Reconstructive surgeries include procedures performed on areas of the body that are abnormal to correct a deformity or defect, such as for women who have had a breast removed.
www.cancer.org

REMISSION

Remission or partial remission indicates a positive response of a cancer to the treatment. It does not mean that a cancer is cured.
www.tirgan.com

SARCOIDOSIS

A multi-system inflammatory disease of unknown etiology that predominantly affects the lungs and intrathoracic lymph nodes. Sarcoidosis manifests with the presence of noncaseating granulomas (NCGs) in affected organ tissues.
www.emedicine.medscape.com

SECOND OPINION

The opinion of a second medical professional that can confirm or comment on a medical opinion already received.

SEPTIC SHOCK

A potentially lethal drop in blood pressure due to the presence of bacteria in the blood. Bacterial toxins, and the immune system response to them, cause a dramatic drop in blood pressure, preventing the delivery of blood to the organs. Septic shock can lead to multiple organ failure including respiratory failure, and may cause rapid death. Toxic shock syndrome is one type of septic shock.
www.medical-dictionary.thefreedictionary.com

SIDE EFFECTS

Undesirable and possibly harmful and unintended effects of medications.

SOMATOSTATIN

First discovered in hypothalamic extracts and identified as a hormone that inhibited secretion of growth hormone.
www.vivo.colostate.edu/hbooks

SONOGRAM

An ultrasound exam that uses high-frequency sound waves to scan the body.
www.americanpregnancy.org

STAGE

See staging.

STAGING

Describes the extent or severity of a cancer diagnosis based on information about the tumor. *Note: The cited website describes all aspects in detail but clearly.*
www.nccn.org

STROKE

A condition where a blood clot or ruptured artery or blood vessel interrupts blood flow to an area of the brain. A lack of oxygen and glucose (sugar) flowing to the brain leads to the death of brain cells and brain damage, often resulting in an impairment in speech, movement and memory.
www.medicalnewstoday.com

TAMOXIFEN

A drug that blocks the actions of estrogen and is used to treat and prevent some types of breast cancer.
www.drugs.com

TARGETED THERAPY

A type of cancer treatment that uses drugs to attack unique aspects of cancer cells with little harm to healthy cells. Targeted therapies can work by blocking the process that changes normal cells into cancer, thereby stopping the abnormal growth behavior of a tumor and/or preventing the formation of blood vessels that bring nutrients to the tumor.
www.pancan.org

TAXOL

A member of the taxane family of drugs made from yew trees (genus Taxus), which is used to treat cancer. It is a clear, colorless fluid that is given as a chemotherapy infusion. Because it is quite thick and sticky, it requires a pump to properly administer the infusion.
www.breastcancer.about.com

TINNITUS

The subjective perception of sound by an individual, in the absence of external sounds.
www.entnet.org

TOMOGRAPHY

The process for generating a tomogram, a two-dimensional image of a slice or section through a three-dimensional object.
www.medterms.com

TUMOR

An abnormal growth of body tissue. Tumors can be cancerous (malignant) or non-cancerous (benign).
www.ncbi.nih.gov

TUMOR BOARD

A treatment planning approach in which a number of doctors who are experts in different specialties (disciplines) review and discuss the medical condition and treatment options of a patient. In cancer treatment, a tumor board review may include that of a medical oncologist (who provides cancer treatment with drugs), a surgical oncologist (who provides cancer treatment with surgery) and a radiation oncologist (who provides cancer treatment with radiation).Also called a multidisciplinary opinion.
www.cancer.gov

ULTRASOUND

See sonogram.

X-RAY

A type of electromagnetic radiation, just like visible light. An X-ray machine sends individual X-ray particles through the body. The images are recorded on a computer or film.

Structures that are dense (such as bone) will block most of the X-ray particles, and will appear white. Metal and contrast media (special dyes used to highlight areas of the body) will also appear white. Structures containing air will be black, and muscle, fat and fluid will appear as shades of gray.
www.nlm.nih.gov

Index

A

abnormal cells, 31, 209
abortion and breast cancer, 214
Academy of Nutrition and Dietetics, 150
acupuncture, 167
Adams, Pamela, 235
adjuvant therapy, 97, 99. *See also* chemotherapy
advice, 45–46, 103–4, 135, 199. *See also* life lessons learned; support, family and friends
advocate, importance of, 28, 83. *See also* support, family and friends; individual organizations
    Dawn M's experience, 70–71
African-Americans, creating community awareness
    Dorothy's experience, 199–200
aging and cancer rates, 222
allergies
    latex, 29
    Rituxan, 35
alternative therapy, 163–68, 221
American Cancer Society, 111
    and health insurance options, 181
    Look Good Feel Better program, 146–47
    Patient Navigation program, 145–46
    Reach to Recovery, 145
    Relay for Life, 201–3, 225
        Pamela S's experience, 200–203
American College of Surgeons, 25
American Society of Clinical Oncology (ASCO), 25
anemia, 120, 152. *See also* fatigue
anti-estrogen therapy, 99, 222–23
anxiety, 61–62, 139, 141, 143–44, 157, 159, 209–10
appointments, companions for, 28, 83, 135
Arimidex, 99
    Anne J's experience, 84–85, 87
    recurrence prevention, 206, 222–23
aromatase inhibitors. 87, *See also* chemotherapy
    adverse symptoms, 133
    nausea with, 103
    overview, 99
    post menopausal treatment, 87
    pros and cons, 125
    recurrence prevention, 222–23
art/sculpture as therapy and encouragement
    Marion's experience, 27, 29–30
Avon Walk for Breast Cancer, 227–30

B

Bach, David: *Smart Women Finish Rich*, 180
Bagle, Meera, 235
Behr, Marion, 235
Belfatto, Deborah Q., 207–8
biopsies
    breast lumps, 49, 61–62
    explained, 30–31, 79–80
    male breast cancer, 69
    microcalcifications, 121
    needle, 61, 77, 105, 207, 227
    results and second opinions, 29
    sentinel node, 106, 107
    stereotactic, 49, 79–80
    surgical, 105–6, 207, 213
    types of, 80
birth control pills. *See* oral contraceptives
bladder cancer, 33
Board certification, importance of, 25
bonding with survivors, 57, 87, 194, 196
    Lucinda's experience, 197, 199
bone marrow transplant, allogenic, 164–65
BRCA gene mutations
    about, 59, 61, 85
    breast cancer in men, 63–66
    other cancer risks in men, 65–66
    ovarian cancer prevention, 50
    testing for, 69, 110–11, 214
breast cancer, early onset, personal experiences of, 26–27, 46–47, 55, 57–58, 61–62, 66–67, 69–70, 70–71
Breast Cancer Prevention Institute, 215, 217
Breast Cancer Prevention Trial, 99
Breast Cancer Resource Center, 194
breast compression and mammograms, 79
Breast Friends support network, 227
breast lumps
    biopsies for, 49, 61–62
    in men, 63–66, 85, 89
breast reconstruction, 47, 87, 110, 205
    about, 111, 113–14
    male breast, 70
    surgeon, 25
breast self-exam, 81, 105
    conflicting advice, 49
    faithfully done, 26, 55, 83, 193, 197
    in men, 70
    Keshia's experience, 83–84
    teens, 203
breast surgeon, 25, 104–7, 109–11.
    See also oncologists: surgical
breasts
    anatomy and physiology, 63–66
    cultural significance of, 157

dense tissue and mammography, 75–76
effect of drugs, legal and street, 65
fibrocystic, 191
    Kathi's experience, 203, 205–6
budgeting, 180
Byrnes-Paul, Diane, 210–11

C

CA 125 test, 52
calcification, 49
Cambodia, health care histories, 91–95
cancer
    defined, 31
    risk factors for. *See* family history and risk; risk factors
Cancer Education and Early Detection (CEED), 183, 185
Cancer Hope Network, 111, 145
    formation of, 210–12
    volunteering, 87
        Linda's experience, 209–10
cancer related fatigue (CRF), 151–53, 155
Cancer Support Community (CSC), 25, 194–96
    free programs, 150, 175
Cancer Trends Progress Report (US), 141
CancerCare, 163, 167
    CancerCare Copay Foundation, 175, 177
    complementary medicine, 167–68
    financial assistance, 176
    free professional services, 139, 141
    palliative care, 163
care comparisons, developing countries
    Cambodia
        Men S's experience, 91
        Naov's experience, 92–93
    a doctor's perspective, 94–95
caregiving and understanding
    Tobias's experience, 126–27, 129
CAT scan. *See* CT scan
CEED. *See* Cancer Education and Early Detection
cellulitis and lymphedema, 115
Centers for Disease Control (CDC), detection programs, 183
cervical cancer, 183, 188–89, 212
chemotherapy
    before and after surgery, 109–10, 223
    coping with, 206
    cure, control or shrink, 118–21
    defined, 27
    examples of, 87, 121, 123, 124–25
    port
        Annelise's experience, 121, 123

side effects, 35, 52, 123, 124–26, 126–27, 129, 170
   systemic control, 97, 99
children
   Cancer Support Community (CSC), 196
   concern for, 55, 57, 61–62
   explaining cancer to, 44, 101, 160
   Monica's experience, 101, 103–4
Chronic Disease Fund's Good Days Program, 175
church as a support network, 199
clinical research/trials
   about, 43
   benefits of, 25, 51, 99–100
   GHRH antagonists, 219–21
   improved survival outcomes, 223
   taking part in
      Sushma's experience, 43–46
COBRA, health insurance after job termination, 179, 186–87
colonoscopies, routine, 133, 222
colorectal cancer, 58, 183, 212
   Evie's experience, 131–33, 135
communication
   essential to care, 100
   nurse navigators, 143–45
   oncology social workers, 139, 141, 159–61, 163
   patient navigators, 145–46
complementary therapies, 163–68, 168–71, 194–96
Complete Decongestive Therapy (CDT), 115–16
Compazine, 127
compression garments for lymphedema, 116–17
conflicting advice, 47, 49
conservative therapy, 130
Consolidated Omnibus Budget Reconciliation Act. See COBRA
constipation, 149, 170
Center for Contemporary Art, 235
coping strategies
   chemotherapy, 35, 37
   courage/strength of character, 26–27
   doctors' visits, 31–33
   graduate school and professional goals, 200–201
   helpful list, 45–46, 135
   independence, 103, 121
   knowledge and positive outlook
      Meera's experience, 55, 57–58
   memories, making good ones, 30
   positive attitude, 121, 123
   psychotherapy, 135

survivors, talking to, 197, 199
counseling and education programs, 160, 196, 208, 212
cradles for radiation therapy, 27, 130
CRF (cancer related fatigue). See cancer related fatigue
CSC. See Cancer Support Community
C.S.O. (Certified Specialist in Oncology Nutrition), 147, 149–51
CT scan, 125, 130
cure rates, breast cancer, 231
cysts, about, 73

D

Dalai Lama as a healing presence
   Mariann's experience, 191, 193–94
DCIS. See ductal carcinoma in situ
death and COBRA, 187
death and dying
   family members, 43, 55, 191
   oncology social worker's role, 161
   thoughts on, 33–34
decision-making, difficulty of, 85
denial, 33–35, 37
Department of Health (DOH), 81
depression, 33, 152, 170, 197
despair as a side effect, 211
detection, early, 61, 131–33, 135
   community-based screening agencies, 183, 185, 208
   Pamela A's experience, 26–27
detection and education programs
   In The Pink Early Cancer Detection and Education, 212–13
   Komen®, Susan G., 208
   National Breast and Cervical Cancer Early Detection (NBCCED), 188–89
   Women's Health & Counseling Center, (now Zufall Health), 183, 185
diagnosis
   after giving birth, 230
   differential, 63–66
   family history, 58–59, 61
   and grieving, 161
   response to, 44–46
   trauma of, 157
   types of breast cancer, 105
diagnostic procedures. See also biopsies
   colonoscopy, 133
   discordant results, 106
   genetic testing, 61, 69, 110–11
   mammograms, 74–75
   MRI (Magnetic Resonance Imaging), 76–77

ultrasound (sonogram), 76, 80–81, 205
Diak, Wanda, 211
diarrhea, 149, 170
diary-keeping, 123–26
diet and cancer risk, 222
diet and nutrition, 147, 149–51
dietitians, 150
divorce and COBRA, 187
doctors, selection of, 25–26, 30, 97, 210
drugs, effect on breast tissue, 65
ductal carcinoma in situ (DCIS)
   cure rates, 231
   discussed, 107, 132, 205
   invasive, 84–85, 87, 107, 132
   regular mammograms, importance of, 214
   staging of, 106–7, 118–19
   treatment options, 132

E

edema. See lymphedema
education and counseling programs, 160, 196, 208, 212
Elixir Fund, 173, 175–77
empathy, 70–71
empowerment and Cancer Support Community, 195–96
encouragement, to never give up, 121, 123
endometrial (uterine) cancer, 58
energy conservation, 153, 155
ERISA employer offered medical plans, 177, 179
estrogen status, 25
   treatment options, 87, 99, 125, 193
   understanding, 85
exercise, 206
   cancer prevention, 151
   fatigue management, 153, 155
   lymphedema management, 117
   walking, 229
experimental care and medical insurance, 179

F

faith and healing, 46–47
   Dalai Lama, 191, 193
   harmony, 193
   meditation, 165–66
   spiritual care providers, 157, 159
   spirituality of, 46–47, 159
false positive, 75
families, concern for, 44, 46–47, 55, 57, 160
family history and risk, 47, 58–59, 61–62.
   See also risk factors

family physicians/doctors, 30–33, 37–39
fatigue, cancer and treatment related
    causes and management, 151–53, 155
    chemotherapy, 69–70, 120–21
        Paula's experience, 123–26
    disruptiveness of, 35
    early symptoms, 92
    and *Jin Shin Jyutsu*, 170
    loving support, 126–27, 129
    nutrition for, 149
    support of friends, 62
    working with, 206
fear as empowering, 57–58, 101, 103, 157,
    159, 197, 199, 205–6
Federal Drug Administration (FDA),
    mammogram regulation, 75, 81
Femara, 99
fibroadenoma, 55
fibrocystic breasts, monitoring, 191, 203,
    205–6
financial assistance, 81
    cancer care costs, resources, 141–42
    non-medical costs, 176
    non-profit organizations, 173, 175–77
    uninsured patients, 183, 185, 188–89
financial counselors, 25
financial planner, personal, 175, 180–81
food, sensitivity to, 121, 126–27, 129, 149
free professional services, 139, 141–42, 153, 176

G

genetic risk, counseling and testing, 47,
    58–59, 61, 69, 110–11
    Nora's experience, 61–62
Gilda's Club, support network, 194, 195, 227
glossary, 252–59
grieving and diagnosis, 161
growth hormone-releasing hormone
    (GHRH) antagonists, 219–21
guided imagery, 157, 159, 166–67
gynecologist, 25
    role of, 47, 49–51
        Pam C's experience, 51–53
gynecomastia
    about, 64–66
    in later life, 89

H

hair loss, 126
    American Cancer Society wig service, 145
    buzz cuts, 52, 55, 57
    Look Good Feel Better program, 146–47
    wigs, 206

Hardy, Cheryl, 235
Hashimoto's disease, 45
healing
    harmony, 193
    spirituality of, 46–47, 159
health insurance (US)
    American Cancer Society information
        about, 181
    Health Insurance Portability and
        Accountability Act (HIPAA), 187
    inadequacies of, 32, 173, 175–77
    insurance, generally, 177–79
    options, 181
    Patient Protection and Affordable Care
        Act (US), (PPACA), 177–79, 186, 187,
        188, 189
    uninsured patients, help for, 183, 185,
        188–89
HER2 and Herceptin clinical trial, 100
Herschli, Lisa, 208
holistic care and approach, 45–46, 163–68,
    168–71, 194–96
hope
    Hope Network, 111, 145, 210–12
    inspirational, 230–31, 233
    as a renewable resource, 121, 123, 126
hormone replacement therapy (HRT) and
    breast cancer, 84, 103, 214, 215, 231
hormone therapy/treatment, 97, 99–100, 125
hormones, effect on breast tissue, 64–65
hospice care, 161, 163
hospitals, breast cancer
        certification of, 25
        teaching, 32
house cleaning, free, 142, 153
HRT. *See* hormone replacement therapy
Hubert-McKenna, Kathleen, 208
hydration and dehydration management, 149
hypothyroidism, 45, 210

I

ileostomy management, 133, 135
immune system and lymphatic system,
    114–15, 130, 171
implants and breast reconstruction, 85, 110,
    111, 113
In The Pink Early Cancer Detection and
    Education Program, 212–13
independence as a coping strategy, 103–4,
    121
Indian Health Service and tribal
    organizations, 188
indigestion, 171
inflammatory breast cancer, 110, 111

information
    culturally appropriate, lack of, 199–200
    gathering, 55, 83, 132, 197
    resources, 236–38
insomnia, 33, 169, 171
insurance, life, 181
insurance, medical (US). *See* health
    insurance (US)
integrative medicine, 163–68
invasive, defined, 107

J

Jin Shin Jyutsu, 168–71
journal-keeping, 123–26, 160
    medical questions and answers,
        20–23, 29
judicial separation and COBRA, 187

K

Komen. *See* Susan G. Komen®

L

Lanfranchi, Angela, 235
LCIS. *See* lobular carcinoma *in situ*
legal documents, personal, updated, 181
lesion, 49
Lidocaine, 80
life celebrated, 37, 55, 57–58, 62, 70, 73–74,
    121, 123, 135, 205–6
life lessons learned, 27, 29–30, 83–84, 131–
    33, 135. *See also* advice; support, family
    and friends
lifestyle choices as cancer prevention, 51,
    214, 215, 217, 222
lobular carcinoma *in situ* (LCIS), 107, 209
    staging of, 118
Look Good Feel Better program, 146–47
loss and mourning, 161
lumpectomy or mastectomy, 71, 83, 85, 97,
    109–10, 132, 193, 203, 205, 207, 209
lumps in the male breast, 63–66
lymph nodes
    axillary, 65, 71, 85, 114, 118, 119, 131, 213
    metastasis, 31, 97
    sentinel, and staging, 85, 106–7, 118–19
lymphatic system and immune system,
    114–15, 130, 171
Lymphazurin (dye), 107
lymphedema, 85, 87, 114–17, 132
lymphoma, non-Hodgkin's. *See* non-
    Hodgkin's lymphoma

M

Magnetic Resonance Imaging (MRI), 76–77
Mammaprint® molecular test, 119
mammograms
    benign findings, 49
    breast self-exam, 81, 83–84
    calcifications, 84–85, 107, 205
    cancers not detected by, 49, 83
    deodorant use, 79
    digital, 74
    importance of, 29, 73–74, 80, 227
        Lori's experience, 225, 227
        Sondra's experience, 73–74
    life saving, 213–14
    National Breast and Cervical Cancer
        Early Detection Program, NBCCEDP-
        funded, 189
    negative result, 207
    radiologist's perspective, 74–77
    radiology technologist's perspective,
        79–81
    recommendations on, 74
    regulation of, 75, 81
    screening and diagnostic, 47, 49, 74–77,
        231
mammography, 79–81
    Jeanette's experience, 213–14
    mathematics of, 233
Mammography Quality Standard Act
    (MQSA), 81
mastectomies
    bilateral, 194
    ductal carcinoma in situ, 231
    or lumpectomies, 109–10
    prophylactic, 205, 209
    and reconstruction, 85, 111, 113
    types of, 109
medical care, lack of in Cambodia, 91–95
    Men S's experience, 91
    Naov's experience, 92–93
medical care team and informed decisions,
    25, 29, 31, 85
Medicare/Medicaid, 32, 161, 177, 187, 188
medications
    chemotherapeutic, 87, 119–20
    dosage and timing, 27, 120
    payment assistance plans, 175–77
meditation, 165–66
melanoma, 65
men and breast cancer, 58–59, 63–66
    Rich L's experience, 66–67, 69–70
    Wilbur's experience, 89
metastasis

bone and liver, 123
cancer in men, 65
defined, 31
risk of, and treatment choices, 97, 99
microcalcification, 75, 121, 205, 213
milk duct, 63, 107, 205
mind-body connection therapy, 163–68,
    168–71
monitoring, post-treatment, 32
MRI (Magnetic Resonance Imaging), 76–77

N

National Breast and Cervical Cancer Early
    Detection Program (NBCCEDP), 188–89
National Center for Complementary and
    Alternative Medicine (NCCAM), 163, 165
National Comprehensive Cancer Network
    (NCCN)
    cancer related fatigue, 151
    testing and monitoring guidelines, 25
National Institutes of Health (NIH), 116
National Naval Medical Center Breast Care
    Center, 116
nausea, management tips, 127, 149, 171
needle breast biopsies, 61, 77, 105, 207, 227
negative thoughts, avoidance of, 125
neoplasm, malignant, 31
neutropenia, 120
nipples
    inversion as a sign of cancer, 92
    reconstruction, 70, 113
Nobel Prize in Physiology and Medicine
    (1977), 219
non-Hodgkin's lymphoma
    Joyce's experience, 33–35, 37
    Richard D's experience, 164–65
non-profit organizations and financial
    assistance, 142, 175–76
nurse navigators, role of, 143–45
nurse practitioners, 25, 32
nurses, oncology, 25, 41–43
nutrition
    during and after treatment, 147, 149–51
    American Cancer Society guidelines, 150

O

Obamacare, 177–79, 186, 187, 188
oncologist
    medical, 25, 58–59, 61, 97, 99–100,
        118–21, 221–23
    radiation, 25, 129–31
    surgical, 25, 104–7, 109–11, 230–31, 233
Oncology Nurses Society, 42

Oncology Nutrition Practice Group, 150
Oncotype DX® molecular test, 109, 119
options. See treatment options
oral contraceptives and breast cancer, 214, 215
    group 1 carcinogens, 231
ovarian cancer, 51–53, 58
    prevention and BRCA gene, 50

P

pancreatic cancer, 58, 65
    and GHRH antagonists, 220
pastoral care. See spiritual care providers
pathologists, 105
Patient Access Network, 175
Patient Advocate Foundation, 176
patient navigators and cancer survivors,
    145–46
Patient Protection and Affordable Care Act
    (US), (PPACA), 177–79, 186, 187, 188, 189
personal control, maintaining, 161, 164–65,
    207
PET scan, 22, 35, 125, 257
physician assistants, 25, 32
Picker, Debbie, 202–3
pink, two perspectives, 123–26
plans, written, 155
pleomorphic, 213
poetry
    Michael's experience, 136–37
port
    ease of use, 121, 123
    in chemotherapy, 119
    positioning of, 119
power of attorney, 181
PPACA (Patient Protection and Affordable
    Care Act), 177–79, 186, 187, 188, 189
prayer and thanksgiving, 101, 157, 159, 197, 199
pregnancy, effect on breast cancer risk, 58,
    217, 231
preventative surgery, 109
prevention, best treatment, 99, 183,
    222, 231, 233. See also Breast Cancer
    Prevention Institute
primary care doctors, 25
    role of, 30–33, 37–39
procrastination, 34, 67
progesterone levels, 25, 193, 254, 258
prostate cancer, 58, 183, 212
    BRCA gene mutations, 65
    hormone dependent, 219–20
psychologists/psychiatrists, for support,
    62, 103
psychotherapists and coping, 135

Q

Qigong, 166, 221
questions, asking, 20–23, 25, 29, 67, 69

R

Race for the Cure, 208
radiation therapy
    after lumpectomy, 97
    ductal carcinoma *in situ*, 231
    explained, 129–31
    for recurrence prevention, 109–10
    sexual intimacy, 131
radiologist, breast, 25, 74–77
radiology technologists, role of, 79–81
Raloxifene, 99
Reach to Recovery, 145
reconstruction. *See* breast reconstruction
reconstruction surgeon, 25, 110, 111, 113–14
    See also breast reconstruction
records, copies of, 21–22, 37
red blood cell counts, 120
referrals, 83, 135
relaxation tapes, 210
Relay for Life, taking part in, 200–203, 225
remission, 32, 34
research studies. *See* clinical research/trials
resources and information, 25, 142, 175–77,
    236–38, 252–59
    complementary therapies, 168–69
risk factors. *See also* family history and risk
    abortion, 214
    breast cancer in men, 63, 65
    different perspective, 104
    family history, 58–59, 61
    hope, cures, prevent, 230–31, 233
    hormone replacement therapy (HRT),
        215, 231
    management of, 47
    smoking, 215, 222

S

Sala, Aviva, 201
sarcoidosis, 45
science, good, and good treatment, 221–23
screening
    avoidance of, 37, 81
    BRCA gene mutations, 59, 61
    breast self-exam, 83–84
    CEED program, 183
    genetic testing, 69
    In The Pink Early Cancer Detection and

Education Program, 212–13
    mammograms, 74–77
second opinions, importance of, 25–26, 29,
    31, 37, 83, 207, 222–23
self-acupressure, 168–71
self-confidence, maintenance of, 146–47
self-esteem and breast reconstruction, 111,
    113–14
selfies. *See* breast self-exam
sentinel nodes. *See* lymph nodes
sexual intimacy and radiation therapy, 131
shamanic journeying, 167
side effects of treatment. *See also* fatigue,
    cancer and treatment related
    anemia, 120
    appetite, loss of, 149
    chemotherapy, 35, 50, 52, 120, 121
    defined, 35
    despair, 210–11
    and *Jin Shin Jyutsu*, 170
    neutropenia, 120
    radiation, 131
Sisters Network of Central New Jersey, 84,
    197, 199–200
skin care products, use of, 131
Smart Women Finish Rich (Bach), 180
smoking and breast cancer, 58, 215, 222
social services, hospital, and financial
    assistance, 142, 173, 175–77, 181
social workers, oncology, 25, 46, 139, 141–
    42, 159–61, 163, 194–96
sonograms (ultrasound), 76, 80–81, 205
spiritual care providers, 47, 157, 159
spirituality and healing, 164–65, 193, 199–200
staging of breast cancer
    cure rates, 231
    defined, 118–19
    lymph nodes, 106–7
statistics, breast cancer, 230–31, 233
stomach cancer, 65
stress management, 153, 155, 168–71
support, family and friends, 31, 35, 62,
    126–27, 129, 133
    accepting help from, 146, 153, 200
    appointments, 38, 83–84, 132, 133, 135
    asking for, 133, 135
    "breast" friends, 85, 87
    buddy, 111
    community, 200–203
    importance of
        Peggy's experience, 46–47
    strong and ever-present, 70–71, 191, 193
support networks and organizations. *See*
    individual organizations

Supportive Care Framework cancer guide, 143
surgery options, 97, 104–7, 109–11, 111,
    113–14, 130, 207
survival rates, 230–31
survivorship and hope, 233
Susan G. Komen®
    Belfatto, Deborah Q., role of, 207–8
    financial assistance, 177
    grant money, 215
    New Jersey Affiliate, formation of, 207–8
    New York Race, 205–6

T

Tai Chi, 166
Tamoxifen (anti-estrogen), 99, 206, 213
taste, changed, 121, 149
tattooing
    family support, 71
    nipple reconstruction, 113
    radiation therapy, 130
Taxol, 124
technicians, breast center, 25
telephone contact, supportive
    Cancer Hope Network, 211
    nurse navigators, 144
testicular cancer, 65
THYCA. *See* Thyroid Cancer Survivors
    Association
thyroid cancer, 58, 209–10
Thyroid Cancer Survivors Association
    (THYCA), 210
thyroid shield and mammograms, 80
Toomey, Kathleen, 235
trauma of diagnosis, 157, 211
treatment options
    medical, 97, 99–100
    surgical, 104–7, 109–11, 111, 113–14, 132
tumor
    benign, 74, 203
    malignant, 31, 46, 121, 211
tumor board, defined, 42

U

ultrasound (sonograms), 76, 80–81, 205
uninsured patients, help for, 183, 185, 188–89

V

violin playing, post treatment exercise, 121,
    123
vitamins, caution, 23
volunteering. *See individual support networks*

W

walks for cancer support
    Avon Walk for Breast Cancer, 228–30
    Relay for Life, 200–203, 225
weight-lifting and lymphedema, 117
Wellness Community (TWC). *See* Cancer
    Support Community (CSC)
white blood cell counts, 120
wigs. *See* hair loss
will, making/updating, 181
Women's Health & Counseling Center
    (WHCC). *See* Zufall Health, Somerville
Women's Health Initiative Study, 215, 231
work/employment and chemotherapy,
    120–21
written plans, have one, 155

Y

yoga, 166
Your Sister's House, 197

Z

Zufall Health, Somerville, 183, 185

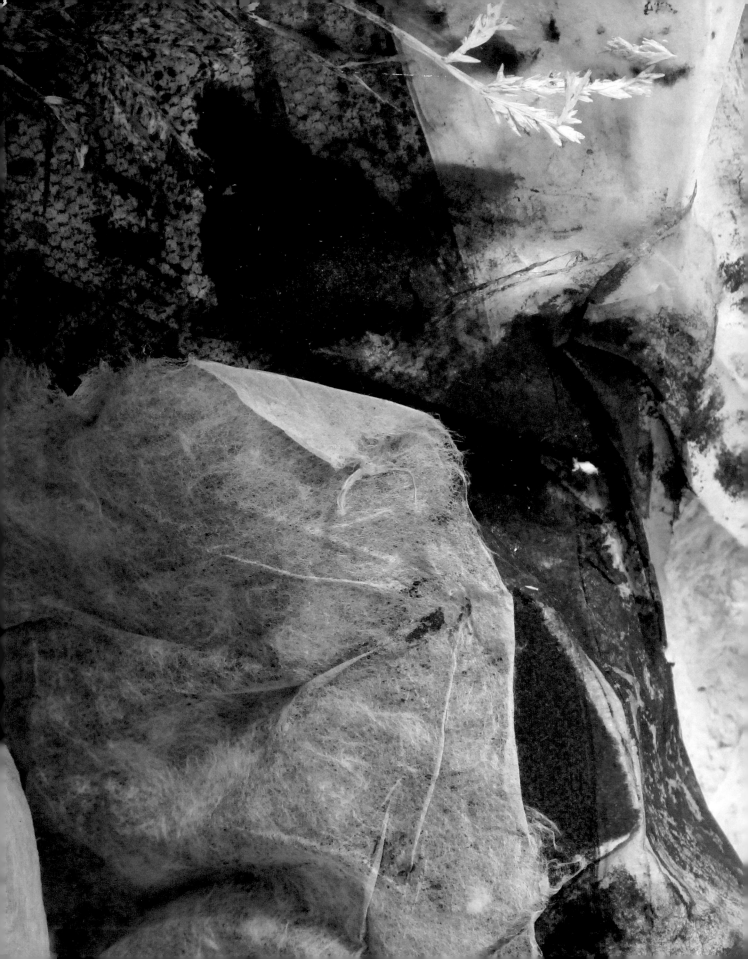